Adolescent and Young Adult Oncology—Ongoing Challenges and Developments in the Future

Contents

Julian Surujballi, Grace Chan, Caron Strahlendorf and Amirrtha Srikanthan
Setting Priorities for a Provincial Adolescent and Young Adult Oncology Program
Reprinted from: *Curr. Oncol.* **2022**, *29*, 4034-4053, doi:10.3390/curroncol29060322 1

Aida Zeckanovic, Philipp Fuchs, Philip Heesen, Nicole Bodmer, Maria Otth and Katrin Scheinemann
Pediatric-Inspired Regimens in the Treatment of Acute Lymphoblastic Leukemia in Adolescents and Young Adults: A Systematic Review
Reprinted from: *Curr. Oncol.* **2023**, *30*, 8612-8632, doi:10.3390/curroncol30090625 21

Carla Vlooswijk, Lonneke V. van de Poll-Franse, Silvie H. M. Janssen, Esther Derksen, Milou J. P. Reuvers and Rhodé Bijlsma et al.
Recruiting Adolescent and Young Adult Cancer Survivors for Patient-Reported Outcome Research: Experiences and Sample Characteristics of the SURVAYA Study
Reprinted from: *Curr. Oncol.* **2022**, *29*, 5407-5425, doi:10.3390/curroncol29080428 42

Nina Francis-Levin, Lauren V. Ghazal, Jess Francis-Levin, Bradley Zebrack, Meiyan Chen and Anao Zhang
Exploring the Relationship between Self-Rated Health and Unmet Cancer Needs among Sexual and Gender Minority Adolescents and Young Adults with Cancer
Reprinted from: *Curr. Oncol.* **2023**, *30*, 9291-9303, doi:10.3390/curroncol30100671 61

Aurelia Altherr, Céline Bolliger, Michaela Kaufmann, Daniela Dyntar, Katrin Scheinemann and Gisela Michel et al.
Education, Employment, and Financial Outcomes in Adolescent and Young Adult Cancer Survivors—A Systematic Review
Reprinted from: *Curr. Oncol.* **2023**, *30*, 8720-8762, doi:10.3390/curroncol30100631 74

Sitara Sharma and Jennifer Brunet
Young Adults' Lived Experiences with Cancer-Related Cognitive Impairment: An Exploratory Qualitative Study
Reprinted from: *Curr. Oncol.* **2023**, *30*, 5593-5614, doi:10.3390/curroncol30060422 117

Moira Rushton, Jessica Pudwell, Xuejiao Wei, Madeleine Powell, Harriet Richardson and Maria P. Velez
Reproductive Outcomes in Young Breast Cancer Survivors Treated (15–39) in Ontario, Canada
Reprinted from: *Curr. Oncol.* **2022**, *29*, 8591-8599, doi:10.3390/curroncol29110677 139

Isabel Baur, Sina Staudinger and Ariana Aebi
Adolescents and Young Adults with Cancer and the Desire for Parenthood—A Legal View from a Swiss Perspective in Consideration of the Relevance of Cancer Support Organizations
Reprinted from: *Curr. Oncol.* **2023**, *30*, 10124-10133, doi:10.3390/curroncol30120736 148

Annelie Voland, Verena Krell, Miriam Götte, Timo Niels, Maximilian Köppel and Joachim Wiskemann
Exercise Preferences in Young Adults with Cancer—The YOUEX Study
Reprinted from: *Curr. Oncol.* **2023**, *30*, 1473-1487, doi:10.3390/curroncol30020113 158

Simon Basteck, Wiebke K. Guder, Uta Dirksen, Arno Krombholz, Arne Streitbürger and Dirk Reinhardt et al.
Effects of an Exercise Intervention on Gait Function in Young Survivors of Osteosarcoma with Megaendoprosthesis of the Lower Extremity—Results from the Pilot Randomized Controlled Trial proGAIT
Reprinted from: *Curr. Oncol.* **2022**, *29*, 7754-7767, doi:10.3390/curroncol29100613 173

Stephanie J. Kendall, Jodi E. Langley, Mohsen Aghdam, Bruce N. Crooks, Nicholas Giacomantonio and Stefan Heinze-Milne et al.
The Impact of Exercise on Cardiotoxicity in Pediatric and Adolescent Cancer Survivors: A Scoping Review
Reprinted from: *Curr. Oncol.* **2022**, *29*, 6350-6363, doi:10.3390/curroncol29090500 187

Karolina Bryl, Suzi Tortora, Jennifer Whitley, Soo-Dam Kim, Nirupa J. Raghunathan and Jun J. Mao et al.
Utilization, Delivery, and Outcomes of Dance/Movement Therapy for Pediatric Oncology Patients and their Caregivers: A Retrospective Chart Review
Reprinted from: *Curr. Oncol.* **2023**, *30*, 6497-6507, doi:10.3390/curroncol30070477 201

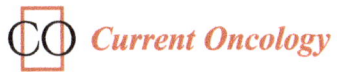 *Current Oncology*

Article

Setting Priorities for a Provincial Adolescent and Young Adult Oncology Program

Julian Surujballi [1,2,3], Grace Chan [4], Caron Strahlendorf [4] and Amirrtha Srikanthan [1,2,3,5,*]

1. The Ottawa Hospital Cancer Centre, Ottawa, ON K1H 8L6, Canada; jsurujballi@toh.ca
2. The Ottawa Hospital Research Institute, Ottawa, ON K1H 8L6, Canada
3. Department of Medicine, University of Ottawa, Ottawa, ON K1N 6N5, Canada
4. BC Children's Hospital, Vancouver, BC V6H 3N1, Canada; gchan@cw.bc.ca (G.C.); cstrahlendorf@cw.bc.ca (C.S.)
5. Department of Medicine, The Ottawa Hospital, Ottawa, ON K1H 8L6, Canada
* Correspondence: asrikanthan@toh.ca; Tel.: +1-613-737-7700

Abstract: Adolescent and young adult (AYA, ages 15–39 years) oncology patients are an underserved population with specialized needs. AYA programs are absent from most Canadian centers. We identified a priority list and sequence for new programs to address. Program goals, priorities, and activities were developed through literature review, national consensus documents, and expert opinion. Health care providers (HCPs) involved in AYA cancer care, administrators, and patient and family representatives were engaged to co-develop program goals and activities. A modified Delphi technique was used through two iterations followed by an in-person meeting to prioritize program implementation. Consensus was defined as a mean score of less than 2.0 (not important) or 4.0 or greater (important). Items without consensus (scored between 2.0 and 3.99) were discussed at the in-person meeting. Sixty provincial stakeholders completed the Delphi survey across multiple disciplines. Twenty-seven stakeholders attended the in-person meeting. All goals were deemed important, except development of a research program. Patient implementation tasks ranked highest. Priority sequence of implementation was: patient care first, followed by HCP education; patient and family education; program sustainability plan; evaluation; research; then a model for multidisciplinary tumor board review. These represent key goals for new AYA oncology programs and a priority sequence of implementation.

Keywords: AYA; oncology; program development

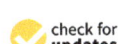

Citation: Surujballi, J.; Chan, G.; Strahlendorf, C.; Srikanthan, A. Setting Priorities for a Provincial Adolescent and Young Adult Oncology Program. *Curr. Oncol.* 2022, 29, 4034–4053. https://doi.org/10.3390/curroncol29060322

Received: 3 May 2022
Accepted: 31 May 2022
Published: 1 June 2022

Publisher's Note: MDPI stays neutral with regard to jurisdictional claims in published maps and institutional affiliations.

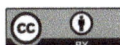

Copyright: © 2022 by the authors. Licensee MDPI, Basel, Switzerland. This article is an open access article distributed under the terms and conditions of the Creative Commons Attribution (CC BY) license (https://creativecommons.org/licenses/by/4.0/).

1. Introduction

Adolescents and young adults (AYA, defined as ages 15–39 years old) with cancer suffer interruption of normative physical, behavioral, cognitive, and emotional development [1–3]. The AYA period includes development of values, personal identity, formation of strong personal relationships, starting families, and attaining financial independence [4,5]. A cancer diagnosis disrupts this development, whether through facing early death, interruption of social life activities, returning to live with parents, and/or fearing for the future due to treatment late effects or recurrence [4]. In addition, AYAs may experience more intense symptom burden, have less-developed coping mechanisms, and exhibit poorly developed autonomy in decision making [4]. Families of AYAs with cancer also experience distress, which may compromise their ability to support AYA patients. Although the most inclusive definition ranges from ages 15–39, programs worldwide vary in patient inclusion, depending on local resources and needs [3,6–8].

Cancer is the leading cause of disease-related death in adolescents and young adults (AYAs) in the US and Canada [9,10]. Despite improving survival among the broader AYA cancer population, survival rates continue to lag behind those observed in younger and older populations for specific cancer types, such as breast cancer, and sarcoma [6,11]. There are deficiencies for AYA in care across the cancer journey, through diagnosis and treatment, to survivorship or palliative care. Multiple factors impact this disparity, including diagnostic delay, more aggressive disease biology, poor treatment adherence, and system issues such as poor processes and structures to address unique AYA needs [12–15].

Recognizing the uniqueness of this population, current recommendations state that AYA cancer therapy be administered by individuals with AYA-specific expertise [16,17]. Despite these recommendations, many oncology programs in Canada lack a dedicated AYA program, and those that exist lack standardization. Thus, AYAs aged 15–21 years may thus receive care in pediatric or adult systems, although neither system is specifically designed for the specific needs of this vulnerable group [18]. This provides the opportunity to design new bespoke programs that meet the needs of health care providers (HCPs), patients, and families specific to the Canadian context. Co-designing programs that meet the needs of all end-users requires involvement of all affected parties, including patients, families, health care providers, and health care administrators. Though AYA programs have been proposed in the past, limited data exist regarding implementation sequencing at the ground level. To that end, we describe the efforts undertaken in the province of British Columbia (BC), Canada to identify the key priorities for patients, families, front-line HCPs, and administrators with and without AYA expertise, in improving AYA patient care delivery. The goal of this work is to identify how various components of an AYA program may be best implemented and in which priority.

For the context of this study, health care in Canada is largely delivered at the provincial level with rules, regulations, funding, and organization differing from province to province. Funding and oversight are provided by provincial organizations, such as BC Cancer in BC, to regional institutions where health care is delivered to patients. Larger academic centers typically receive more provincial funding and more staff that could be allocated to specific programs. As such, a provincial "umbrella" program is feasible through collaboration between provincial organizations and academic centers. Resources developed through this program could then be shared with regional centers.

2. Materials and Methods

2.1. Study Design

Proposed AYA program goals, priorities, components, and activities (79 distinct items) were developed through literature review, national consensus documents, and provincial expert opinion (via the BC Cancer/BC Children's provincial AYA Joint Steering Committee). A modified Delphi survey technique with two iterations was used to gather stakeholder input and feedback prior to a stakeholder meeting [19,20]. Consensus was defined as a mean score of less than 2.0 (indicating not important) or 4.0 or greater (indicating important). Items without consensus (scored between 2.0 and 3.99) after round one were discussed in-person by stakeholders.

2.2. Program Components

The following program components were pre-identified by the BC AYA Joint Steering Committee. These components were: (1) program mission and goals; (2) patient care implementation; (3) health care provider (HCP) education strategy and needs assessment process; (4) patient and family education strategy; (5) program evaluation strategy; (6) model for multidisciplinary tumor boards; (7) model for program expansion and sustainability; and (8) AYA research priorities. For each component, program objectives, criteria, processes, and strategies were developed prior to the in-person stakeholder session. This was done using existing resources, expert opinion, national consensus, and peer-reviewed research (see Appendix B for a complete list of components).

2.3. Participant Identification and In-Person Session Format

Key stakeholders involved in AYA cancer care from each health authority in BC were identified by contacting medical directors in each health authority, provincial heads of nursing, patient and family counseling, and pain and symptom management services. Participants who completed the online survey were invited to participate in the in-person session. Individuals were recruited for participation if they had at least 5 years of clinical oncology experience post terminal degree training, and 10% of their adult clinical practice included AYA cancer patients. For the health care provider participants based out of pediatric institutions, a percentage of AYA clinical practice was not pre-specified. Additionally, regional leaders who are aware of early-career staff recognized as AYA champions were provided the opportunity to put additional names forward. See Appendix D for the in-person session agenda.

For the in-person meeting, participants were assigned to groups of 5–6 individuals. Groups were provided with discussion guides and first-round Delphi survey results and asked to discuss each component. Results of these discussions were summarized narratively. Due to the size of the small groups, the multidisciplinary conference tumor board review and AYA research priority components were not discussed at the stakeholder session, as these components were ranked lowest for prioritization.

2.4. Data Analysis

Descriptive statistics were generated for participant demographics and Delphi responses. Mean Delphi results were presented. Survey respondents were asked to prioritize program component implementation, ranking each component on a scale of 1 to 7 (first to last). The frequencies of participant rankings for each item were summed. Items were ranked according to weighted mean rankings from lowest to highest.

3. Results

3.1. Respondent Characteristics

A total of 100 participants were invited to participate. Sixty participants completed the Delphi survey. Twenty-seven individuals attended the in-person session. Appendix A (Table A1) provides demographic details on survey respondents and session participants. Respondents included administration (6.7%), patient and family representatives (1.7%), oncology physicians (26.7%), nursing (26.7%), counseling (21.7%), pain and symptom management (6.7%), psychiatry (1.7%), nurse practitioners (1.7%), speech–language pathology (1.7%), nutrition (1.7%), and unspecified (1.7%)

3.2. Delphi Survey and Round Table Discussion Results

After two rounds of the Delphi survey, consensus was reached on 84% of items. All items on which consensus was reached were deemed important. Full details of Delphi survey results and the discussion guide are available in Appendix B. The top 10 highest rated items across all components are listed in Table 1. Average scores per program component are shown in Figure 1 and the proportion of items rated "important" per component is shown in Figure 2. A complete list of items rated "important" is provided in Appendix C.

All program goals were endorsed as important, except the development of an AYA research program. Priority of program implementation was ranked as patient care first, followed by: HCP education; patient and family education; research; program sustainability plan; evaluation; then model for multidisciplinary tumor board review. Of the various program activities, patient implementation tasks ranked highest. Common themes that emerged from table discussions during the in-person meeting are categorized and summarized narratively below.

Table 1. Top 10 highest rated items across all components.

Domain	Score	Description
Patient care implementation	4.67	Establish referral pathways for pre-defined high problem issues (such as suicide, psychosocial distress, fertility preservation, urgent end of life symptom management)
Patient care implementation	4.66	Develop referral pathways for patients referred to BC Cancer, BCCH, VGH based on age and diagnosis
Patient care implementation	4.64	Create process so all AYA patients offered AYA program consultation with advanced practice nurse (APN) and counselor
Program mission and goals	4.61	Program mission: create a provincial interdisciplinary cancer program for AYA aged 15–29 years that will regionally implement recommendations across all BC Cancer sites in partnership with BCCH
Patient care implementation	4.57	Create process so all AYA patients offered follow-up with APN or counselor during treatment trajectory
Program expansion and sustainability	4.56	Foster relationships with motivated survivors, patients, and families for ongoing advocacy
Patient care implementation	4.53	Ensure all AYA patients screened for distress at intake
HCP education	4.53	HCP needs assessment survey topic: the unique psychosocial needs of AYA
Patient and family education	4.5	Develop patient education materials on survivorship and late effects for AYA
Patient and family education	4.48	Develop patient education materials on fertility preservation and counseling

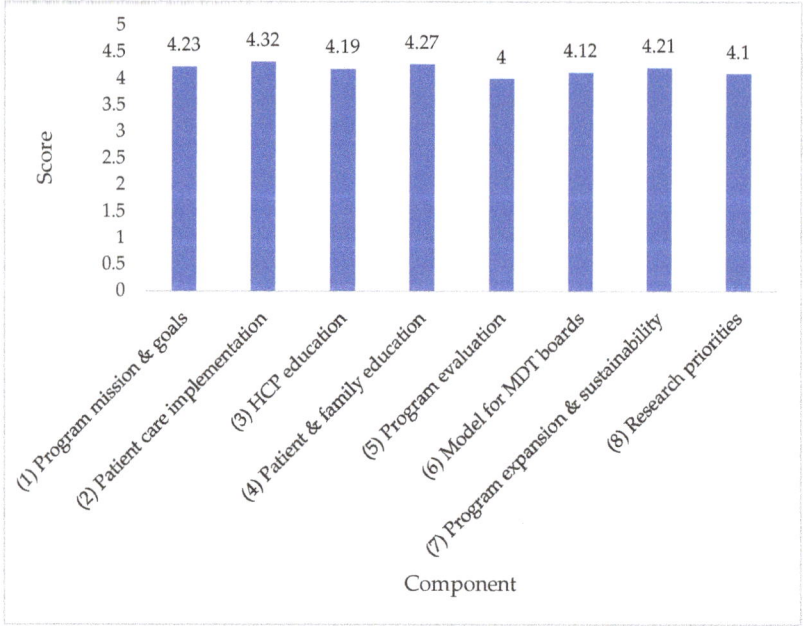

Figure 1. Average score per component.

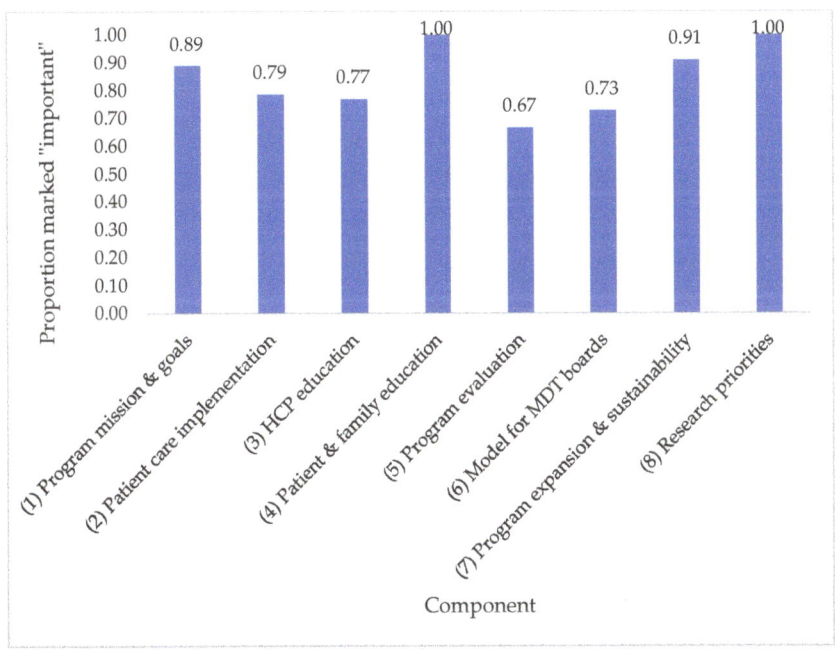

Figure 2. Proportion of items rated "important" per component.

3.2.1. Scope of Program

Groups highlighted the importance of creating a provincial AYA program, with a provincial umbrella to provide consistent information, resources, and guidelines to regional programs (five of five groups). Regional centers should consider regional context and link to local resources (five of five groups). The need for integration of alternative ways of care delivery (such as telemedicine, or virtual care) to expand provincial reach was noted (three of five groups).

The age range of 15–29 years versus 39 years as the upper age limit was debated. The 15–29 age range was suggested for pilot programs, with increased eligibility to age 39 for a provincial program (five of five groups), with flexible age cutoffs depending on the tumor group. Program components thought to be missing from the original program goals include AYA survivorship integration (three of five groups), focused fertility resources (two of five groups), and focused palliative care resources (one of five groups).

Participants recommended having an AYA "champion" or clinical lead in each tumor group, bone marrow transplant programs, diagnostic imaging, fertility services, and palliative care services. Implementation of the program would vary based on regional resources, including human health resources, and local demand for services. Discussions suggested that the most sustainable and impactful model would be to develop AYA regional hubs in major urban centers with higher resource capacity (for example, in Vancouver through the BC Cancer—Vancouver Centre), and the development of local AYA champions in less resourced areas, or the provision of virtual services. As regional volumes grow, capacity for multiple AYA regional hubs could be developed throughout a province (for example, the Fraser Health Authority including Surrey could be targeted for AYA resource development).

3.2.2. Psychosocial Services

Groups recommended development of an AYA-specific distress screening, with regular distress screening throughout the care trajectory (four of five groups). Similarly, items pertaining to psychosocial services scored highly across all domains (Table 2). It was agreed that psychosocial wellbeing should be measured and tracked as a program evaluation strategy, though there was no consensus on what metrics should be evaluated.

Table 2. Item ratings relating to psychosocial services across all program components.

Score	Program Item	Component
4.67	Establish pathways for high problem issues (such as suicide, psychosocial distress, fertility preservation, urgent end of life symptom management)	Patient Care
4.66	Create referral pathways at each institution based on age and diagnosis	Patient Care
4.64	Ensure all AYA patients offered AYA program consultation with advanced practice nurse (APN) and counselor	Patient Care
4.57	Create process so all AYA patients offered follow-up with APN or counselor during treatment trajectory	Patient Care
4.56	Foster relationships with motivated survivors, patients, and families for ongoing advocacy	Sustainability
4.53	HCP education topic: the unique psychosocial needs of AYA	HCP Education
4.50	Patient education materials on survivorship and late effects for AYA	Patient/Family Education

3.2.3. Care Pathways

Participants noted the importance of clearly defined care pathways, with identified contact points throughout the care trajectory (three of five groups). Definitions of what a care pathway entailed were not specified, with recognition that disease groups would likely have different needs. To assist AYA patients with system navigation, an AYA resource person could be appointed (two of five groups). One group suggested that psychosocial screening should be done initially and on an ongoing basis, with the first screening and assessment within 48 h of the first oncology appointment, and thereafter every 2 weeks during active medical care.

3.2.4. Role of AYA Team

There were mixed opinions as to whether an AYA clinical specialist (such as an advanced practice nurse (APN) or counselor) should provide direct patient care (two of five groups) versus helping existing providers to deliver AYA care (three of five groups). Suggested possible roles for the APN included staff education, direct patient care, building AYA program capacity, and survivorship care. The importance of using communications technology (email, patient portal, apps, virtual support groups) was highlighted by two of the five groups. All five groups throughout discussions mentioned the need for AYA-specific screening tools to help address the unique psychosocial needs of this group.

3.2.5. Health Care Provider Education Delivery

The group suggested that HCP education delivery could include rounds, newsletters, emails, champions, modules (with dedicated time or incentives), general practitioner in oncology (GPO) training, nursing lunch and learns, and by adding resources to institutional websites.

3.2.6. Priorities for Education

Top priorities were HCP education, needs assessments and educating family physicians on the survivorship needs of AYA patients (including sending care plans to family physicians). It was agreed that creation of an AYA fellowship program should be a long-term priority and should not be included in the pilot.

Suggested priority topics for patient and family education included palliative care, sexuality and sexual health, vocational rehabilitation, returning to work or school, survivorship and late effects including psychosocial needs, and transitioning to a new normal.

The group agreed that all resources developed should be evidence-based and supported by literature. Proposed education delivery methods included web-based, patient portal, podcasts, Facebook live, webinars, YouTube, and at the point of care. Communication could occur using social media and posters with AYA images, and ideally be interactive. Proposed methods for peer support delivery were online, face to face, through peer volunteers, and through local organizations. Peer support can be social in nature, psychoeducational, or focus on expressive arts.

3.2.7. Patients and Family Engagement

The group agreed that engagement should be on an ongoing basis and include asking patients and families for feedback, questionnaires and follow-up in individualized ways that are meaningful to the person, and communications from individual AYA programs. There was emphasis to ensure staff are informed regarding patient engagement strategies, and that the process to engage is transparent. In addition, patient and family involvement should be incorporated in program evaluation.

3.2.8. Program Expansion and Sustainability

The group suggested building an inventory of available resources and adjusting as needed over time, as well as developing a separate website and app. The team should provide education to build capacity within each center. An AYA peer navigator should be identified to support patients in navigating the system during active treatment and beyond. It was agreed that dedicated funding is needed for the AYA team. A sustainable program requires support to liaise with the community and community resources. One suggestion was that a patient and family advisory council with regional representation should provide input into the program.

3.2.9. Implementation Prioritization

Eighteen of 27 participants completed this section of the survey. Of these, 15 participants ranked all seven items while three did not (see Appendix E for individual results). Priority of program implementation was ranked as patient care first, followed by: HCP education; patient and family education; program expansion and sustainability; evaluation; research; then model for multidisciplinary tumor board review. Of the various program activities, patient implementation tasks ranked highest.

3.2.10. Potential Program Tasks

Actual delivery of the program will vary regionally based on local constraints, resources, and patient volumes, and final implementation will need to be negotiated with regional and provincial leaders, and adapted over time. The recommendations provided by the stakeholders provide an overview of the principles that should be in place and priority targets for development and implementation. Example tasks that could be undertaken at the provincial and regional level for the top ten high priority items that were discussed are highlighted (Table 3).

Table 3. Example tasks of the proposed AYA program.

Domain Priority	Description of Priority Item	Provincial Task	Regional Task
Patient care implementation	Establish referral pathways for pre-defined high problem issues (such as suicide, psychosocial distress, fertility preservation, urgent end of life symptom management)	Establish provincial working group to create best practice standard operating procedures, including appropriate screening tools and timelines for access to care	Identify available local resources
			Establish locations for alternate care when local resources lacking
	Develop referral pathways for patients referred to different locations based on age and diagnosis		Clarify and establish local limitations through process mapping
			Establish human resource targets for optimal staffing
	Create process so all AYA patients offered AYA program consultation with advanced practice nurse (APN) and counselor	Develop human resource job descriptions for AYA program staff and establish number of staff needed per population	Determine if referral will happen at new patient registration or after first consultation
	Create process so all AYA patients offered follow-up with APN or counselor during treatment trajectory	Create standards for timelines to referral, and frequency of follow-up assessments based on disease site	Automate and deliver routine screening for AYA-specific distress factors
	Ensure all AYA patients screened for distress at intake		
Health care provider education	HCP needs assessment survey topic: the unique psychosocial needs of AYA	Establish funding and education opportunities for various AYA HCPs	Create local standards for continuing education opportunities
Patient and family education	Develop patient education materials on survivorship and late effects for AYA	Create electronic and written resources	Tailor individual education to patient needs by front-line staff
	Develop patient education materials on fertility preservation and counseling	Provide easily identifiable mechanism for navigating to resource (i.e., provincial website)	Local referrals to appropriate regional centers
Program expansion and sustainability	Foster relationships with motivated survivors, patients, and families for ongoing advocacy	Support and maintain patient and family advisory mechanisms	Promote engagement among motivated AYA patients and family
		Identify and recruit ongoing participants specific to AYA cancer	Direct individuals to available opportunities

4. Discussion

AYA program development is of value to a wide range of stakeholders. Herein, we present the first provincial efforts of developing priorities for ground-level implementation. This work is transferrable to other jurisdictions, as the highest ranked program components and discussion points raised are relevant to other institutions. Of the program components, patient care implementation was ranked as the highest priority for stakeholders, followed by health care provider education. Implementation of a multidisciplinary tumor board ranked lowest.

Based on round table discussion, while individual regional programs should be developed to suit the needs of each center, regional "umbrella" programs are required to ensure that information, resources, and guidelines are consistent. This model allows for sharing of limited resources between centers and increases consistency of care regardless of geographic location. While the groups recommended this "umbrella" program be developed at the provincial level, alternatively this can be done at a national level for certain items (such as standards of care and guidelines) to avoid duplication of work between provinces while still allowing regional centers to grow as per their unique needs.

Items relating to referrals, direct patient care, and psychosocial support scored higher than those relating to research, quality improvement, or formation of tumor board case reviews. These findings are logical in the context of a pilot AYA program as patients, families, and front-line HCPs are more likely to benefit from these tangible interventions. This is consistent with existing evidence that communication between AYA patients and their HCPs remains poor, and distress support remains inadequate [21–23]. Pilot AYA programs focusing on patient care and psychosocial support resonate with front-line staff and patients. This is consistent with grassroots clinics that have developed thus far in various jurisdictions including Toronto, Montreal, and Alberta. Fertility preservation screening and referral were identified as specific issues that could be easily targeted as initial steps. This is consistent with national and international priorities in the AYA population [2,4,5,16,17].

While items pertaining to QI, research, and indirect patient care such as holding tumor board discussions did not score as highly, many did still reach the threshold for consensus and were deemed important. As a strategy to prevent detraction of resources away from direct patient care and psychosocial support, implementation of items that do not have immediate impact on patient care can be deferred until an institution's AYA program is more established. Items pertaining to patient care implementation scored the highest of items across all domains, comprising the top three highest rated items and five of the top 10. Items relating to psychosocial support, automatic referrals, and follow-up through the AYA program, APN, or counselor were especially highly rated. It must be acknowledged, however, that AYA patients with cancer are an understudied population and thus establishing a research program will be essential for the future of AYA treatment and survivorship. Even if not implemented immediately, establishing a research program should be part of any AYA program and cannot be forgotten.

Despite consensus to create an AYA APN and counselor with whom patients would be offered consultation and follow-up, there was lack of consensus regarding their workflow. This represents the variation in needs of individual institutions even within similar jurisdictions. Recommendations ranged from the AYA staff seeing all AYA patients, instituting a referral-based process for high risk AYA, to no direct patient care responsibilities and capacity building among front-line staff alone. The majority felt some direct patient care would be beneficial, particularly for higher needs patients. In addition, the need to identify an AYA resource clinician with clinical expertise in AYA cancer care at each cancer center to support high needs patients, in addition to the AYA-specific APN and counselor, was identified. There is need for further clarification of these roles at the level of both umbrella and institutional program levels.

Although the average rating of items under HCP education was not as high as in other domains, the number of important items (10) was second highest, behind only patient care implementation (11). Based on consensus, completing HCP needs assessment surveys including the following topics is recommended: survivorship and late effects for AYA, the unique psychosocial needs of AYA, navigating interpersonal relationships for patients in treatment, palliative care needs for AYA, and coaching lifestyle changes, healthy diet, and exercise for AYA patients on treatment. These needs assessments would serve to ask HCPs what they need to succeed, in addition to providing evidence-based information on best practices in AYA oncologic care. This could include annual grand rounds on AYA oncology, development of online modules, and establishing partnerships with other organizations.

There was unanimous consensus for a strong focus on HCP education and capacity building, regardless of the future direct patient care role of the AYA-specific APN and counselor. Although patient care implementation was identified as the highest priority, HCP education is inherent to the provision of patient care [24] and requires less infrastructure to begin. Moving forward with HCP education either as an initial step or concurrently with patient care implementation based on each center's resources will impact patient care. Focusing on HCP education will improve direct patient care through existing personnel and staff by improving knowledge and skill sets. By providing such continuing education opportunities, each program will also conform with best practices to ensure ongoing development of staff skills. It was evident that staff and patient and family partners recognize that providing care to this demographic is challenging, particularly when raising distressing topics, such as loss of fertility, ongoing and long-term toxicity, and incurable diagnoses. Providing direct support to HCPs and patients during these higher stress interactions will improve delivery of care and improve HCP and patient satisfaction.

Existing AYA clinical programs exist to varying degrees in Canada. In Toronto, for example, the Princess Margaret Cancer Centre provides a local AYA program which patients and health care providers can refer into. With this program, a clinical nurse specialist provides counseling, and referrals and direction to various resources in the tertiary centers and community that would be relevant to the individual patient's concerns [25]. Alberta Health Services (AHS) is another example. The AHS program provides AYA patient navigators, who are specially trained registered nurses, at the Edmonton and Calgary cancer sites to provide individualized support to patients, facilitate referrals to appropriate services, and link patients to available resources [26]. Although differing in regional scope, both programs prioritized clinical delivery of care through AYA-specific health care providers who can help navigate health care systems and provide direction towards psychosocial support. The current study identifies how to further expand on existing programs by suggesting proposed next steps for implementation of more comprehensive AYA programs.

Limitations

This work has limitations. Despite initial invitations, limited responses from patient and family partners were received during the online iterations. However, despite this set-back, the overall findings are consistent with national guidelines which were developed with patient and family representatives and feedback from national AYA advocacy groups. As the primary goal was to develop an implementation strategy within local centres, diverse feedback from front-line clinicians, administrators, and clinicians in managerial roles was needed and successfully obtained.

5. Conclusions

Improving AYA delivery of care is an important priority for stakeholders. This body of work provides practical steps to support cancer centers in the development of local programs. Recruiting AYA clinicians to develop and deliver programs and improving health care provider competencies through education endeavors serves as the initial next step institutions can undertake.

Author Contributions: Conceptualization, A.S., G.C. and C.S.; methodology, A.S., G.C. and C.S.; validation, A.S. and J.S.; formal analysis, A.S. and J.S.; investigation, A.S. and J.S.; resources, A.S.; data curation, A.S.; writing—original draft preparation, A.S. and J.S.; writing—review and editing, A.S., G.C, C.S. and J.S.; visualization, J.S.; supervision, A.S.; project administration, A.S.; funding acquisition, A.S. All authors have read and agreed to the published version of the manuscript.

Funding: This research was funded through the Specialist Services Committee of BC Cancer.

Institutional Review Board Statement: Not applicable.

Informed Consent Statement: Not applicable.

Data Availability Statement: The data presented in this study are available in this article.

Acknowledgments: Funding was made available through the Specialist Services Committee to bring together representatives from BC Cancer and BC Children's Hospital. We thank the MSES for their financial support in this endeavor. We thank and acknowledge Avril Ullett, program manager at BC Cancer, and Bernice Budz, also from BC Cancer, who contributed to this work at the time of its development. We also thank our patient and family partners, who continue to advocate to improve the delivery of care to our AYA patients. This work was presented as an oral presentation titled "Setting Priorities for a Provincial Adolescent and Young Adult Oncology Program" at the Global Adolescent and Young Adult Congress, December 2018, in Sydney, Australia. This work was presented as a poster presentation titled "Setting Priorities for a Provincial Adolescent and Young Adult Oncology Program" at the Canadian Centre for Applied Research in Cancer Control Conference, May 2019 in Halifax, Nova Scotia, Canada.

Conflicts of Interest: The authors declare no conflict of interest.

Appendix A

Table A1. Delphi survey respondent and engagement session participant areas of work.

	Round 1		Round 2	
Area of Work	Responses (*n*)	%	Participants (*n*)	%
Administration	4	6.7%	1	3.7%
Oncology	16	26.7%	10	37.0%
Nursing	16	26.7%	4	14.8%
Psychosocial and Therapeutic Services	13	21.7%	5	18.5%
Radiation Therapy	1	1.7%	0	0%
Pain and Symptom Management	4	6.7%	0	0%
Nutrition	1	1.7%	0	0%
Patient/Caregiver Advisor	1	1.7%	3	11.1%
Psychiatry	1	1.7%	1	3.7%
Nurse Practitioner	1	1.7%	1	3.7%
Speech Language Pathology	1	1.7%	0	0%
Vocational Rehabilitation	0	0%	1	3.7%
Other—Patient Advocate	0	0%	1	3.7%
No Response	1	1.7%	0	0%
Total	60	100%	27	100%

Appendix B

Note: those items scored <2.00 or >3.99 in round one of the survey were interpreted as either unimportant and excluded from program development, or important and included in program development. Those items that scored from 2.01–3.99 were interpreted as inconclusive, and rescored in the second survey iteration. The table below shows the weighted mean for rounds one and two of the survey. Those items in yellow in round one were inconclusive and rescored, and, if green in round two, are important and should be included in the program.

Appendix B.1. Discussion Guides

Program Mission and Goals—Discussion Guide

Program mission: Create a provincial interdisciplinary cancer program for adolescents and young adults aged 15–29 years that will regionally implement recommendations across all BC Cancer sites in partnership with BC Children's Hospital

- Is this mission appropriate?
- Is the age range appropriate?
- Are there others who should be involved?

Review program goals with the following questions in mind:

- Are these goals comprehensive enough for a provincial program?
- Is there anything missing? Anything that should be omitted?
- What are the priority goals for implementation?

Patient Care Implementation—Discussion Guide

- Should all AYA patients receive a consult with AYA program advanced practice nurse (APN) or counselor? If not, what are the ideal consultation criteria?
- The new AYA program will hire an APN and counselor to take on the following activities/roles:
    - ○ Introduce AYA program to patients and families
    - ○ Administer AYA distress screen to identify immediate needs
    - ○ Patient and family counseling and education
    - ○ Provide access to AYA specific information
    - ○ Facilitate referral to speciality services
    - ○ Fertility counseling and referral
    - ○ Links to community resources
    - ○ Links to family counseling and support services
- ■ Based on the above, are there any additional activities the APN and counselor should engage in with patients and families?
    - Should the APN or counselor see patients during existing oncology appointments?
    - How frequently should APN or counselor check in with patients throughout treatment trajectory and post treatment?
    - What AYA-specific screening tools are needed?
    - What role should the AYA APN and counselor play in capacity building of BC Cancer staff?

Health Care Provider Education—Discussion Guide

- Is the list of education topics exhaustive? Are there other education topics that should be included?
- How can health care provider education be best delivered?
- How can primary care providers be involved in AYA oncology education?
- What would partnerships with various organizations, such as FPON, CON sites, Divisions of Family Practice, look like for health care provider education?

Program Evaluation Strategy—Discussion Guide

- How can we collect patient reported outcomes from AYA patients across all tumor groups?
- Review the proposed measures in the draft evaluation strategy—are these the right things to collect?
- How should evaluation updates be shared with patients, families, and senior leadership on a regular basis?

Patient and Family Education and Engagement—Discussion Guide

- Review the list of patient education material topics in the Delphi survey below. Is this list exhaustive? Are other topics needed?
- What is the best way to provide patient and family education? (e.g., printed materials, new AYA website, etc.)
- What would an AYA peer support network look like for BC?
- How can we engage patients and families on an ongoing basis to inform program development?

Program Expansion and Sustainability—Discussion Guide

- What is the best way to expand the program? (for example, increase age range to 39; have AYA specialist APNs/counselors at each center; capacity building with existing BC Cancer staff and have AYA APN and counselor as specialists available for consultation)
- What needs to be in place to sustain this program?
- What is currently feasible at each center?

Appendix B.2. Delphi Survey Results Summary

Item	Round 1 Weighted Mean	Round 2 Weighted Mean
Program Mission and Goals		
Program mission: Create a provincial interdisciplinary cancer program for adolescents and young adults aged 15–29 years that will regionally implement recommendations across all BC Cancer sites in partnership with BCCH	4.61	-
Goal 1: Develop health care provider education curriculum based on a formal learning needs assessment with clinical teams	4.08	-
Goal 2: Facilitate clinical consults with referral pathways to other services and flexible access to interventions	4.45	-
Goal 3: Integrate access to AYA-specific psychosocial distress screening and fertility preservation screening and referral	4.41	-
Goal 4: Develop multidisciplinary tumor board case reviews supported at BCCH and BC Cancer	3.78	4.04
Goal 5: Create evidence-based quality improvement and program evaluation plans	4.02	-
Goal 6: Develop a comprehensive AYA research program	3.83	3.81
Goal 7: Introduce patient reported outcome measurement to improve patient experience	4.18	-
Goal 8: Support patients and families through education and peer support network	4.43	-
Patient Care Implementation		
Develop referral pathways for patients referred to BC Cancer, BCCH, VGH based on age and diagnosis	4.66	-
Ensure all AYA patients screened for distress at intake	4.53	-
Create process so all AYA patients offered AYA program consultation with advanced practice nurse (APN) and counselor	4.64	-
Create process so all AYA patients offered follow-up with APN or counselor during treatment trajectory	4.57	-
Create process so all AYA patients routinely contacted at pre-specified times during care trajectory for follow-up of clinical issues	4.30	-
AYA APN and/or counselor to see patients referred into the program only (referral-based program)	3.98	3.91
AYA APN and/or counselor meet with all AYA patients at least once after new patient intake appointment	4.38	-
AYA APN and counselor to work out of a dedicated space separate from current oncology clinics	3.15	3.70
AYA APN and counselor to see patients during pre-existing oncology clinic appointments	3.79	3.96
Develop/adapt and implement AYA-specific screening tools (psychological distress, fertility screening)	4.33	-
Establish referral pathways for pre-defined high problem issues (such as suicide, psychosocial distress, fertility preservation, urgent end of life symptom management)	4.67	-
Establish transition pathways between BCCH, BC Cancer, and VGH	4.45	-
Develop/adapt tumor-specific treatment guidelines	4.05	-
Develop/adapt AYA-specific supportive care guidelines	4.35	-
Health Care Provider Education Strategy		
Conduct health care provider (HCP) education needs assessment through surveys of nursing, counseling, and physicians at BCCH and BC Cancer asking respondents to rank education priorities	3.98	3.79
Conduct education needs assessment among GPOs via survey asking respondents to rank education priorities	3.23	4.04
Conduct education needs assessment among primary care providers via survey asking respondents to rank education priorities	3.88	

Item	Round 1 Weighted Mean	Round 2 Weighted Mean
HCP needs assessment survey topic: fertility preservation and counseling	4.40	-
HCP needs assessment survey topic: survivorship and late effects for AYA	4.44	-
HCP needs assessment survey topic: the unique psychosocial needs of AYA	4.53	-
HCP needs assessment survey topic: navigating interpersonal relationships for patients in treatment	4.38	-
HCP needs assessment survey topic: palliative care needs for AYA	4.47	-
HCP needs assessment survey topic: coaching lifestyle changes, healthy diet, and exercise for AYA patients on treatment	4.20	-
Development of online continuing medical education accredited module in AYA oncology targeted to all health care providers involved in AYA care	3.91	4.13
Development of AYA fellowship program with Royal College diploma for Focused Competency in Adolescent and Young Adult Oncology	3.80	3.67
Annual grand rounds on AYA oncology	3.65	4.42
Establish formal partnerships between various organizations for ongoing HCP education (i.e., Family Practice Oncology Network, Community Oncology Network sites)	3.96	4.09
Patient and Family Education and Engagement Strategy		
Conduct environmental scan to determine top educational needs of AYA patients and families	4.38	-
Conduct environmental scan to identify existing AYA patient and family education resources to be adapted to BC context	4.05	-
Gather BC Cancer and BCCH new patient materials to adapt to AYA needs	4.06	-
Develop patient education materials on fertility preservation and counseling	4.48	-
Develop patient education materials on survivorship and late effects for AYA	4.50	-
Develop patient education materials on healthy lifestyle including nutrition and exercise	4.24	-
Develop an AYA peer support network	4.30	-
Develop a long-term patient and family engagement strategy for ongoing feedback into program development	4.14	-
Program Evaluation Strategy		
Ensure collection of adequate baseline outputs and outcomes prior to program implementation	4.00	-
Identify opportunities for data collection within existing resources	4.00	-
Identify additional resources required (including staff) for ongoing data collection	3.95	4.23
Establish frequency of data collection and frequency of review by oversight committee	3.85	3.73
Establish outputs and outcomes of relevance for data collection	4.24	-
Determine how evaluation updates will be shared with patients, family, and senior leadership on a regular basis	3.86	3.82
Model for Multidisciplinary Conference (MDC) Tumor Board Review		
Identify required team members for tumor board attendance and optional attendees	3.79	4.05
Representatives from medical oncology, radiation oncology, surgery/surgical oncology, pathology, diagnostic radiology, nursing, and patient and family counseling should be present to provide the complete range of expert opinion appropriate for the disease site and appropriate for the hospital	4.45	-
Representatives for BCCH and BC Cancer oncology services will attend conference	4.23	-
Establish ideal frequency, date, and timing of tumor boards and how notification will be undertaken—MDC should occur for a minimum of 1 h every 2 weeks	3.82	3.89
Identify electronic/online tumor board opportunities and platforms	4.21	-
All new AYA patient treatment plans should be forwarded to AYA MDC coordinator	4.04	-
Not all cases forwarded to the MDC coordinator need to be discussed at the AYA MDC	3.82	3.80
The individual physician and the MDC chair can determine which cases are discussed in detail at the MDC	3.94	4.15
Other cases (e.g., recurrent or metastatic cancer) can be forwarded to the MDC coordinator for discussion, at the discretion of the individual physician	3.89	3.80
AYA MDC will primarily serve to identify all suitable treatment options, and ensure the most appropriate treatment recommendations are generated for each cancer patient discussed prospectively in a multidisciplinary forum	4.43	-

Item	Round 1 Weighted Mean	Round 2 Weighted Mean
Secondary functions of AYA MDC will include: a forum for the continuing education of medical staff and health professionals, contributing to the development of standardized patient management protocols, and contributing to linkages among regions to ensure appropriate referrals and timely consultation	4.22	-
AYA Research Priorities		
Form an AYA research and evaluation working group	4.15	-
Identify platforms for data collection	4.05	-
Develop and implement a program evaluation strategy through research	4.00	-
Identify patient reported outcomes and clinical outcomes for collection	4.29	-
Develop a quality improvement plan and strategy	4.14	-
Identify key stakeholders for AYA research	4.00	-
Identify and implement an AYA research agenda	3.95	4.05
Develop an AYA research education plan (e.g., fellowship training for HCPs)	3.76	4.10
Model for Program Expansion and Sustainability		
Identify key clinical and operations stakeholders for ongoing expansion	4.23	-
Develop website content and create a program email address	4.42	-
Develop social media strategies	4.00	-
Foster and develop online platform and app development	4.26	-
Review different models of expansion (spoke and hub; health authority-specific champions)	4.11	-
Identify available resources for de-centralized telemedicine expansion capacity	4.09	-
Identify available resources (including HCP compensation) for physical expansion capacity	4.13	-
Identify and explore operations and infrastructure limitations to expanding AYA program	3.84	4.38
Identify BC Cancer Foundation long-term funding opportunities	4.49	-
Identify AYA "champions" in regional centers to for ongoing program development	4.29	-
Foster relationships with motivated survivors, patients, and families for ongoing advocacy	4.56	-

Appendix C. All Items Rated Important across All Domains

Program Item	Score	Component
Program mission: Create a provincial interdisciplinary cancer program for adolescents and young adults aged 15–29 years that will regionally implement recommendations across all BC Cancer sites in partnership with BCCH	4.61	Program Mission and Goals
Goal 1: Develop health care provider education curriculum based on a formal learning needs assessment with clinical teams	4.08	Program Mission and Goals
Goal 2: Facilitate clinical consults with referral pathways to other services and flexible access to interventions	4.45	Program Mission and Goals
Goal 3: Integrate access to AYA-specific psychosocial distress screening and fertility preservation screening and referral	4.41	Program Mission and Goals
Goal 4: Develop multidisciplinary tumor board case reviews supported at BCCH and BC Cancer	4.04	Program Mission and Goals
Goal 5: Create evidence-based quality improvement and program evaluation plans	4.02	Program Mission and Goals
Goal 7: Introduce patient reported outcome measurement to improve patient experience	4.18	Program Mission and Goals
Goal 8: Support patients and families through education and peer support network	4.43	Program Mission and Goals
Develop referral pathways for patients referred to BC Cancer, BCCH, VGH based on age and diagnosis	4.66	Patient Care Implementation

Program Item	Score	Component
Ensure all AYA patients screened for distress at intake	4.53	Patient Care Implementation
Create process so all AYA patients offered AYA program consultation with advanced practice nurse (APN) and counselor	4.64	Patient Care Implementation
Create process so all AYA patients offered follow-up with APN or counselor during treatment trajectory	4.57	Patient Care Implementation
Create process so all AYA patients routinely contacted at pre-specified times during care trajectory for follow-up of clinical issues	4.30	Patient Care Implementation
AYA APN and/or counselor meet with all AYA patients at least once after new patient intake appointment	4.38	Patient Care Implementation
Develop/adapt and implement AYA-specific screening tools (psychological distress, fertility screening)	4.33	Patient Care Implementation
Establish referral pathways for pre-defined high problem issues (such as suicide, psychosocial distress, fertility preservation, urgent end of life symptom management)	4.67	Patient Care Implementation
Establish transition pathways between BCCH, BC Cancer, and VGH	4.45	Patient Care Implementation
Develop/adapt tumor-specific treatment guidelines	4.05	Patient Care Implementation
Develop/adapt AYA-specific supportive care guidelines	4.35	Patient Care Implementation
Conduct education needs assessment among GPOs via survey asking respondents to rank education priorities	4.04	Health Care Provider Education Strategy
HCP needs assessment survey topic: fertility preservation and counseling	4.40	Health Care Provider Education Strategy
HCP needs assessment survey topic: survivorship and late effects for AYA	4.44	Health Care Provider Education Strategy
HCP needs assessment survey topic: the unique psychosocial needs of AYA	4.53	Health Care Provider Education Strategy
HCP needs assessment survey topic: navigating interpersonal relationships for patients in treatment	4.38	Health Care Provider Education Strategy
HCP needs assessment survey topic: palliative care needs for AYA	4.47	Health Care Provider Education Strategy
HCP needs assessment survey topic: coaching lifestyle changes, healthy diet, and exercise for AYA patients on treatment	4.20	Health Care Provider Education Strategy
Development of online continuing medical education accredited module in AYA oncology targeted to all health care providers involved in AYA care	4.13	Health Care Provider Education Strategy
Annual grand rounds on AYA oncology	4.42	Health Care Provider Education Strategy
Establish formal partnerships between various organizations for ongoing HCP education (i.e., Family Practice Oncology Network, Community Oncology Network sites)	4.09	Health Care Provider Education Strategy
Conduct environmental scan to determine top educational needs of AYA patients and families	4.38	Patient and Family Education and Engagement Strategy
Conduct environmental scan to identify existing AYA patient and family education resources to be adapted to BC context	4.05	Patient and Family Education and Engagement Strategy
Gather BC Cancer and BCCH new patient materials to adapt to AYA needs	4.06	Patient and Family Education and Engagement Strategy
Develop patient education materials on fertility preservation and counseling	4.48	Patient and Family Education and Engagement Strategy
Develop patient education materials on survivorship and late effects for AYA	4.50	Patient and Family Education and Engagement Strategy

Program Item	Score	Component
Develop patient education materials on healthy lifestyle including nutrition and exercise	4.24	Patient and Family Education and Engagement Strategy
Develop an AYA peer support network	4.30	Patient and Family Education and Engagement Strategy
Develop a long-term patient and family engagement strategy for ongoing feedback into program development	4.14	Patient and Family Education and Engagement Strategy
Ensure collection of adequate baseline outputs and outcomes prior to program implementation	4.00	Program Evaluation Strategy
Identify opportunities for data collection within existing resources	4.00	Program Evaluation Strategy
Identify additional resources required (including staff) for ongoing data collection	4.23	Program Evaluation Strategy
Establish outputs and outcomes of relevance for data collection	4.24	Program Evaluation Strategy
Identify required team members for tumor board attendance and optional attendees	4.05	MDC Tumor Board Review
Representatives from medical oncology, radiation oncology, surgery/surgical oncology, pathology, diagnostic radiology, nursing, and patient and family counselling should be present to provide the complete range of expert opinion appropriate for the disease site and appropriate for the hospital	4.45	MDC Tumor Board Review
Representatives for BCCH and BC Cancer oncology services will attend conference	4.23	MDC Tumor Board Review
Identify electronic/online tumor board opportunities and platforms	4.21	MDC Tumor Board Review
All new AYA patient treatment plans should be forwarded to AYA MDC coordinator	4.04	MDC Tumor Board Review
The individual physician and the MDC chair can determine which cases are discussed in detail at the MDC	4.15	MDC Tumor Board Review
AYA MDC will primarily serve to identify all suitable treatment options, and ensure the most appropriate treatment recommendations are generated for each cancer patient discussed prospectively in a multidisciplinary forum	4.43	MDC Tumor Board Review
Secondary functions of AYA MDC will include: a forum for the continuing education of medical staff and health professionals, contributing to the development of standardized patient management protocols, and contributing to linkages among regions to ensure appropriate referrals and timely consultation	4.22	MDC Tumor Board Review
Form an AYA research and evaluation working group	4.15	AYA Research Priorities
Identify platforms for data collection	4.05	AYA Research Priorities
Develop and implement a program evaluation strategy through research	4.00	AYA Research Priorities
Identify patient reported outcomes and clinical outcomes for collection	4.29	AYA Research Priorities
Develop a quality improvement plan and strategy	4.14	AYA Research Priorities
Identify key stakeholders for AYA research	4.00	AYA Research Priorities
Identify and implement an AYA research agenda	4.05	AYA Research Priorities
Develop an AYA research education plan (e.g., fellowship training for HCPs)	4.10	AYA Research Priorities
Identify key clinical and operations stakeholders for ongoing expansion	4.23	Model for Program Expansion and Sustainability
Develop website content and create a program email address	4.42	Model for Program Expansion and Sustainability
Develop social media strategies	4.00	Model for Program Expansion and Sustainability
Foster and develop online platform and app development	4.26	Model for Program Expansion and Sustainability

Program Item	Score	Component
Review different models of expansion (spoke and hub; health authority-specific champions)	4.11	Model for Program Expansion and Sustainability
Identify available resources for de-centralized telemedicine expansion capacity	4.09	Model for Program Expansion and Sustainability
Identify available resources (including HCP compensation) for physical expansion capacity	4.13	Model for Program Expansion and Sustainability
Identify and explore operations and infrastructure limitations to expanding AYA program	4.38	Model for Program Expansion and Sustainability
Identify BC Cancer Foundation long-term funding opportunities	4.49	Model for Program Expansion and Sustainability
Identify AYA "champions" in regional centers to for ongoing program development	4.29	Model for Program Expansion and Sustainability
Foster relationships with motivated survivors, patients, and families for ongoing advocacy	4.56	Model for Program Expansion and Sustainability

Appendix D. Agenda

BC Adolescent and Young Adult Oncology Program
Create the Program You Need

Time	Item Number	Items
8:30 a.m.	1.0	Registration, Coffee & Continental Breakfast
9:00 a.m.	2.0	Welcome & Opening Remarks
	2.1	A Family's Experience with AYA Cancer Care
	2.2	Cancer Care for AYA in BC—Current Situation
	2.3	BC AYA Oncology Program—Program Development to Date
10:00 a.m.	3.0	Table Discussion & Report Back: Program Mission & Goals
11:30 a.m.		-Lunch-
12:30 p.m.	4.0	Table Discussion & Report Back: Patient Care Implementation
2:30 p.m.		-Break-
3:00 p.m.	5.0	Breakout Sessions
	5.1	Health Care Provider Education Strategy
	5.2	Patient & Family Education Strategy
	5.3	Program Evaluation Strategy
	5.4	Model for Multidisciplinary Tumour Review Board
	5.5	Program Sustainability & Expansion Plan
4:30 p.m.	6.0	Breakout Session Report Back & Large Group Discussion
5:00 p.m.	7.0	Closing Remarks & Next Steps

Appendix E. Program Implementation Prioritization—Individual Results

	Health Care Provider Education	Patient and Family Education	Patient Care Implementation	Program Expansion and Sustainability	Research Priorities	MDC Tumor Board Review	Evaluation Strategy
	Respondent			Rank in order of prioritization 1–7			
1	-	-	-	1	-	3	2
2	3	2	1	6	4	5	7
3	4	5	1	3	2	6	7
4	2	1	3	4	6	7	5
5	2	3	1	4	5	-	6
6	3	2	1	-	-	4	-
7	2	1	3	4	5	6	7
8	3	1	2	5	4	7	6
9	1	2	3	7	4	5	6
10	3	2	1	5	6	7	4
11	3	6	5	7	2	4	1
12	5	4	1	3	6	7	2
13	5	2	1	4	3	6	7
14	2	3	1	4	5	6	7
15	1	2	3	6	7	5	4
16	2	3	1	7	6	4	5
17	1	3	2	5	7	6	4
18	2	3	1	6	7	5	4

References

1. Canadian Parternship Against Cancer Framework for the Care and Support for Adolescents and Young Adults with Cancer. Available online: https://www.partnershipagainstcancer.ca/topics/framework-adolescents-young-adults/ (accessed on 12 November 2021).
2. Coccia, P.F.; Pappo, A.S.; Beaupin, L.; Borges, V.F.; Borinstein, S.C.; Chugh, R.; Dinner, S.; Folbrecht, J.; Frazier, A.L.; Goldsby, R.; et al. Adolescent and Young Adult Oncology, Version 2.2018, NCCN Clinical Practice Guidelines in Oncology. *J. Natl. Compr. Cancer Netw.* **2018**, *16*, 66–97. [CrossRef] [PubMed]
3. National Cancer Institute Adolescents and Young Adults (AYAs) with Cancer. Available online: https://www.cancer.gov/types/aya (accessed on 29 November 2021).
4. Canadian Parternship Against Cancer Adolescents & Young Adults with Cancer: A System Performance Report Toronto, ON, Canada. 2017. Available online: https://s22457.pcdn.co/wp-content/uploads/2019/01/Adolescents-and-young-adults-with-cancer-EN.pdf (accessed on 12 November 2021).
5. Canadian Parternship Against Cancer Person-Centred Perspective Indicators in Canada: A Reference Report. Adults and Young Adults with Cancer. Toronto, ON, Canada. 2017. Available online: https://s22457.pcdn.co/wp-content/uploads/2019/10/Adolescents-and-Young-Adults-with-Cancer-Reference-Report-EN.pdf (accessed on 12 November 2021).
6. Barr, R.; Rogers, P.; Schacter, B. Adolescents and Young Adults with Cancer: Towards Better Outcomes in Canada. Preamble. *Cancer* **2011**, *117*, 2239–2240. [CrossRef] [PubMed]
7. Youth Cancer Service: Canteen Australian Youth Cancer Framework for Adolescents and Young Adults with Cancer. Available online: https://www.canteen.org.au/health-education/measures-manuals/australian-youth-cancer-framework (accessed on 29 November 2021).
8. NHS England NHS Commissioning Children and Young People's Cancer. Available online: https://www.england.nhs.uk/commissioning/spec-services/npc-crg/group-b/b05/ (accessed on 29 November 2021).
9. Bleyer, A.; Barr, R. Cancer in Young Adults 20 to 39 Years of Age: Overview. *Semin. Oncol.* **2009**, *36*, 194–206. [CrossRef] [PubMed]
10. Leading Causes of Death in Canada-2009 Ten Leading Causes of Death by Selected Age Groups, by Sex, Canada 1-15 to 24 Years. 2009. Available online: https://www150.statcan.gc.ca/n1/pub/84-215-x/84-215-x2012001-eng.htm (accessed on 25 February 2009).

11. Lewis, D.R.; Siembida, E.J.; Seibel, N.L.; Smith, A.W.; Mariotto, A.B. Survival Outcomes for Cancer Types with the Highest Death Rates for Adolescents and Young Adults, 1975-2016. *Cancer* **2021**, *127*, 4277–4286. [CrossRef] [PubMed]
12. Bisogno, G.; Compostella, A.; Ferrari, A.; Pastore, G.; Cecchetto, G.; Garaventa, A.; Indolfi, P.; De Sio, L.; Carli, M. Rhabdomyosarcoma in Adolescents: A Report from the AIEOP Soft Tissue Sarcoma Committee. *Cancer* **2012**, *118*, 821–827. [CrossRef]
13. Bhatia, S.; Landier, W.; Shangguan, M.; Hageman, L.; Schaible, A.N.; Carter, A.R.; Hanby, C.L.; Leisenring, W.; Yasui, Y.; Kornegay, N.M.; et al. Nonadherence to Oral Mercaptopurine and Risk of Relapse in Hispanic and Non-Hispanic White Children with Acute Lymphoblastic Leukemia: A Report from the Children's Oncology Group. *J. Clin. Oncol.* **2012**, *30*, 2094–2101. [CrossRef] [PubMed]
14. Brasme, J.F.; Morfouace, M.; Grill, J.; Martinot, A.; Amalberti, R.; Bons-Letouzey, C.; Chalumeau, M. Delays in Diagnosis of Paediatric Cancers: A Systematic Review and Comparison with Expert Testimony in Lawsuits. *Lancet Oncol.* **2012**. [CrossRef]
15. Canner, J.; Alonzo, T.A.; Franklin, J.; Freyer, D.R.; Gamis, A.; Gerbing, R.B.; Lange, B.J.; Meshinchi, S.; Woods, W.G.; Perentesis, J.; et al. Differences in Outcomes of Newly Diagnosed Acute Myeloid Leukemia for Adolescent/Young Adult and Younger Patients: A Report from the Children's Oncology Group. *Cancer* **2013**, *119*, 4162–4169. [CrossRef] [PubMed]
16. Identifying and Addressing the Needs of Adolescents and Young Adults with Cancer: Workshop Summary. Available online: https://pubmed.ncbi.nlm.nih.gov/24479202/ (accessed on 1 May 2022).
17. Ferrari, A.; Stark, D.; Peccatori, F.A.; Fern, L.; Laurence, V.; Gaspar, N.; Bozovic-Spasojevic, I.; Smith, O.; De Munter, J.; Derwich, K.; et al. Adolescents and Young Adults (AYA) with Cancer: A Position Paper from the AYA Working Group of the European Society for Medical Oncology (ESMO) and the European Society for Paediatric Oncology (SIOPE). *ESMO Open* **2021**, *6*, 100096. [CrossRef] [PubMed]
18. Albritton, K.H.; Wiggins, C.H.; Nelson, H.E.; Weeks, J.C. Site of Oncologic Specialty Care for Older Adolescents in Utah. *J. Clin. Oncol.* **2007**, *25*, 4616–4621. [CrossRef] [PubMed]
19. Powell, C. The Delphi Technique: Myths and Realities. *J. Adv. Nurs.* **2003**, *41*, 376–382. [CrossRef] [PubMed]
20. Hsu, C.; Sandford, B. The Delphi Technique: Making Sense of Consensus. *Pract. Assess. Res. Eval.* **2007**, *12*, 10. [CrossRef]
21. Smith, A.W.; Parsons, H.M.; Kent, E.E.; Bellizzi, K.; Zebrack, B.J.; Keel, G.; Lynch, C.F.; Rubenstein, M.B.; Keegan, T.H.M.; Cress, R.; et al. Unmet Support Service Needs and Health-Related Quality of Life among Adolescents and Young Adults with Cancer: The AYA HOPE Study. *Front. Oncol.* **2013**, *3*, 75. [CrossRef] [PubMed]
22. Barr, R.D.; Ferrari, A.; Ries, L.; Whelan, J.; Bleyer, W.A. Cancer in Adolescents and Young Adults: A Narrative Review of the Current Status and a View of the Future. *JAMA Pediatr.* **2016**, *170*, 495–501. [CrossRef] [PubMed]
23. Zebrack, B.J.; Corbett, V.; Embry, L.; Aguilar, C.; Meeske, K.A.; Hayes-Lattin, B.; Block, R.; Zeman, D.T.; Cole, S. Psychological Distress and Unsatisfied Need for Psychosocial Support in Adolescent and Young Adult Cancer Patients during the First Year Following Diagnosis. *Psychooncology* **2014**, *23*, 1267–1275. [CrossRef] [PubMed]
24. Hayes-Lattin, B.; Mathews-Bradshaw, B.; Siegel, S. Adolescent and Young Adult Oncology Training for Health Professionals: A Position Statement. *J. Clin. Oncol.* **2010**, *28*, 4858–4861. [CrossRef] [PubMed]
25. Princess Margaret Cancer Centre AYA Program, Princess Margaret Cancer Centre. Available online: https://www.uhn.ca/PrincessMargaret/Clinics/Adolescent_Young_Adult_Oncology (accessed on 1 May 2022).
26. Alberta Health Services; CancerControl Alberta Adolescent and Young Adult (AYA) Patient Navigation. Available online: https://www.albertahealthservices.ca/assets/info/cca/if-cca-adolescent-young-adult-patient-navigation.pdf (accessed on 1 May 2022).

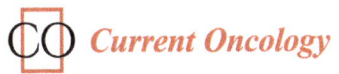

Systematic Review

Pediatric-Inspired Regimens in the Treatment of Acute Lymphoblastic Leukemia in Adolescents and Young Adults: A Systematic Review

Aida Zeckanovic [1,2,*], Philipp Fuchs [1,2], Philip Heesen [3], Nicole Bodmer [1,2], Maria Otth [1,2,4,5,†] and Katrin Scheinemann [4,5,6,†]

1. Department of Oncology, University Children's Hospital Zurich, 8032 Zurich, Switzerland; philipp.fuchs@kispi.uzh.ch (P.F.); nicole.bodmer@kispi.uzh.ch (N.B.); maria.otth@kispisg.ch (M.O.)
2. Children's Research Center, University Children's Hospital Zurich, 8032 Zurich, Switzerland
3. Faculty of Medicine, University of Zurich, 8006 Zurich, Switzerland; philip.heesen@uzh.ch
4. Division of Hematology/Oncology, Children's Hospital of Eastern Switzerland, 9006 St. Gallen, Switzerland; katrin.scheinemann@kispisg.ch
5. Faculty of Health Sciences and Medicine, University of Lucerne, 6000 Lucerne, Switzerland
6. Department of Pediatrics, McMaster Children's Hospital and McMaster University, Hamilton, ON L8S 4L8, Canada
* Correspondence: aida.zeckanovic@kispi.uzh.ch; Tel.: +41-44-266-74-55
† These authors contributed equally to this work.

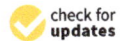

Abstract: Adolescents and young adults (AYA) with acute lymphoblastic leukemia (ALL) have significantly worse outcomes than their younger counterparts. Current treatment guidelines rely mostly on non-randomized retrospective studies. We performed a systematic review of studies published within the last 15 years comparing pediatric-inspired regimens (PIR) versus adult-type regimens or performing an age-stratified analysis of outcomes in the AYA population. Due to the heterogeneity of data, a meta-analysis was not possible. However, the gathered data show a trend toward improvement in outcomes and an acceptable toxicity profile in patients treated with PIRs compared to conventional adult-type regimens. There is still room for further improvement, as older patients within the AYA population tend to perform poorly with PIR or conventional adult-type chemotherapy. Further randomized studies are needed to develop an optimal treatment strategy for AYA with ALL.

Keywords: acute lymphoblastic leukemia; adolescents and young adult; protocol; pediatric-inspired; survival

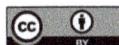

1. Introduction

While the long-term prognosis of children with acute lymphoblastic leukemia (ALL) has improved in recent decades, the outcome of adolescents and young adults (AYA) patients aged from 15 to 39 years remains markedly worse than that of their younger counterparts [1]. Based on population-based data from the EUROCARE-5 study, which monitors the survival of cancer patients in Europe, the 5-year relative survival of children aged 0–14 years is 85.8%. In comparison, the relative survival rates in the adolescent (15–19 years) and young adult (20–39 years) age groups were 62.2% and 52.8%, respectively [2].

Due to the broad age range of the AYA population, these patients are treated in pediatric as well as adult settings with a myriad of different protocols. However, treating ALL in this age group is a challenge not only due to an increased incidence of unfavorable cytogenetic aberrations but also due to unique psychosocial circumstances as well as higher treatment-related toxicity compared to younger children [3]. Based on the current data and expert opinion guidelines, the best therapeutic approach for an AYA patient with ALL is to use a pediatric-inspired regimen (PIR) [3–7]. Compared to conventional adult-type protocols, PIRs tend to have more therapy elements and encompass higher cumulative doses of asparaginase, vincristine, and steroids, in addition to a generally longer maintenance phase [5]. The most prominent examples of PIR are protocols incorporating a Dana–Farber Cancer Institute (DFCI) or Berlin–Frankfurt–Münster (BFM) study group backbone. However, data on treatment strategies in AYA and ALL are limited due to the lack of randomized comparative studies and thus prone to bias, making interpretation and comparison difficult.

The purpose of this systematic review is to provide a comprehensive synthesis of published comparative studies examining the outcomes and toxicity of AYA patients treated for ALL with PIR versus conventional adult regimens. Furthermore, we would like to summarize the available data on age-stratified outcomes and adverse events (AE) in AYA patients receiving PIR treatment.

2. Materials and Methods

We conducted the systematic literature search according to the PRISMA guidelines in PubMed in November 2022 [8]. The search strategy was built around the following three concepts: "acute lymphoblastic leukemia", "adolescents and young adults", and "treatment protocol/strategy" (Supplementary Data). Publications on myeloid leukemia and those with animal models were omitted through the search strategy. We restricted the search to studies published between November 2007 and November 2022. The inclusion criteria were given through the PICO framework [8]. The population included AYA cancer patients diagnosed with ALL. The AYA population was defined as patients diagnosed between the ages of 15 and 39 years, or at least 75% of the study population had to be within this range. The intervention corresponded to the treatment protocol, either a pediatric, pediatric-inspired, or adult protocol. Depending on the data provided in the eligible publications, we aimed to compare either adult-type versus pediatric/pediatric-inspired protocols or pediatric/pediatric-inspired protocols stratified by different age categories. The envisaged outcomes included survival (e.g., overall (OS) or event-free survival (EFS)), toxicity (e.g., toxic death, admission to the ICU), or reasons for the protocols used. However, the final reporting of these outcomes depended on whether the data were provided in the eligible publications or not.

Two authors performed the title and abstract screening (MO, AZ) and full-text screening (AZ, PF) each. Discrepancies between reviewers one and two were solved by a third reviewer (KS) using the same criteria. We extracted the data from the eligible studies onto a standard sheet, including the first author, year of publication, study design, patients' characteristics, information on the treatment protocol, and the outcomes assessed. We assessed the quality, relevance, and reliability of each included study by using the appropriate critical appraisal tool from the Joanna Briggs Institute (JBI) (https://jbi.global/critical-appraisal-tools) (accessed on 15 October 2022), including the checklists for cohort studies. Since the tools from the Joanna Briggs Institute do not have predefined categorizations, we defined a classification with three categories. If all criteria of the respective checklist were fulfilled, we assigned the study "Quality 1". If one or two criteria were not fulfilled, we assigned the study to "Quality 2". If three or more criteria were not fulfilled, the study was assigned "Quality 3".

The protocol for this review was published on Prospero (https://www.crd.york.ac.uk/prospero; ID: CRD42022384667) (accessed on 27 December 2022).

3. Results

3.1. Description of Studies and Regimens

The literature search identified 5132 publications. A total of 168 potentially relevant full-text articles were retrieved for further evaluation. Among these, 26 met the inclusion criteria for our systematic review (Figure 1, Table 1, Supplementary Data) [9–34]. Fifteen of the included studies (57%) had a prospective design [9,14,16,19,20,22,23,25–30,32,33].

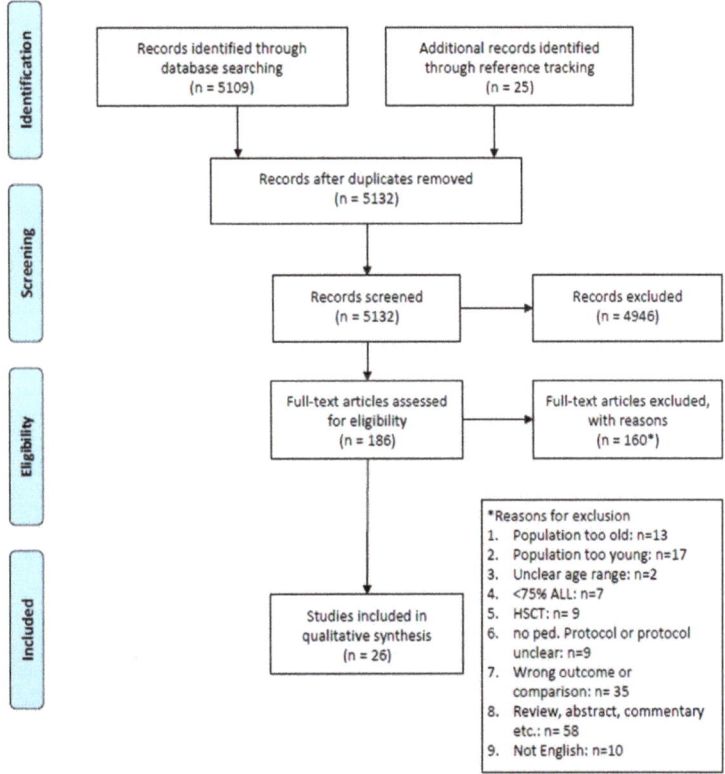

Figure 1. PRISMA flow diagram.

Twelve studies comparing the outcomes and/or toxicity of PIR vs. conventional adult-type regimens are summarized in Table 2 [10–12,15,17,18,21,22,24,29–31]. None of the studies were randomized controlled trials. Four studies included patients given PIR that were compared with historical controls receiving conventional adult regimens [12,24,29,30]. Others compared patients treated with PIR and adult protocols during approximately the same time periods. One study did not use any risk-adapted treatment for PIR; the others used some sort of risk stratification of patients [18].

Five studies had a median follow-up shorter than two years for at least one analyzed group [12,15,17,18,31], and one study did not specify the duration of follow-up [21]. Additionally, two studies had significantly longer follow-ups for the patients treated with conventional adult protocols [12,24], whereas another had significantly longer follow-ups for the patients treated with PIR [15]. In most studies, the compared groups had well-matched age distributions. However, in two studies, the group receiving the conventional adult treatment was slightly older than the PIR group [21,31], whereas the opposite was true for one study [12].

Nineteen studies, summarized in Table 3, describe the treatment outcomes or toxicities in different age groups, either within the defined AYA range or as a comparison to younger or older patients. Three studies have a shorter follow-up than 2 years [12,17,19], while one has a significantly shorter follow-up for the oldest analyzed age group [32]. Two studies contain data gathered during two different periods [9,12].

Table 1. Characteristics of the studies included in this review.

Author, Year, Country	Years of Recruitment	Diagnosis	PIR	Adult Protocol	N of Pediatric Patients (%)	N of Adult Patients (%)	Median Age (Range) in Years	JBI Score
Studies comparing adolescents and young adult patients receiving a PIR or adult regimen								
Al-Khabori, 2010 Canada [11]	January 1990–March 2007	T-ALL	DFCI regimen	9203ALL, Protocol C, Hyper-CVAD, MRC UKALL XII/ECOG E2993	32 (44)	40 (56)	30.8 (17–69)	1
Alacacioglu, 2014 Turkey [10]	March 2006–October 2012	ALL	BFM-Like	Hyper-CVAD	20 (40)	30 (60)	Overall: 27.5 (18–59) PIR: 25 Hyper-CVAD: 30.5	2
Almanza-Huante, 2021 Mexico [12]	PIR: March 2016–June 2019 hyper-CVAD: February 2009–June 2015	BCR–ABL negative ALL	modified ALL-BFM 90, modified CALGB C10403	Hyper-CVAD	73 (30)	173 (70)	Overall: 22 (14–43) PIR: 24 Hyper-CVAD: 20	1
Cheng, 2022 Taiwan [15]	2008–2019	VHR-ALL	TPOG-ALL-2002 protocol	Hyper-CVAD/HD-Methotrexate and Cytarabine	16 (59)	11 (41)	PIR: 24.3 (18–36) Hyper-CVAD: 33 (20–40)	1
Ganesan 2021 India [17]	2012–2017	ALL (including MPAL)	MCP-841, BFM-90, -95 or -2000, COG Protocols	GMALL, Hyper-CVAD, UKALL	1002 (88)	139 (12)	Overall: range 15–29 PIR: 20 Adult: 23	1
Ganesan, 2018 India [18]	January 2000–December 2014	BCR–ABL negative ALL	BFM 95, SR arm	MCP-841 (22%) GMALL (9%) INCTR (4%) UKALL (2%)	147 (63)	85 (37)	Overall: 21 (18–30) PIR: 21.8 Adult: 22.4	2
Gupta, 2019, Canada [21]	1992–2011	ALL	DFCI Protocol 91-01	Not specified	123 (54)	106 (46)	Range 15–21 Pediatric centers: mean 16 ± 1 Adult centers: mean 19 ± 1	1
Hayakawa, 2014, Japan [22]	August 2002–October 2009	BCR–ABL negative B-ALL	ALL202	ALL97-U	139 (57)	104 (43)	19 (15–24)	1

Table 1. Cont.

Author, Year, Country	Years of Recruitment	Diagnosis	PIR	Adult Protocol	N of Pediatric Patients (%)	N of Adult Patients (%)	Median Age (Range) in Years	JBI Score
Tantiworawit, 2019, Thailand [31]	January 2007–December 2017	ALL	TPOG protocol	Hyper-CVAD or GMALL protocol	35 (33)	75 (67)	Overall: 26 (15–63) Adult: 29.5 (16–63) PIR: 24 (15–39)	2
Rytting, 2014 USA [30]	October 2006–April 2012	BCR–ABL negative ALL	Augmented BFM regimen	Historic Hyper-CVAD cohort	85	71	PIR: 21 (13–39) Adult: 26 (16–40)	1
Rytting, 2016, USA [29]	October 2006–March 2014	BCR–ABL negative ALL	Augmented BFM regimen	Historic Hyper-CVAD cohort	106	102	PIR: 22 (13–39) Adult: 27 (15–40)	1
Kliman, 2017, Canada [24]	PIR: February 2008–November 2014 Adult: February 2003–July 2008	SR BCR–ABL negative ALL	Modification of DFCI 01–175	Comparative adult ALL protocols (not exactly specified)	22	25	Overall: 24.5 (18–40) PIR: 27.6 Adult: 23.5	2

Studies comparing age-stratified outcomes and toxicity in adolescents and young adult patients receiving a PIR or adult regimen

Ref.	Years of recruitment	Diagnosis	Protocol	Age groups and N of patients	JBI score
Advani, 2021, USA [9]	CALGB 10403: 2007–2012 COG AALL0232: 2004–2011	B- or T-precursor ALL	PIR: CALGB 10403 and COG AALL0232 (arm identical to CALGB 10403)	CALGB 10403: - 16–21 years: n = 94 (33%) - 22–30 years: n = 131 (45%) - 31–39 years: n = 64 (22%) COG AALL0232: - 16–21 years: n = 146 (92%) - 22–30 years: n = 12 (8%)	1
Almanza-Huante, 2021 Mexico [12]	PIR: March 2016–June 2019 Adult: February 2009–June 2015	BCR–ABL negative ALL	PIR: modified ALL-BFM 90, modified CALGB C10403 Adult: Hyper-CVAD	14–20 years: - PIR: n = 23; Hyper-CVAD: n = 69 21–43 years: - PIR n = 50; Hyper-CVAD n = 68	1

Table 1. Cont.

Author, Year, Country	Years of Recruitment	Diagnosis	PIR	N of Pediatric Patients (%) Adult Protocol	N of Adult Patients (%)	Median Age (Range) in Years	JBI Score
Brandwein, 2014 Canada [13]	June 2000–June 2011	BCR–ABL negative ALL	PIR: DFCI 91-01	17–<34 years: n = 73 (47%) 34–<50 years: n = 54 (35%) 50–60 years: n = 29 (19%)			1
Burke, 2022, USA [14]	January 2004–January 2011	HR B-ALL, excluding DS patients	PIR: COG AALL0232	<16 years: n = 2443 (=younger children) 16–30 years: n = 597 (=AYA population)			1
Cheng, 2022, Taiwan [15]	2008–2019	VHR-ALL	PIR: TPOG-ALL-2002 protocol	18–25 years: n = 7 26–34 years: n = 9			1
De Angelo, 2015, USA and Canada [16]	August 2002–February 2008	ALL (excl. mature B-cell ALL)	PIR: DFCI Pediatric ALL Consortium regimen/DFCI Adult: ALL Consortium Protocol 01-175	18–29 years: n = 48 (52%) 30–50 years: n = 44 (48%)			2
Ganesan, 2021, India [17]	2012–2017	ALL (including MPAL)	PIR: MCP-841[7], BFM-90, -95 or -2000), COG Adult: GMALL, Hyper-CVAD, UKALL	15–17 years: n = 403 (29.1%) 18–24 years: n = 688 (49.7%) 25–29 years: n = 292 (21.2%)			1
Gómez-De León, 2022, Mexico [19]	2016–2020	BCR–ABL negative B-ALL	PIR: Modified BFM protocol	16–19 years: n = 31 20–29 years: n = 33 30–39 years: n = 16 ≥40 years: n = 11			2
Greenwood, 2021, Australia [20]	July 2012–June 2018	ALL	PIR: ANZCHOG Study 8 protocol	Median 22.7 years (16–38 years), analyzed as a continuous variable			1
Hough, 2016 UK, Ireland [23]	October 2003–June 2011	BCR–ABL negative B-ALL	PIR: UKALL2003	16–24 years: n = 2287 10–15 years: n = 610 <10 years: n = 229			1

Table 1. *Cont.*

Author, Year, Country	Years of Recruitment	Diagnosis	PIR	N of Pediatric Patients (%) Adult Protocol	N of Adult Patients (%)	Median Age (Range) in Years	JBI Score
Valtis, 2022, USA [34]	2000–2018	ALL	PIR: DFCI ALL Consortium 00-001, 05-001, 01-175, 06-254	15-19 years: *n* = 138 (38%) 20-29 years: *n* = 110 (30%) 30-39 years: *n* = 62 (17%) 40-50 years: *n* = 57 (16%)			1
Toft, 2018, Denmark, Estonia, Finland, Iceland, Lithuania, Norway, Sweden [32]	July 2008–December 2014	T-ALL or BCR–ABL negative B-ALL, excluding patients with DS	PIR: NOPHO ALL2008 protocol	1-9 years: *n* = 1022 (68%) 10-17 years: *n* = 266 (18%) 18-45 years: *n* = 221 (14%)			1
Toft, 2016, Countries see above [33]	July 2008–April 2013	T-ALL or BCR–ABL negative B-ALL, excluding patients with DS	PIR: NOPHO ALL2008 protocol	1-9.9 years: *n* = 733 (69%) 10-14 years: *n* = 118 (11%) 15-17 years: *n* = 77 (7%) 18-26 years: *n* = 70 (7%) 27-45 years: *n* = 64 (6%)			1
Rytting, 2014, USA [30]	October 2006–April 2012	BCR–ABL negative ALL	PIR: Augmented BFM regimen	12-21 years: *n* = 44 (52%) 22-40 years: *n* = 41 (48%)			1
Rytting, 2016, USA [29]	October 2006–March 2014	BCR–ABL negative ALL	PIR: Augmented BFM regimen Adult: Historical cohort (treated with Hyper-CVAD)	13-21 years: - PIR *n* = 99 (50%); adult *n* = 100 (50%) 22-40 years: - PIR *n* = 53; adult *n* = 81			1
Ribera, 2008, Spain [28]	June 1996–June 2005	SR ALL	PIR: PETHEMA ALL-96 protocol	15-18 years: *n* = 35 (43%) 19-30 years: *n* = 46 (57%)			1

Table 1. Cont.

Author, Year, Country	Years of Recruitment	Diagnosis	PIR	Adult Protocol	N of Pediatric Patients (%)	N of Adult Patients (%)	Median Age (Range) in Years	JBI Score
Ribera, 2020, Spain [27]	August 2008–April 2018	SR BCR-ABL negative ALL	PIR: PETHEMA ALLRE08		15-18 years: n = 38 (43%) 19-30 years: n = 51 (57%)			1–2
Quist-Paulsen, 2020, Countries as Toft et al. [25]	July 2008–March 2016	T-ALL	PIR: NOPHO ALL2008 protocol		1-9: n = 117 (42%) 10-17: n = 78 (28%) 18-45: n = 83 (30%)			1
Rank, 2018, Countries same as Toft et al. [26]	July 2008–February 2016	BCR-ABL negative ALL	PIR: NOPHO ALL2008 protocol		1-9.9 years: n = 1192 (67%) 10-17.9 years: n = 306 (17%) 18-45 years: n = 274 (16%)			1

ALL: Acute lymphoblastic leukemia; DFCI: Dana-Faber Cancer Institute; Hyper-CVAD: Hyperfractionated cyclophosphamide, vincristine, doxorubicin, dexamethasone; BFM: Berlin-Frankfurt-Münster Study Group; CALGB: Cancer and Leukernia Group B Study Group; MPAL: Mixed phenotype acute leukemia; SR: Standard risk; HR: High risk; VHR: Very high risk; BCR-ABL: positive ALL: ALL with BCR-ABL translocation; TPOG: Taiwan Pediatric Oncology Group; MCP-841: Multicentre protocol 841; COG: Children's Oncology Group; GMALL: German Multicentre ALL Protocol; INCTR: International Network for Cancer Treatment and Research; ANZCHOG: Australian and New Zealand Children's Haematology/Oncology Group; NOPHO: Nordic Society of Paediatric Haematology and Oncology; PETHEMA: Programa Español de Tratamientos en Hematologia.

Table 2. Main findings of studies comparing outcomes and toxicity in adolescents and young adult patients receiving a pediatric/pediatric-inspired (PIR) or adult regimen.

Ref.	CR Rate after Induction (PIR vs. Adult)	EFS/RFS/DFS/Relapse Rate (PIR vs. Adult)	OS (PIR vs. Adult)	Toxicity (PIR vs. Adult)	The Median Duration of Follow-Up in Months (Range)
AL-Khabouri, 2010 [11]	84% vs. 93%	3-year RFS: 89% vs. 24%; p < 0.0001	3-year OS 81% vs. 44%; p = 0.0003 5-year OS 75% (85% CI: 55–88%) vs. 25% (95% CI:13–39%); p = 0.0003	NA	54 (13–238)
Alacacioglu, 2014 [10]	95% vs. 96%	Mean RFS: 53.9 ± 5.4 vs. 39.1 ± 6.8 months; p = 0.009	Mean OS: 55.1 ± 4.9 vs. 41.5 ± 6.4 months; p = 0.012 5-year OS: 59% vs. 34%	No anaphylactic reactions to E. coli L-ASP, no pancreatitis, or venous complications. Mild elevation of liver enzymes. No complications caused a delay in either protocol.	37

Table 2. Cont.

Ref.	CR Rate after Induction (PIR vs. Adult)	EFS/RFS/DFS/Relapse Rate (PIR vs. Adult)	OS (PIR vs. Adult)	Toxicity (PIR vs. Adult)	The Median Duration of Follow-Up in Months (Range)
Almanza-Huante, 2021 [12]	79.5% vs. 64.2%; $p = 0.02$	Relapse rate: 44.1% vs. 60%; $p = 0.04$	OS: 18.5 [95% CI, 13.61–23.43] vs. 11.08 months [95% CI, 7.33–14.83]) 2-year OS: 41.5% vs. 28.1%; $p = 0.01$	IRM: 1.4% PIR vs. 8% hyper-CVAD ($p = 0.04$) TRD due to infection: 3.3% PIR vs. 28.1% hyper-CVAD	Hyper-CVAD: 101 BFM: 32 CALGB: 22
Cheng, 2022 [15]	NA	5-year EFS: 71.6 ± 12.2% vs. 45.5 ± 15.0%; $p = 0.152$ HR: 0.42; $p = 0.16$ 5-year EFS (untransplanted patients): 83.3% ± 10.8% vs. 28.6% ± 17.1%; $p = 0.039$ HR 4.19, $p < 0.05$	NA	Toxic death: $n = 1$ in both groups	PIR: 60 months (6–108) Adult: 20 months (2–127)
Ganesan, 2021 [17]	NA	2-year EFS: 56.6% vs. 52.1%; $p = 0.730$ HR with 95% CI: 1.05 (0.81–1.35); $p = 0.736$ 2-year RFS: 75.1% vs. 75.4%; $p = 0.702$	2-year OS: 75.4% vs. 59.0%; $p < 0.001$ HR with 95% CI: 1.72 (1.29–2.29; $p < 0.001$ (univariate) 3.19 (1.95–5.22); $p < 0.001$ (multivariate)	NA	23 months (95% CI 6–38)
Ganesan, 2018 [18]	84% vs. 82%	5-year RFS: 51% vs. 35%; $p = 0.027$ 5-year EFS: 40% vs. 27% $p = 0.054$	5-year OS: 43% vs. 33%; $p = 0.2$	IRM: 10% vs. 1% $p = 0.001$; major causes: sepsis, L-ASP associated thrombotic complications TRD: 12% vs. 2%; $p = 0.031$	21 months (0.3–165)
Gupta, 2019 [21]	NA	5-year EFS, treated between 2006 and 2011: pediatric center AYA 80.8 ± 5.8% vs. adult center with PIR 71.8% ± 7.2% vs. adult centers with adult protocols 60.0% ± 11.0%; $p = 0.02$	5-year OS, treated between 2006 and 2011: pediatric center 90.9 ± 4.3%, adult center with PIR 76.9 ± 6.82%, adult centers with adult protocols 65.0 ± 10.7.0%; $p = 0.004$	NA	NA
Hayakawa, 2014 [22]	94% (95% CI 88–97%) vs. 84% (75–90%)	5-year DFS: 67% (95% CI 58–75%) vs. 44% (33–55%), not statistically significant, but the p-value has not been shown	5-year OS: 73% (95% CI 64–80%) vs. 45% (35–55%) not statistically significant, but the p-value has not been shown	Sepsis, hepatic toxicity, and neuropathy were more frequent in PIR. No toxic deaths occurred during post-remission therapy due to severe adverse events.	PIR: 61 Adult: 67

Table 2. Cont.

Ref.	CR Rate after Induction (PIR vs. Adult)	EFS/RFS/DFS/Relapse Rate (PIR vs. Adult)	OS (PIR vs. Adult)	Toxicity (PIR vs. Adult)	The Median Duration of Follow-Up in Months (Range)
Tantiworawit, 2019 [31]	88.2% vs. 79.2%, $p = 0.23$	2-year DFS: 47.1% vs. 24.7% (HR 1.73, 1.22–3.03, $p = 0.04$) Relapse rate: 34.3% vs. 54.2%, $p < 0.01$ DFS for BCR–ABL negative ALL: 46.8% vs. 18.7% (HR 2.16, 1.16–4.01, $p = 0.01$)	2-year OS 50.8% vs. 31.2% (HR 1.52, 0.83–2.78, $p = 0.16$) For BCR–ABL negative ALL 2-year OS of 59.4% vs. 31.8% (HR 2.03, 1.04–3.96, $p = 0.03$)	IRM: 2.9 vs. 5.6%, $p = 0.53$	11.6 (1–120)
Rytting, 2014 [30]	94% vs. 99%, $p = 0.14$	NA	3-year OS rate: 74% vs. 71%, not statistically significant, but the p-value has not been shown	See Table 3	40 (4–75)
Rytting, 2016 [29]	93% vs. 98%, p-value not shown	NA	5-year OS: 60% vs. 60%	Toxicity (PIR vs. adult): No significant difference for allergic reactions, liver enzyme and bilirubin elevation, ON, thrombosis, stroke-like events, neuropathy, bleeding, or deaths in CR Hypofibrinogenemia 35% vs.14%, $p < 0.001$ Pancreatitis 11% vs. 3%, $p = 0.02$ Induction infections grade 3–4: 22% vs. 45%, $p < 0.001$ Infections in CR in the first 60 days: 30% vs. 60%, $p < 0.001$	PIR: 66 months (17–107) Adult: 88 (1–152)
Kliman, 2017 [24]	100% vs. 86%, $p = 0.095$	3-year EFS: 80% vs. 45%, $p = 0.019$	3-year OS: 80% vs. 59%, $p = 0.12$	There were no significant differences between the incidence of candidemia, severe infection, thrombosis, pancreatitis, or toxic death.	Overall: 40.1 PIR: 36.8 Adult: 73.1

CR: Complete remission; EFS: Event-free survival; RFS: Relapse-free survival; DFS: Disease-free survival; OS: Overall survival; L-ASP: L-Asparaginase; Hyper-CVAD: Hyperfractionated cyclophosphamide, vincristine, doxorubicin, dexamethasone; BFM: Berlin–Frankfurt–Münster Study Group; NA: Not applicable; CI: Confidence interval; HR: Hazard ratio; AYA: Adolescents and young adults; TRD: Treatment-related deaths; IRM: Induction-related mortality.

Table 3. Main results of studies comparing age-stratified outcomes and toxicity in adolescents and young adult patients receiving a pediatric-inspired (PIR) or adult regimen.

Ref.	CR Rate after Induction	EFS/RFS/Relapse Rate	OS	Toxicity	Median Follow-Up in Months (Range)
Advani, 2021 [9]	NA	NA	NA	IRM with CALGB 10403 and COG AALL0232: 3.1% and 1.3%. Main Grade 3 and 4 toxicities with an incidence > 15%: hyperglycemia, bilirubin and ALT increases, febrile neutropenia, and infection. Post-induction mortality with CALGB 10403 and COG AALL0232: 1.3% and 0.8%. Main Grade 3 and 4 post-induction toxicities with an incidence > 15%: febrile neutropenia, infection, sensory neuropathy, hyperglycemia, bilirubin, AST and ALT increases, anaphylaxis. Increased age correlated with a decreased fibrinogen level and ALT increase in induction (OR 1.103; $p = 0.0001$ and OR 1.111; $p = 0.0002$) and post-induction therapy (OR 1.037; $p = 0.039$ and OR 1.045; $p = 0.011$).	NA
Almanza-Huante, 2021 [12]	Age group 14–20 years 71.0% PIR vs. 69.6% hyper-CVAD; $p = 1.0$	NA	Median OS 27.4 months (95% CI 9.5–45.3) in PIR vs. 15.4 months (8.5–22.3) in hyper-CVAD ($p = 0.30$)	IRM: 0% PIR vs. 10.1% hyper-CVAD ($p = 0.18$)	Hyper-CVAD: $n = 101$ BFM: $n = 32$ CALGB. N = 22
	Age group 21–43 years 84% PIR vs. 57.4% hyper-CVAD $p = 0.02$	NA	Median OS 16.9 months (95% CI 13.1–20.6) PIR vs. 9.2 months (95% CI 6–12.5) in hyper-CVAD ($p < 0.01$)	IRM: 2% PIR vs. 6.9% hyper-CVAD and 2% ($p = 0.39$)	
Brandwein, 2014 [13]	17–<34 years: 99% 34–50 years: 87% 50–60 years: 26% ($p = 0.02$)	NA	5-year OS (95% CI), univariate: 17–<34 years: 80% (67–88%) 34–50 years: 50% (35–63%) 50–60 years: 62% (42–77%) $p = 0.001$ Age (cont. variable) as a predictor of OS ($p = 0.0046$)	NA	42 months (range 0.3–135 months)

Table 3. Cont.

Ref.	CR Rate after Induction	EFS/RFS/ Relapse Rate	OS	Toxicity	Median Follow-Up in Months (Range)
Burke, 2022 [14]	NA	5-year EFS: 65.4 ± 2.2% for AYA vs. 78.1 ± 0.9% for younger patients ($p < 0.0001$) Age as a significant predictor of EFS as categorical (<16 vs., >16) and continuous variable in univariate and multivariable analysis (categorical univariate: $p < 0.0001$; continuous univariate: $p < 0.0001$; categorical multivariable: $p = 0.018$; continuous multivariable: $p < 0.0001$ respectively)	5-year OS: 77.4 ± 2.0% for AYA vs. 87.3 ± 0.7% for younger patients ($p < 0.0001$)	IRM 2.2% in AYA versus 1.6% in younger patients ($p = 0.366$) Toxicity Grade ≥ 3 in induction (AYA vs. younger): Hyperglycemia: 23.6% vs. 15.4% ($p < 0.0001$) Hyperbilirubinemia: 6.9% vs. 3.7% ($p = 0.0007$) Febrile neutropenia: 7.4% vs. 13.8% ($p < 0.0001$) There was no significant difference in thrombosis or pancreatitis. Toxicity Grade ≥ 3 in post-induction (AYA vs. younger): Mucositis: 18.2% vs. 11.7% ($p = 0.0002$) Peripheral neuropathy: 12.1% vs.7.8% ($p = 0.001$) Febrile neutropenia: 45.2% vs. 56.8% ($p < 0.0001$) Hyperbilirubinemia: 17.3% vs. 9.5% ($p < 0.0001$) Hepatic failure: 1.3% vs. 0.3% ($p = 0.009$) Deaths in remission: 5.7% vs. 2.4% ($p < 0.0001$), mostly Grade 5 infections.	NA
Cheng, 2022 [15]	NA	5-year EFS: 64.3 ± 21.0% for 18-25 years vs. 76.2 ± 14.8% for older group; $p = 0.265$	NA	NA	60 months (6-108)
DeAngelo, 2015 [16]	NA	4-year EFS (95% CI) age 18-29 vs. 30-50: 55% (39-69%) vs. 61% (44-74%), $p = 0.61$	4-year OS (95% CI) age 18-29 vs. 30-50: 68% (52-80%) vs. 65% (49-77%), $p = 0.93$	NA	54 (95% CI 49-60)
Ganesan, 2021 [17]	NA	2-year EFS, HR (95% CI) 15-17 years: 56.7%, ref. 18-24 years: 55.9%, 1.01 (0.83-1.23), $p = 0.937$ 25-29 years: 55.4% 1.02 (0.80-1.30); $p = 0.862$ 2-year RFS: 15-17 years: 74.8% 18-24 years: 75.3% 25-29 years: 75.4% $p = 0.948$ (log-rank)	2-year OS; HR (95% CI) 15-17 years: 75.6%, ref. 18-24 years: 73.0%; 1.20 (0.91-1.58), $p = 0.203$ 25-29 years: 69.3%; 1.37 (0.99-1.89); $p = 0.057$	NA	23 (95% CI 6-38)

Table 3. Cont.

Ref.	CR Rate after Induction	EFS/RFS/Relapse Rate	OS	Toxicity	Median Follow-Up in Months (Range)
Gomez, 2022 [19]	NA	≥40 years with lower EFS: 8.3 months (95% CI 0–21.2; $p = 0.006$); no difference in the AYA groups Age as continuous variable HR (95% CI): 1.93 (0.99–1.07)	There was no statistically significant difference in OS between age groups. Age as continuous variable HR (95% CI): 1.03 (0.9–1.07)	Induction deaths: bleeding ($n = 4$), severe pancreatitis ($n = 1$), and a sudden unwitnessed event ($n = 1$)	18 (1–52.8)
Greenwood, 2021 [20]	NA	NA	HR: 0.85 (95% CI 0.36–2.10) for OS ($p = 0.751$)		44 (1–96)
Hough, 2016 [23]	NA	5-year EFS 16–24 years: 72.3% (66.2–78.4) 10–15 years: 83.6% (80.5–86.7) <10 years: 89.8% (88.4–91.2) OR = 2.1 (95% CI: 1.7–2.4), p (trend) < 0.00005, p (10–15 vs. ≥16) = 0.00004	5-year OS 16–24 years: 76.4% (70.5–82.3) 10–15 years: 87.5% (84.8–90.2) <10 years: 94.2% (93.2–95.2) OR = 2.7 (2.2–3.4), p (trend) < 0.00005, p (10–15 vs. ≥16) = 0.0004	5-year risk of DIR 16–24 years: 6.1% (2.8–9.4) 10–15 years: 3.4% (1.8–5.0) <10 years: 2.1% (1.5–2.7) OR = 2.0 (1.4–3.9), p (trend) = 0.0007 SAE incidence < 10 years vs. 10–24 years 2.58 (95% CI: 2.24–2.95), $p < 0.00005$ The time to first SAE was significantly shorter, and the cumulative incidence of SAEs was significantly higher in >10 years.	70 (1–121)
Valtis, 2022 [34]	NA	NA	NA	ON 5-year cumulative incidence (95% CI) < 30 years vs. 30–50 years: 21% (95% CI, 16–27) vs. 8% (CI, 4–14); univariate HR 2.77 (95% CI, 1.35–5.65); $p = 0.004$ ON 5-year cumulative incidence (95% CI) with peg-asparaginase vs. E. coli asparaginase 24% (95% CI, 18–30) vs. 5% (95% CI, 2–10); HR 5.28 (95% CI, 2.24–12.48); $p = 0.001$ ON 5-year cumulative incidence (95% CI): 15–19 years: 18 (12–25) 20–29 years: 25 (17–36) 30–39 years: 12 (5–23) 40–50 years: 4 (1–11) $p = 0.003$ (Gray test)	59 (1–169)

Table 3. *Cont.*

Ref.	CR Rate after Induction	EFS/RFS/ Relapse Rate	OS	Toxicity	Median Follow-Up in Months (Range)
Toft, 2018 [32]	NA	5-year EFS (HR, 95% CI) 1–9 years: 0.89 ± 0.01 (ref.) 10–17 years: 0.80 ± 0.03 (2.0; 1.4–2.8) $p < 0.001$ 18–45 years: 0.74 ± 0.04 (2.8; 2.0–4.0) $p < 0.001$	5-years OS (HR, 95% CI) 1–9 years: 0.94 ± 0.01 (ref.) 10–17 years: 0.87 ± 0.02 (2.3; 1.5–3.5) $p < 0.001$ 18–45 years: 0.78 ± 0.03 (3.8; 2.5–5.7) $p < 0.001$	IRM 0.01 in all groups; $p = 0.87$ Adverse events in 1–9 vs. 10–17 vs. 18–45 years: No sig. difference in ICU[14] admission, peripheral paralysis, anaphylactic reaction to ASP, invasive fungal infection, pancreatitis, hyperlipidemia, seizures Thrombosis: 3.6% vs. 15.3% vs.17.5% ($p < 0.001$) ON: 2.3% vs. 13.4% vs.8.5% ($p < 0.001$) Increasing incidence of at least one toxic event ($p < 0.0001$): 1–9.9 years: 44.5% 10–14 years: 57.6% 15–17 years: 62.3% 18–26 years: 64.0% 27–45 years: 64.2% Toxic events during induction: There was no significant difference in ICU admissions, septic shock, heart failure, anaphylactic reactions, pancreatitis, seizures, coma, VOD, PRES, abdominal surgery, ON, liver or kidney dysfunction, bleeding, or peripheral paralysis.	55 (36–77) 1–9 years: 59 10–17 years: 55 18–45 years: 38
Toft, 2016 [33]	NA	NA	NA	Hyperglycemia was more common >9 years (overall $p < 0.0001$) and 18–28 years (OR = 11.3 (95% CI: (2.9;43.5); $p = 0.0002$). Thrombosis was more frequent in 15–17 years (OR 10.2 (2.6;39.1), $p = 0.0004$) and 18–28 years (OR 7.3 (1.5;31.7), $p = 0.007$). Toxic events after induction: There was no significant difference in heart failure, pancreatitis, hyperglycemia, abdominal catastrophe, CNS catastrophe/bleeding, anaphylactic reaction, VOD, liver or kidney dysfunction, hypertension, *Pneumocystis jiroveci* pneumonia, PRES, coma, seizures, peripheral paralysis, or ICU admission. Increasing incidence of ON, thrombosis, and fungal	40 (12–71)

Table 3. Cont.

Ref.	CR Rate after Induction	EFS/RFS/ Relapse Rate	OS	Toxicity	Median Follow-Up in Months (Range)
				infections with age ($p < 0.0001$, $p < 0.0001$, $p = 0.006$, respectively). OR (95% CI) for thrombosis was 5.4 (2.6–11.0), 5.1 (2.4–10.4), and 5.0 (2.2–10.8) for patients 15–17, 18–26, and 27–45 years, respectively, compared with children 1–9 years (all $p < 0.0001$). OR (95% CI) for avascular osteonecrosis for patients 10–14, 15–17, 18–26, and 27–45 years 10.4 (4.4–24.9, $p < 0.0001$), 6.3 (1.9–18.3, $p = 0.001$), 4.9 (1.3–15.0; $p = 0.009$), and 6.6 (1.8–21.2, $p = 0.003$) compared to 1–9 years, respectively.	
Tantiworawit, 2019 [30]	NA	NA	3-year OS ($\leq$21 years vs. >21 years): 85% vs. 60%, $p = 0.055$	Toxicity ($\leq$21 years vs. >21 years): There was no significant difference in the incidence of allergic reactions to ASP, pancreatitis, elevated liver enzymes or bilirubin, ON, thrombosis, stroke-like events, or neuropathy. Grade 3 hypofibrinogenemia: 10 vs. 21%, $p = 0.006$	40 (4–75)
Rytting, 2016 [29]	NA	NA	5-year OS $\leq$ 21 years (PIR vs. adult): 65% vs. 68%	NA	PIR: 66 months (17–107) Adult: 88 (1–152)
			5-year OS > 21 years (PIR vs. adult): 57% and 58% Differences between protocols were not statistically significant, and the p-value was not shown.		
Ribera, 2008 [28]	NA	EFS 15–18 vs. 19–30 years : 60% (95% CI : 43%–77%) vs. 63% (48%–78%), $p = 0.97$	OS 15–18 vs. 19–30 years: 77% (95% CI: 63%–91%) vs. 63% (46%–80%) $p = 0.44$	Toxicity (15–18 vs. 19–30 years): Grade 1 infections: 2.9 vs. 28%, $p = 0.007$ Grade 4 neutropenia: 44% vs. 59% Grade 4 thrombocytopenia: 10% vs. 33% Delays during reinduction were significantly more frequent in young adults than in adolescents, $p = 0.04$ Modifications in L-ASP or VCR were performed in 19% of cycles in adolescents vs. 33% in young adults, $p = 0.03$	50 (24–120)

Table 3. Cont.

Ref.	CR Rate after Induction	EFS/RFS/Relapse Rate	OS	Toxicity	Median Follow-Up in Months (Range)
Ribera, 2020 [27]	NA	5-year EFS 15–18 vs. 19–30 years: 78% (95% CI: 59–89) vs. 49% (31–65%), $p = 0.151$	5 years OS 15–18 vs. 19–30 years: 87% (95% CI: 74%–100%) vs. 63% (46%–80%), $p = 0.021$	There were no differences between adolescents and YA in drug modifications and delays	50 (0.5–114)
Quist-Paulsen, 2020 [25]	NA	5-year EFS (increasing age groups): 0.80 (95% CI: 0.72–0.88, ref.) vs. 0.75 (0.65–0.85) vs. 0.64 (0.52–0.76), p-values not shown	5-year OS (increasing age groups): 0.82 (95% CI: 0.74–0.88, ref.) vs. 0.76 (0.66–0.86, $p = 0.3$) vs. 0.65 (0.55–0.75, $p = 0.01$)	NA	Overall: 71 1–9 years: 76 (48–100) 10–17 years: 71 (53–91) 18–45 years: 68 (56–82)
Rank, 2018 [26]	NA	NA	NA	2.5-year cumulative incidence of any TE 1–9.9 years: 3.7% (2.64–4.8) 10–17.9 years: 15.5% (11.3–19.4) 18–45 years: 18.1% (13.2–22.8) $p < 0.0001$ The adjusted TE-specific hazard significantly increased in patients aged 6.0 to 14.9 years (HRa, 2.0; 95% CI, 1.2–3.5; $p = 0.01$), 15.0 to 20.9 years (HRa, 7.74; 95% CI, 4.52–13.2; $p < 0.0001$), and 21.0 to 45.9 years (HRa, 6.54; 95% CI, 3.69–11.6; $p < 0.0001$), using 1.0 to 5.9 years as reference. Patients aged 18.0–45.9: increased hazard of PE compared with children younger than 10.0 years (HRa, 11.6, 95% CI: 4.02–33.7; $p < 0.0001$). Adolescents aged 10.0 to 17.9 years: increased hazard of CSVT compared with children younger than 10.0 years (HRa 3.3, 95% CI: 1.5–7.3; $p = 0.003$).	52

CR: Complete remission; EFS: Event-free survival; RFS: Relapse-free survival; OS: Overall survival; IRM: Induction-related mortality; SAE: Severe adverse event; CALGB: Cancer and Leukemia Group B Study Group; DFCI: Dana–Farber Cancer Institute; DIR: Deaths in remission; ON: Osteonecrosis; ICU: Intensive care unit; PRES: Posterior reversible encephalopathy syndrome; VOD: Veno-occlusive disease/sinusoid obstruction syndrome; PE: Pulmonary embolism; CSVT: Cerebral venous thrombosis; COG: Children's Oncology Group; L-ASP: L-Asparaginase; VCR: Vincristine; AST: Aspartate aminotransferase; ALT: Alanine aminotransferase; NA: Not applicable; CI: Confidence interval; HR: Hazard ratio; AYA: Adolescents and young adults.

The regimens of both PIR and conventional adult protocols were different between the studies. The dosing regimens are described in detail in the corresponding articles. However, in general, PIR had higher cumulative dosages of chemotherapeutic agents such as corticosteroids, vincristine, and methotrexate and incorporated more asparaginase. Regarding the studied populations, the type of ALL (B-ALL, T-ALL, or BCR–ABL positive ALL) differed between the studies but was consistent within each study (Table 1). Quality appraisal according to the JBI quality assessment scale for cohort studies is shown in Table 1.

3.2. Treatment Outcomes and Toxicity in AYA Patients When Treated with PIR versus Conventional Adult Regimens

A statistically significant improvement in OS in patients given PIR compared to conventional adult protocols was reported in 6 out of 11 studies (Table 2) [10–12,17,21,22]. Even in the five studies that found that OS did not statistically significantly differ between the two types of treatment strategies, the reported OS for PIR tended to be higher than in the adult-type regimens [18,24,29–31].

The limited data and their accuracy did not allow us to perform a meta-analysis to assess the impact of the treatment strategy used. Even the consultation with the guidance of Tierney JF et al. did not allow a calculation of the hazard ratios (HR) [35]. Only three studies report HRs, but the HRs were given for different time points (2 years, 3 years, and 5 years), which further impeded performing a meta-analysis [17,21,31].

The clinical endpoints other than OS were very heterogeneous among the studies (Table 2). Nevertheless, a similar trend can be seen with the reported relapse rates, event-free survival (EFS), relapse-free survival (RFS), and disease-free survival (DFS), which were described in 10/12 studies. Three studies demonstrate an improvement in EFS, two in RFS, and two in DFS for the entire analyzed group [10–12,18,21,22,24,31]. Additionally, Cheng et al. report a significant improvement in 5-year EFS for a sub-group of untransplanted patients, and Ganesan et al. report, in addition to the improvement in the relapse rate and RFS, a trend toward improvement of EFS ($p = 0.054$) in the analyzed ALL patients [15,18].

Altogether, nine out of twelve studies report an improvement in either OS or EFS/RFS/ relapse rate or both, while three studies found equivalent results. No study reported statistically significant superior outcomes with conventional adult-type chemotherapy.

The results are less impressive for post-induction complete remission rate (CR), reported by nine studies, with only two showing a statistically significant increase in CR rate in patients given PIR compared to patients given conventional adult protocols (Table 2) [10–12,18,22,24,29–31].

Regarding toxicity, the studies show increased toxicity with PIR compared to conventional adult protocols. Most commonly, an increased incidence of pancreatitis, hypofibrinogenemia, neuropathy, hepatic toxicity, and infections was reported by the studies [10,22,24,29] (Table 2). However, most toxicities were described as mild and manageable with supportive care [10,24]. Most importantly, except for one study from India, no other studies reported significantly increased induction-related mortality (IRM) or treatment-related deaths [15,17,24,29,31]. Almanza-Huante et al. report a decrease in IRM and TRD with a modified pediatric protocol [12].

3.3. Age-Stratified Analysis of Outcomes and Toxicities in AYA Patients Treated with PIR

Nineteen studies were included in this section. These studies examine outcomes between different age groups of AYA ALL patients treated with PIR (Tables 1 and 3). For two studies, an age-stratified PIR vs. adult-type protocol comparison is available. Almanza-Huante et al. found a significant increase in CR at the end of induction and OS in patients aged 21–43 years treated with PIR as opposed to an adult-type protocol, with no increase in IRM. However, the follow-up duration was significantly shorter in patients who were treated with PIR, which might impact the reported OS. Conversely, Rytting et al. found no difference in OS between patients aged ≥21 and <21 years treated with PIR versus an adult-type protocol.

The remaining studies examined age-stratified outcomes or toxicity in patients treated exclusively with PIR (Table 3). Six of these studies report a significantly superior OS in younger age groups [13,14,23,25,27], with two additional studies also showing a trend towards inferior OS with increasing age ($p = 0.057$ and $p = 0.055$) [17,30]. On the contrary, four studies found no significant difference in OS between different age groups [16,19,20,28]. Similarly, heterogeneous results can be found for EFS, with four studies showing better outcomes for younger age groups [14,23,25,32] and five studies showing no significant difference between the age groups [15–17,27,28]. However, the studies identifying age as a significant predictor of EFS belong to those with the largest number of enrolled patients and thus the largest statistical power [14,23,25,32].

Furthermore, there are several adverse events (AE) whose incidence seems to be increasing with age (Table 3). Hough et al. report an overall increased cumulative incidence of AEs for patients aged >10 years and a significantly shorter time to the first AE after the start of treatment [23]. The AEs most commonly reported with increasing age are thrombosis, hypofibrinogenemia, hepatic injury, and infectious complications [9,14,26,28,30,32,33]. The risk of ICU admission and IRM does not seem to increase with age [14,32,33]. However, two studies report an increased incidence of toxic deaths in remission in older age groups [14,23]. Several studies show that the incidence of avascular osteonecrosis (ON) reaches its peak in the AYA age group, with a decrease in frequency in younger children and adults [32–34]. Furthermore, Valtis et al. show an increased risk for ON with the use of pegylated asparaginase, which is used with increasing frequency in new generations of PIR [34].

4. Discussion

This systematic review of 26 published comparative studies reporting outcomes of AYA patients with ALL shows a trend towards improvement in outcomes and an acceptable toxicity profile in patients treated with PIRs, compared to conventional adult-type regimens. While direct comparison and analysis were difficult due to heterogeneous study populations, treatment settings, treatment eras, and treatment protocols, most of the included studies nevertheless reported an increase in survival with the use of PIR.

Despite PIRs quickly becoming the standard of care for ALL treatment in the AYA population, further improvements are necessary. Our systematic review demonstrates a clear trend towards poorer survival with increasing age, even when using PIRs [13,14,23,25,27]. This is most likely due to a combination of higher therapy-related toxicity, requiring dose reductions and protocol adjustments and causing treatment delays, as well as disease biology [14,23].

Since PIRs are expected to be more intensive than adult-type regimens, an increase in treatment-related toxicity and adverse events is expected. However, our data show that while certain AEs increase with age, their toxicity is mostly manageable. Furthermore, PIRs also showed good results even in lower- and middle-income countries [10,12,17–19,31]. Yet, setting the age limit for the feasibility of these protocols is crucial so that the added toxicity and mortality do not surpass the positive effect of PIR on survival. With our analysis of age-stratified outcomes, we were unable to identify the optimal upper age limit for PIR.

Some of the included studies report low completion rates, high treatment abandonment rates, and large proportions of patients requiring dose reductions and treatment delays with increasing age [9,19,22,28]. In the study by Ribera et al., there were significantly more delays during reinductions and dose modifications for vincristine or asparaginase in young adults than in adolescents ($p = 0.04$ and $p = 0.03$, respectively). Adjustments to the protocol or alterations in the treatment strategy are more likely if the physician is unfamiliar with the protocol [9]. This is highlighted by the study by Gupta et al., which found a trend towards inferior EFS in patients treated with PIR in adult centers versus pediatric centers (HR 1.92, 95% CI 0.99–3.75, $p = 0.06$). The magnitude of the disparity between the two types of treatment centers persisted over time and even after adjusting for sociodemographic factors. This may be partially explained by a larger proportion of AYA patients treated in pediatric centers being registered on clinical trials (86/123 (69.9%) vs. 7/152 (4.6%), $p < 0.001$) or by better psychosocial support [21].

However, it is also well documented that treatment completion in the AYA age group is often low despite the physicians' familiarity with the protocol. In the study by Advani et al., 57% of the AYA patients completed all therapy according to the COG AALL0232 PIR protocol versus 74% of the patients below 18 years of age [9]. Furthermore, Hayakawa et al. also report frequent terminations due to AEs or patients' wishes. The latter happened predominantly during maintenance therapy [22]. This is presumably due to long, arduous PIR treatment programs resulting in low motivation. An alternative explanation for treatment termination in some low- and middle-income countries is socioeconomic factors, such as needing to pay for treatment out of pocket [19].

All these factors make translating the conclusions of this systematic review into clinical practice a precarious endeavor. The main limitations of our systematic review are based on the limited available data, including the lack of randomized studies and the heterogeneity in reporting the outcomes.

Randomized studies are needed to establish international treatment standards for AYA patients with ALL, improve risk stratification, and evaluate treatment response assessment using minimal disease measurements. Such studies would also ensure better data collection, adherence to the treatment dosing and schedule, integrated management of the most common AEs, and better support for physicians unfamiliar with the pediatric-inspired treatment protocols. Without them, we may not be able to definitively elucidate the magnitude of the influence of various treatment elements on improved outcomes (the prescribed regimen, locus of care, physicians´ experience with the protocol, compliance, socioeconomic and psychosocial factors, etc.).

5. Conclusions

Unfortunately, the gathered data do not allow for clear conclusions about the best treatment protocols to use in the AYA population. The trend towards improved outcomes with PIR must be viewed with caution, as non-randomized trials are prone to bias and difficult to compare and interpret. We should strive to enroll AYAs with ALL in randomized controlled trials of PIR vs. conventional adult-type protocols to definitively elucidate the best treatment strategy.

Supplementary Materials: The supporting information about our search strategy and extracted data from each article can be downloaded at: https://www.mdpi.com/article/10.3390/curroncol30090625/s1. Supplementary S1: Search strategy; Supplementary S2: Extracted data of each included study.

Author Contributions: Conceptualization, M.O. and K.S.; methodology, M.O. and K.S.; formal analysis, P.H.; title and abstract screening, A.Z. and M.O.; full-text screening and data extraction, A.Z. and P.F.; data curation, A.Z., P.F. and M.O.; writing—original draft preparation, A.Z.; writing—review and editing, P.F., P.H., N.B., M.O. and K.S.; supervision, N.B. and K.S.; project administration, M.O.; funding acquisition, N.B. and K.S. All authors have read and agreed to the published version of the manuscript.

Funding: This research was funded by Swiss Cancer Research Foundation, Grant Number: HSR-5219-11-2020 and Palatin Stiftung 0069/2021.

Institutional Review Board Statement: Not applicable.

Informed Consent Statement: Not applicable.

Conflicts of Interest: The authors declare no conflict of interest.

References

1. Ferrari, A.; Stark, D.; Peccatori, F.A.; Fern, L.; Laurence, V.; Gaspar, N.; Bozovic-Spasojevic, I.; Smith, O.; De Munter, J.; Derwich, K.; et al. Adolescents and young adults (AYA) with cancer: A position paper from the AYA Working Group of the European Society for Medical Oncology (ESMO) and the European Society for Paediatric Oncology (SIOPE). *ESMO Open* **2021**, *6*, 100096. [CrossRef]
2. Trama, A.; Botta, L.; Foschi, R.; Ferrari, A.; Stiller, C.; Desandes, E.; Maule, M.M.; Merletti, F.; Gatta, G. Survival of European adolescents and young adults diagnosed with cancer in 2000-07: Population-based data from EUROCARE-5. *Lancet Oncol.* **2016**, *17*, 896–906. [CrossRef] [PubMed]
3. Mohan, S.R.; Advani, A.S. Treatment of Acute Lymphoblastic Leukemia in Adolescents and Young Adults. *J. Adolesc. Young Adult Oncol.* **2011**, *1*, 19–24. [CrossRef] [PubMed]
4. Ram, R.; Wolach, O.; Vidal, L.; Gafter-Gvili, A.; Shpilberg, O.; Raanani, P. Adolescents and young adults with acute lymphoblastic leukemia have a better outcome when treated with pediatric-inspired regimens: Systematic review and meta-analysis. *Am. J. Hematol.* **2012**, *87*, 472–478. [CrossRef] [PubMed]
5. Boissel, N.A.-O.; Baruchel, A.A.-O. Acute lymphoblastic leukemia in adolescent and young adults: Treat as adults or as children? *Blood* **2018**, *132*, 351–361. [CrossRef]
6. Rizzari, C.; Putti, M.C.; Colombini, A.; Casagranda, S.; Ferrari, G.M.; Papayannidis, C.; Iacobucci, I.; Abbenante, M.C.; Sartor, C.; Martinelli, G. Rationale for a pediatric-inspired approach in the adolescent and young adult population with acute lymphoblastic leukemia, with a focus on asparaginase treatment. *Hematol. Rep.* **2014**, *6*, 5554. [CrossRef]
7. Schafer, E.S.; Hunger, S.P. Optimal therapy for acute lymphoblastic leukemia in adolescents and young adults. *Nat. Rev. Clin. Oncol.* **2011**, *8*, 417–424. [CrossRef] [PubMed]
8. Liberati, A.; Altman, D.G.; Tetzlaff, J.; Mulrow, C.; Gøtzsche, P.C.; Ioannidis, J.P.A.; Clarke, M.; Devereaux, P.J.; Kleijnen, J.; Moher, D. The PRISMA statement for reporting systematic reviews and meta-analyses of studies that evaluate health care interventions: Explanation and elaboration. *PLoS Med.* **2009**, *6*, e1000100. [CrossRef]
9. Advani, A.S.; Larsen, E.; Laumann, K.; Luger, S.M.; Liedtke, M.; Devidas, M.; Chen, Z.; Yin, J.; Foster, M.C.; Claxton, D.; et al. Comparison of CALGB 10403 (Alliance) and COG AALL0232 toxicity results in young adults with acute lymphoblastic leukemia. *Blood Adv.* **2021**, *5*, 504–512. [CrossRef] [PubMed]
10. Alacacioglu, I.; Medeni, S.S.; Ozsan, G.H.; Payzin, B.; Sevindik, O.G.; Acar, C.; Katgi, A.; Ozdemirkan, F.; Piskin, O.; Ozcan, M.A.; et al. Is the BFM Regimen Feasible for the Treatment of Adult Acute Lymphoblastic Leukemia? A Retrospective Analysis of the Outcomes of BFM and Hyper-CVAD Chemotherapy in Two Centers. *Chemotherapy* **2014**, *60*, 219–223. [CrossRef] [PubMed]
11. Al-Khabori, M.; Minden, M.D.; Yee, K.W.L.; Gupta, V.; Schimmer, A.D.; Schuh, A.C.; Xu, W.; Brandwein, J.M. Improved survival using an intensive, pediatric-based chemotherapy regimen in adults with T-cell acute lymphoblastic leukemia. *Leuk. Lymphoma* **2010**, *21*, 61–65. [CrossRef] [PubMed]
12. Almanza-Huante, E.; Espinosa-Bautista, K.; Rangel-Patiño, J.; Demichelis-Gómez, R. Comparison of Two Pediatric-Inspired Regimens to Hyper-CVAD in Hispanic Adolescents and Young Adults With Acute Lymphoblastic Leukemia. *Clin. Lymphoma Myeloma Leuk.* **2021**, *21*, 55–62. [CrossRef]
13. Brandwein, J.M.; Atenafu, E.G.; Schuh, A.C.; Yee, K.W.; Schimmer, A.D.; Gupta, V.; Minden, M.D. Predictors of outcome in adults with BCR-ABL negative acute lymphoblastic leukemia treated with a pediatric-based regimen. *Leuk. Res.* **2014**, *38*, 532–536. [CrossRef] [PubMed]
14. Burke, M.A.-O.; Devidas, M.; Chen, Z.; Salzer, W.L.; Raetz, E.A.; Rabin, K.R.; Heerema, N.A.; Carroll, A.A.-O.X.; Gastier-Foster, J.M.; Borowitz, M.J.; et al. Outcomes in adolescent and young adult patients (16 to 30 years) compared to younger patients treated for high-risk B-lymphoblastic leukemia: Report from Children's Oncology Group Study AALL0232. *Leukemia* **2022**, *36*, 648–655. [CrossRef]
15. Cheng, C.N.; Li, S.S.; Hsu, Y.T.; Chen, Y.P.; Chen, T.Y.; Chen, J.S. Outcome of young adult patients with very-high-risk acute lymphoblastic leukemia treated with pediatric-type chemotherapy—A single institute experience. *J. Formos. Med. Assoc.* **2022**, *121*, 694–702. [CrossRef]
16. DeAngelo, D.J.; Stevenson, K.E.; Dahlberg, S.E.; Silverman, L.B.; Couban, S.; Supko, J.G.; Amrein, P.C.; Ballen, K.K.; Seftel, M.D.; Turner, A.R.; et al. Long-term outcome of a pediatric-inspired regimen used for adults aged 18–50 years with newly diagnosed acute lymphoblastic leukemia. *Leukemia* **2015**, *29*, 526–534. [CrossRef] [PubMed]
17. Ganesan, P.A.-O.; Jain, H.A.-O.; Bagal, B.; Subramanian, P.G.; George, B.A.-O.; Korula, A.A.-O.; Mehra, N.; Kalaiyarasi, J.P.; Bhurani, D.A.-O.; Agrawal, N.A.-O.; et al. Outcomes in adolescent and young adult acute lymphoblastic leukaemia: A report from the Indian Acute Leukaemia Research Database (INwARD) of the Hematology Cancer Consortium (HCC). *Br. J. Haematol.* **2021**, *193*, e1. [CrossRef]
18. Ganesan, P.A.-O.; Sagar, T.G.; Kannan, K.; Radhakrishnan, V.; Dhanushkodi, M.; Swaminathan, R.; Sundersingh, S.; Ganesan, T.S. Acute Lymphoblastic Leukemia in Young Adults Treated with Intensive "Pediatric" Type Protocol. *Indian J. Hematol. Blood Transfus.* **2018**, *34*, 422–429. [CrossRef] [PubMed]
19. Gómez-De León, A.; Varela-Constantino, A.L.; Colunga-Pedraza, P.R.; Sánchez-Arteaga, A.; García-Zárate, V.; Rodríguez-Zúñiga, A.C.; Méndez-Ramírez, N.; Cantú-Rodríguez, O.G.; Gutiérrez-Aguirre, C.H.; Tarín-Arzaga, L.; et al. Treatment of Ph-Negative Acute Lymphoblastic Leukemia in Adolescents and Young Adults with an Affordable Outpatient Pediatric Regimen. *Clin. Lymphoma Myeloma Leuk.* **2022**, *22*, 883–893. [CrossRef] [PubMed]

20. Greenwood, M.A.-O.; Trahair, T.A.-O.X.; Sutton, R.A.-O.; Osborn, M.A.-O.; Kwan, J.; Mapp, S.; Howman, R.; Anazodo, A.A.-O.; Wylie, B.; D'Rozario, J.; et al. An MRD-stratified pediatric protocol is as deliverable in adolescents and young adults as in children with ALL. *Blood Adv.* **2021**, *5*, 5574–5583. [CrossRef]
21. Gupta, S.A.-O.; Pole, J.D.; Baxter, N.A.-O.; Sutradhar, R.A.-O.; Lau, C.; Nagamuthu, C.; Nathan, P.C. The effect of adopting pediatric protocols in adolescents and young adults with acute lymphoblastic leukemia in pediatric vs adult centers: An IMPACT Cohort study. *Cancer Med.* **2019**, *8*, 2095–2103. [CrossRef] [PubMed]
22. Hayakawa, F.; Sakura, T.; Yujiri, T.; Kondo, E.; Fujimaki, K.; Sasaki, O.; Miyatake, J.; Handa, H.; Ueda, Y.; Aoyama, Y.; et al. Markedly improved outcomes and acceptable toxicity in adolescents and young adults with acute lymphoblastic leukemia following treatment with a pediatric protocol: A phase II study by the Japan Adult Leukemia Study Group. *Blood Cancer J.* **2014**, *4*, e252. [CrossRef] [PubMed]
23. Hough, R.; Rowntree, C.; Goulden, N.; Mitchell, C.; Moorman, A.; Wade, R.; Vora, A. Efficacy and toxicity of a paediatric protocol in teenagers and young adults with Philadelphia chromosome negative acute lymphoblastic leukaemia: Results from UKALL 2003. *Br. J. Haematol.* **2016**, *172*, 439–451. [CrossRef]
24. Kliman, D.; Barnett, M.; Broady, R.; Forrest, D.; Gerrie, A.; Hogge, D.; Nantel, S.; Narayanan, S.; Nevill, T.; Power, M.; et al. Comparison of a pediatric-inspired treatment protocol versus standard-intensity chemotherapy for young adults with standard-risk BCR-ABL negative acute lymphoblastic leukemia. *Leuk. Lymphoma* **2017**, *58*, 909–915. [CrossRef]
25. Quist-Paulsen, P.; Toft, N.; Heyman, M.; Abrahamsson, J.; Griškevičius, L.; Hallböök, H.; Jónsson, Ó.G.; Palk, K.; Vaitkeviciene, G.; Vettenranta, K.; et al. T-cell acute lymphoblastic leukemia in patients 1–45 years treated with the pediatric NOPHO ALL2008 protocol. *Leukemia* **2020**, *34*, 347–357. [CrossRef]
26. Rank, C.A.-O.; Toft, N.; Tuckuviene, R.; Grell, K.; Nielsen, O.J.; Frandsen, T.L.; Marquart, H.V.H.; Albertsen, B.K.; Tedgård, U.; Hallböök, H.; et al. Thromboembolism in acute lymphoblastic leukemia: Results of NOPHO ALL2008 protocol treatment in patients aged 1 to 45 years. *Blood* **2018**, *131*, 2475–2484. [CrossRef] [PubMed]
27. Ribera, J.A.-O.; Morgades, M.; Montesinos, P.A.-O.; Tormo, M.; Martínez-Carballeira, D.; González-Campos, J.; Gil, C.; Barba, P.; García-Boyero, R.; Coll, R.; et al. A pediatric regimen for adolescents and young adults with Philadelphia chromosome-negative acute lymphoblastic leukemia: Results of the ALLRE08 PETHEMA trial. *Cancer Med.* **2020**, *9*, 2317–2329. [CrossRef]
28. Ribera, J.M.; Oriol, A.; Sanz, M.-A.; Tormo, M.; Fernández-Abellán, P.; del Potro, E.; Abella, E.; Bueno, J.; Parody, R.; Bastida, P.; et al. Comparison of the results of the treatment of adolescents and young adults with standard-risk acute lymphoblastic leukemia with the Programa Español de Tratamiento en Hematología pediatric-based protocol ALL-96. *J. Clin. Oncol.* **2008**, *26*, 1843–1849. [CrossRef]
29. Rytting, M.E.; Jabbour, E.J.; Jorgensen, J.L.; Ravandi, F.; Franklin, A.R.; Kadia, T.M.; Pemmaraju, N.; Daver, N.G.; Ferrajoli, A.; Garcia-Manero, G.; et al. Final results of a single institution experience with a pediatric-based regimen, the augmented Berlin-Frankfurt-Münster, in adolescents and young adults with acute lymphoblastic leukemia, and comparison to the hyper-CVAD regimen. *Am. J. Hematol.* **2016**, *91*, 819–823. [CrossRef]
30. Rytting, M.E.; Thomas, D.A.; O'Brien, S.M.; Ravandi-Kashani, F.; Jabbour, E.J.; Franklin, A.R.; Kadia, T.M.; Pemmaraju, N.; Daver, N.G.; Ferrajoli, A.; et al. Augmented Berlin-Frankfurt-Münster therapy in adolescents and young adults (AYAs) with acute lymphoblastic leukemia (ALL). *Cancer* **2014**, *120*, 3660–3668. [CrossRef]
31. Tantiworawit, A.; Rattanathammethee, T.A.-O.; Chai-Adisaksopha, C.; Rattarittamrong, E.; Norasetthada, L. Outcomes of adult acute lymphoblastic leukemia in the era of pediatric-inspired regimens: A single-center experience. *Int. J. Hematol.* **2019**, *110*, 295–305. [CrossRef] [PubMed]
32. Toft, N.; Birgens, H.; Abrahamsson, J.; Griškevičius, L.; Hallböök, H.; Heyman, M.; Klausen, T.W.; Jónsson, Ó.G.; Palk, K.; Pruunsild, K.; et al. Results of NOPHO ALL2008 treatment for patients aged 1–45 years with acute lymphoblastic leukemia. *Leukemia* **2018**, *32*, 606–615. [CrossRef] [PubMed]
33. Toft, N.; Birgens, H.; Abrahamsson, J.; Griškevičius, L.; Hallböök, H.; Heyman, M.; Klausen, T.W.; Jónsson, Ó.G.; Palk, K.; Pruunsild, K.; et al. Toxicity profile and treatment delays in NOPHO ALL2008-comparing adults and children with Philadelphia chromosome-negative acute lymphoblastic leukemia. *Eur. J. Haematol.* **2016**, *96*, 160–169. [CrossRef] [PubMed]
34. Valtis, Y.A.-O.; Stevenson, K.E.; Place, A.A.-O.; Silverman, L.B.; Vrooman, L.M.; Gotti, G.A.-O.; Brunner, A.M.; Nauffal, M.; DeAngelo, D.A.-O.; Luskin, M.A.-O. Orthopedic toxicities among adolescents and young adults treated in DFCI ALL Consortium Trials. *Blood Adv.* **2022**, *6*, 72–81. [CrossRef] [PubMed]
35. Tierney, J.F.; Stewart, L.A.; Ghersi, D.; Burdett, S.; Sydes, M.R. Practical methods for incorporating summary time-to-event data into meta-analysis. *Trials* **2007**, *8*, 16. [CrossRef] [PubMed]

Disclaimer/Publisher's Note: The statements, opinions and data contained in all publications are solely those of the individual author(s) and contributor(s) and not of MDPI and/or the editor(s). MDPI and/or the editor(s) disclaim responsibility for any injury to people or property resulting from any ideas, methods, instructions or products referred to in the content.

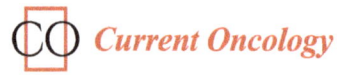

Article

Recruiting Adolescent and Young Adult Cancer Survivors for Patient-Reported Outcome Research: Experiences and Sample Characteristics of the SURVAYA Study

Carla Vlooswijk [1], Lonneke V. van de Poll-Franse [1,2,3], Silvie H. M. Janssen [2,4], Esther Derksen [1], Milou J. P. Reuvers [4], Rhodé Bijlsma [5], Suzanne E. J. Kaal [6,7], Jan Martijn Kerst [4], Jacqueline M. Tromp [8], Monique E. M. M. Bos [9], Tom van der Hulle [10], Roy I. Lalisang [11], Janine Nuver [12], Mathilde C. M. Kouwenhoven [13], Winette T. A. van der Graaf [4,9] and Olga Husson [2,4,14,15,*]

1 Research and Development, Netherlands Comprehensive Cancer Organisation, 3511 DT Utrecht, The Netherlands; c.vlooswijk@iknl.nl (C.V.); l.vandepoll@iknl.nl (L.V.v.d.P.-F.); e.derksen@iknl.nl (E.D.)
2 Department of Psychosocial Research and Epidemiology, Netherlands Cancer Institute, 1066 CX Amsterdam, The Netherlands; sh.janssen@nki.nl
3 Department of Medical and Clinical Psychology, Tilburg University, 5037 AB Tilburg, The Netherlands
4 Department of Medical Oncology, Netherlands Cancer Institute-Antoni van Leeuwenhoek, 1066 CX Amsterdam, The Netherlands; m.reuvers@nki.nl (M.J.P.R.); j.kerst@nki.nl (J.M.K.); w.vd.graaf@nki.nl (W.T.A.v.d.G.)
5 Department of Medical Oncology, University Medical Center, 3584 CX Utrecht, The Netherlands; r.m.bijlsma@umcutrecht.nl
6 Department of Medical Oncology, Radboud University Medical Center, 6525 GA Nijmegen, The Netherlands; suzanne.kaal@radboudumc.nl
7 Dutch AYA 'Young and Cancer' Care Network, Netherlands Comprehensive Cancer Organisation, 3511 DT Utrecht, The Netherlands
8 Department of Medical Oncology, Amsterdam University Medical Centers, 1105 AZ Amsterdam, The Netherlands; j.m.tromp@amsterdamumc.nl
9 Department of Medical Oncology, Erasmus MC Cancer Institute, Erasmus University Medical Center, 3015 GD Rotterdam, The Netherlands; m.bos@erasmusmc.nl
10 Department of Medical Oncology, Leiden University Medical Center, 2333 ZA Leiden, The Netherlands; t.van_der_hulle@lumc.nl
11 Department of Internal Medicine, GROW-School of Oncology and Reproduction, Maastricht UMC+ Comprehensive Cancer Center, 6229 HX Maastricht, The Netherlands; roy.lalisang@mumc.nl
12 Department of Medical Oncology, University Medical Center Groningen, 9713 GZ Groningen, The Netherlands; j.nuver@umcg.nl
13 Department of Neurology, Amsterdam UMC, Amsterdam University Medical Centers, Location VUmc, 1081 HV Amsterdam, The Netherlands; m.kouwenhoven@amsterdamumc.nl
14 Department of Surgical Oncology, Erasmus MC Cancer Institute, Erasmus University Medical Center, 3015 GD Rotterdam, The Netherlands
15 Division of Clinical Studies, Institute of Cancer Research and Royal Marsden NHS Foundation Trust, London SM2 5PT, UK
* Correspondence: o.husson@nki.nl; Tel.: +31-20-512-9111

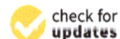

Citation: Vlooswijk, C.; Poll-Franse, L.V.v.d.; Janssen, S.H.M.; Derksen, E.; Reuvers, M.J.P.; Bijlsma, R.; Kaal, S.E.J.; Kerst, J.M.; Tromp, J.M.; Bos, M.E.M.M.; et al. Recruiting Adolescent and Young Adult Cancer Survivors for Patient-Reported Outcome Research: Experiences and Sample Characteristics of the SURVAYA Study. *Curr. Oncol.* **2022**, *29*, 5407–5425. https://doi.org/ 10.3390/curroncol29080428

Received: 10 June 2022
Accepted: 26 July 2022
Published: 29 July 2022

Publisher's Note: MDPI stays neutral with regard to jurisdictional claims in published maps and institutional affiliations.

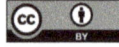

Copyright: © 2022 by the authors. Licensee MDPI, Basel, Switzerland. This article is an open access article distributed under the terms and conditions of the Creative Commons Attribution (CC BY) license (https:// creativecommons.org/licenses/by/ 4.0/).

Abstract: Background: Participation of Adolescents and Young Adults with cancer (AYAs: 18–39 years at time of diagnosis) in patient-reported outcome studies is warranted given the limited knowledge of (long-term) physical and psychosocial health outcomes. We examined the representativeness of AYAs participating in the study, to observe the impact of various invitation methods on response rates and reasons for non-participation. Methods: A population-based, cross-sectional cohort study was performed among long-term (5–20 years) AYA cancer survivors. All participants were invited using various methods to fill in a questionnaire on their health outcomes, including enclosing a paper version of the questionnaire, and sending a reminder. Those who did not respond received a postcard in which they were asked to provide a reason for non-participation. Results: In total, 4.010 AYAs (response 36%) participated. Females, AYAs with a higher socio-economic status (SES), diagnosed more than 10 years ago, diagnosed with a central nervous system tumor, sarcoma, a lymphoid malignancy, stage III, or treated with systemic chemotherapy were more likely to participate.

Including a paper questionnaire increased the response rate by 5% and sending a reminder by 13%. AYAs who did not participate were either not interested (47%) or did want to be reminded of their cancer (31%). Conclusions: Study participation was significantly lower among specific subgroups of AYA cancer survivors. Higher response rates were achieved when a paper questionnaire was included, and reminders were sent. To increase representativeness of future AYA study samples, recruitment strategies could focus on integrating patient-reported outcomes in clinical practice and involving AYA patients to promote participation in research.

Keywords: adolescents and young adults with cancer (AYAs); population-based research; health-related outcomes; non-participation; recruitment strategies; patient-reported outcomes

1. Introduction

Adolescents and young adults (AYAs) are recognized as a distinct population within the oncology community due to the unique challenges they encounter, including delayed diagnosis, lack of progress in treatment, and psychosocial issues [1–5]. The US National Cancer Institute proposed defining AYAs as those aged 15–39 years at initial diagnosis, but also concluded that this age range should be flexibly applied, depending on specific research questions and the health care delivery system [4]. In the Netherlands, care for cancer patients is categorized into centralized pediatric oncology for children (0–18 years) and medical oncology for adults ($\geq$18 years). Therefore, in the Netherlands, AYAs are defined as those aged 18 to 39 years at initial cancer diagnosis and can make use of the age-specific care provided in AYA expert centers nationally coordinated by the Dutch AYA health care network. Although cancer is a disease predominantly affecting older adults, on average 3500 AYAs were diagnosed with cancer in the Netherlands annually in the period between 2010 and 2016 [6]. Survival has been increasing in the AYA population. With a 5-year relative survival of >80%, most AYAs have a long life ahead of them.

In past decades, more and more attention has been paid to the unique clinical needs of AYA cancer patients and, in parallel, the development of specialized AYA guidelines and cancer centers internationally [7–11]. The unique needs of AYAs with cancer include dealing with issues such as fertility, social isolation, family functioning, employment, and financial toxicity [10–12]. Studies that address long-term health issues show that AYA cancer survivors are at greater risk for late effects, such as cardiomyopathy, hearing loss, stroke, thyroid disorders, and diabetes than the general population [13]. Additionally, regarding psychological aspects, AYA cancer survivors are at greater risk of worse mental health than their counterparts, even more than 6 years after completion of treatment [14].

To increase knowledge about the long-term health issues among AYAs, it is important to perform studies among AYAs. However, research has shown that AYA cancer patients have participated less often in clinical trials than younger and older patients [15]. Although the reasons for low clinical trial enrollment among AYAs are not well understood, it will likely be a combination of treatment setting and provider factors (community settings with limited access to trials; knowledge of available trials), with patient-(concerns, knowledge, attitudes, personal conflicts, and socioeconomic factors including underinsurance) and system-level factors (age restrictions; trial availability) [15–17]. Clinical trial participation of AYAs is very important, because currently there is limited knowledge about the effectiveness of treatments for AYA, which has been described as one of the reasons for the limited progress in survival in this age group [18].

Next to clinical trials, patient-reported outcome (PRO) studies can provide relevant information on health outcomes; however, participation of AYAs in PRO studies is often low, with response rates ranging from 25% to 52% [19–24].

In these previously conducted PRO studies, response rates improved by using personal invitation methods and patients preferred paper-pencil rather than online questionnaires [19]. These studies also showed that certain AYA subgroups were less likely to participate. For instance, males and Hispanics less often participate in PRO research than females and non-Hispanic whites [25,26]. In addition, AYAs diagnosed with a melanoma or gynecologic cancer were slightly underrepresented. Reasons for non-participation in observational PRO studies among AYA were not studied before and therefore remain largely unknown.

The burden of adverse long-term health outcomes of cancer and its treatment in AYA cancer survivors highlighted the importance to get more insight into AYA patient subgroups that are more susceptible to specific poor long-term health issues [10]. Therefore, we conducted an observational population-based, cross-sectional cohort study among 5–20-year survivors of AYA cancer; the SURVAYA study (health-related quality of life and late effects among SURVivors of cancer in Adolescence and Young Adulthood). Most research focusing on response rates has been done among AYA in treatment or shortly after. The SURVAYA study provides an optimal opportunity to examine the best way to approach long-term AYA cancer survivors for PRO research.

The secondary aims of the SURVAYA study were to (1) examine representativeness of the study sample regarding sociodemographic and clinical characteristics; (2) examine the impact of different invitation methods on response rate; and (3) describe reasons for non-participation.

2. Materials and Methods

2.1. Setting and Population

An observational population-based, cross-sectional cohort study was performed among AYA patients (18–39 years old at time of cancer diagnosis) registered within the Netherlands Cancer Registry (NCR). The NCR is a population-based registry that covers the total Dutch population of more than 17 million people. Patients diagnosed with cancer between 2000 and 2015 (except stated otherwise between brackets) and treated in the Netherlands Cancer Institute (1999–2014) or one of the university medical centers (University Medical Center Utrecht (1999–2014), Academic Medical Center (1999–2014), Erasmus Medical Center, Maastricht University Medical Center, Radboud University Medical Center, VU University Medical Center, Leiden University Medical Center, and University Medical Center Groningen (1999–2015) were included.

Patients with clinically diagnosed cancer (without histological diagnosis) were excluded. In addition, the following diagnoses were excluded for multifactorial reasons, mainly, based on very good prognosis or extreme rarity of the tumor in this age group (and therefore it is sometimes unclear to the patient that he/she has a form of cancer): neuroendocrine tumors of the gastrointestinal tract, unknown primary site, skin adnexal carcinoma, unspecified skin carcinoma, squamous cell carcinoma of skin, basal cell carcinoma, dermatofibrosarcoma, Kaposi sarcoma, atypical lipoma, atypical chondroma, placental trophoblast tumors, cutaneous lymphomas, and unknown tumor types. The SURVAYA study was approved by the Netherlands Cancer Institute Institutional Review Board (IRB-IRBd18122) and registered within clinical trial registration (NCT05379387).

2.2. Data Collection

Data collection was conducted between May 2019 and June 2021 within PROFILES (Patient Reported Outcomes Following Initial treatment and Long-term Evaluation of Survivorship) [27]. PROFILES is a registry to study the physical and psychosocial impact of cancer and its treatment from a dynamic, growing population-based cohort of both short- and long-term cancer survivors. A linkage with the Dutch municipal records database was established to obtain up-to-date addresses and to know patients are alive at the moment of inviting.

All participants were informed about the study via a letter from their (ex-) attending medical specialist. Three various ways of invitation methods were used and categorized into the following groups: the paper-optional group, no reminder group, and paper-included group.

2.2.1. Paper-Optional Group ($N = 8291$)

The study invitation consisted of a letter with a secure link to a web-based informed consent form, online questionnaire, and log-in instructions. A reply card with a pre-stamped return envelope was also included, to give participants the option to request a paper version of the questionnaire. A reminder was sent to the paper-optional group.

2.2.2. No Reminder Group ($N = 1671$)

The study invitation was the same as for the paper-optional group; however, no reminder was sent to assess the impact of a reminder.

2.2.3. Paper Included Group ($N = 1334$)

This group received the same invitation letter with a secure link to a web-based informed consent, online questionnaire and log-in instructions, but with a paper questionnaire and a pre-stamped return envelope also included. A reminder was sent.

The reminder for the paper-optional group and paper-included group was anticipated to be sent within 3 months after the first invitation; however, due to COVID-19, it was not possible to send invitations in the hospitals and therefore the reminder was sent within a timeframe of 2–7 months. The reminder letter consisted of a link to a web-based informed consent form and online questionnaire, and a postcard which could be used to indicate their reason(s) if patients did not want to participate in the study.

2.3. Measures

Sociodemographic and clinical characteristics were available from the NCR.

Sociodemographic data included gender, age and social-economic status (SES). SES scores arise from the standardized income per household, extracted from four numbers and letters of the Dutch postal code of the Netherlands Institute for Social Research [20]. The scores were decoded into deciles, which were consequently classified as low (deciles 1,2,3), medium (deciles 4,5,6), and high (deciles 7,8,9) SES.

Clinical data included tumor type, tumor stage, primary treatments received, and time since diagnosis. Tumor type was classified according to the third International Classification of Diseases for Oncology (ICDO-3) [28]. Cancer stage was classified according to TNM or Ann Arbor Code (Hodgkin lymphoma and Non-Hodgkin lymphoma) [29]. TNM 5 was used for patients diagnosed from 1999 to 2002, TNM 6 for patients diagnosed from 2003 to 2009, and TNM 7 was used for patients diagnosed from 2010 to 2015. For tumors in the central nervous system, neuroblastomas, paraganglioma, extragonadal / extracerebral germ cell tumors, plasma cell tumors, myeloid hematological malignancies such as acute and chronic myeloid leukemia, myeloproliferative neoplasms, and myelodysplastic syndrome, tumor stage was not determined nor registered.

Information on marital status and educational level were patient-reported via the questionnaire (data only available for respondents).

Reasons for not wanting to participate in the study were patient-reported. AYAs could give multiple answers via the following given response categories (determined a priori with input from AYAs with cancer): I am not interested in the research, I don't want to think about cancer, I prefer an in person invitation, I have never considered myself as an AYA young adult cancer patient, I don't see the added value of this research, I see no incentive or benefit of participating in this research, the questionnaire is too long, I have participated in research too many times, I am too busy, or an open-answer option.

2.4. Statistical Analyses

Statistical analyses were conducted using SAS version 9.4. (SAS Institute, Cary, NC, USA). All differences with a *p*-value < 0.05 were considered statistically significant. For the baseline characteristics, frequencies with percentages and means with standard deviations were used to describe the variables, and Chi-square tests and independent t-tests were used to test the differences between participants and non-respondents. In a multivariable logistic regression, associations between socio-demographic (age, gender, SES) and tumor characteristics (cancer type, stage, primary treatments received and time since diagnosis), and response were determined. Frequencies with percentages were used to describe the self-reported reasons of AYA non-responders and response rate of the paper-optional group, paper-included group, and no reminder group.

3. Results

In total, 17,098 AYA cancer patients were identified via the Netherlands Cancer Registry, whereof 11,296 were invited to participate in the study (Figure 1). Reasons to exclude patients ($n = 5802$) were not having permission from the hospital to invite patients for the study (55%), or not being able to obtain up-to-date vital status and addresses because it was not possible or not allowed to link with municipal personal records database (18%). A total of 4,010 AYAs completed the questionnaire, which resulted in an overall response rate of 36%.

Table 1 describes the characteristics of the total AYA cancer population. Of the total population-based study population, 59% were females, average age of diagnosis was 31.5 years, and time since diagnosis was 12.2 years. Breast cancer (20%), germ cell tumors (16%) and lymphoid hematological malignancies (14%) were the most common tumor types. The supplementary materials (Table S1) shows the different tumor types divided into smaller subgroups.

Table 1. Socio-demographic and tumor characteristics of the total population-based population, and divided in respondents, non-respondents, and excluded.

		Total Population-Based Population		Respondents		Non-Respondents		Excluded		P-Value (Non-Respondents vs. Respondents)
		N = 17,098		N = 4010		N = 7286		N = 5802		
		n	%	n	%	n	%	n	%	
Gender	Male	6997	41	1549	39	3082	42	2366	41	0.0001
	Female	10,101	59	2461	61	4204	58	3436	59	
Age (at diagnosis), (mean (sd))		31.5 (5.9)		31.6 (5.9)		31.4 (5.9)		31.5 (5.8)		0.1354
	18-24 years	2672	16	613	15	1168	16	891	15	
	25-34 years	7782	46	1786	45	3328	46	2668	46	
	35-39 years	6644	39	1611	40	2790	38	2243	39	
Time since diagnosis, (mean (sd))		12.2 (4.6)		12.4 (4.5)		11.6 (4.4)		12.8 (4.8)		0.0001
	5-10 years	6362	37	1386	35	2990	41	1986	34	
	≥11-15 years	558	33	1397	35	2496	34	1687	29	
	≥16-20 years	5156	30	1231	31	1806	25	2119	37	
Social economic status	Low	3161	19	544	14	1510	21	1107	19	0.0001
	Intermediate	5427	32	1236	31	2354	32	1837	32	
	High	8456	50	2220	56	3417	47	2819	49	
Type of cancer	Head and neck	570	3	124	3	305	4	141	2	0.0001
	Colon and rectal	368	2	82	2	151	2	135	2	
	Digestive tract, other	262	2	31	1	63	1	168	3	
	Respiratory tract	166	1	30	1	71	1	65	1	
	Melanoma	1221	7	290	7	617	8	314	5	
	Skin, other	105	1	0	0	0	0	105	2	
	Breast	3346	20	944	24	1553	21	849	15	
	Female genitalia	2073	12	445	11	878	12	750	13	
	Male genitalia	24	0	6	0	12	0	6	0	
	Urinary tract	190	1	46	1	105	1	39	1	
	Thyroid gland	1054	6	248	6	468	6	338	6	
	Central nervous system	545	3	150	4	231	3	164	3	
	Bone or soft tissue sarcoma	1256	7	172	4	291	4	793	14	
	Germ cell tumors	2743	16	692	17	1394	19	657	11	

Table 1. Cont.

		Total Population-Based Population		Respondents		Non-Respondents		Excluded		P-Value (Non-Respondents vs. Respondents)
		N = 17,098		N = 4010		N = 7286		N = 5802		
		n	%	n	%	n	%	n	%	
	Lymphoid hematological malignancies	2339	14	591	15	903	12	845	15	
	Myeloid hematological malignancies	671	4	148	4	226	3	297	5	
	Other	165	1	11	0	18	0	136	2	
Tumor stage	I	7758	45	1726	43	3480	48	2552	44	0.0001
	II	388	23	1053	27	1850	25	967	17	
	III	1994	12	573	14	923	13	498	9	
	IV	618	4	179	4	298	4	141	2	
	Missing	2848	17	469	12	735	10	1644	28	
Primary treatment modality	Surgery	13,145	77	3126	78	5863	81	4156	72	0.0017
	Chemotherapy	8199	48	2239	56	3632	50	2328	40	0.0001
	Radiotherapy	7681	45	1902	47	3293	45	2486	43	0.0213
	Hormone therapy	1734	10	484	12	786	11	464	8	0.0382
	Targeted therapy	1119	7	308	8	514	7	297	5	0.2178
	Stem cell therapy	523	3	142	4	207	3	174	3	0.0392
Marital status (at time of questionnaire)	Partner	NA	NA	NA	3333	83	NA	NA	NA	NA
Education level	No education or primary education	NA	NA	28	1	NA	NA	NA	NA	
	Secondary education			266	7					
	Secondary (vocational) education			1455	36					
	Higher (vocational) education			1374	34					
	University education			878	22					
Mode of completion	Paper	NA	NA	647	16	NA	NA	NA	NA	
	Online			3363	84					

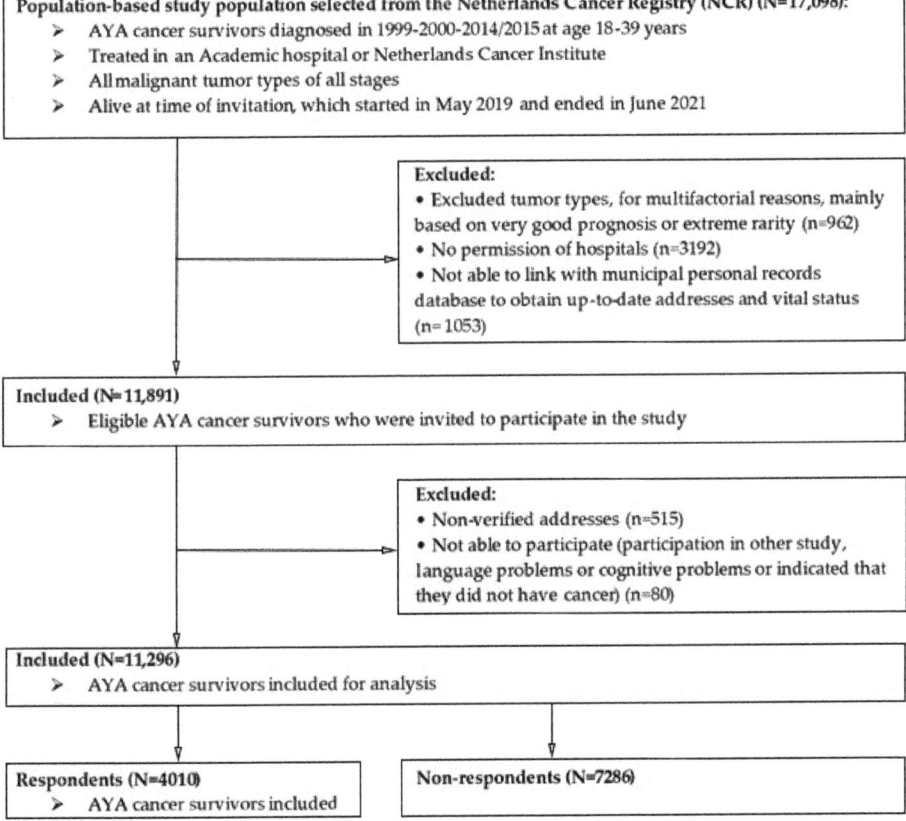

Figure 1. Flowchart of study participants in the SURVAYA study.

3.1. Representativeness Study Sample

In multivariable logistic regression analysis, females were more likely to participate than males (Table 2). AYAs who were diagnosed more than 10 years ago were more likely to participate compared with AYAs who were diagnosed 5–10 years ago. AYAs with an intermediate or high SES were more likely to participate, compared with AYAs with a low SES. Moreover, compared with AYAs with breast cancer, AYAs diagnosed with cancer in the central nervous system, bone and soft tissues, or with a lymphoid hematological malignancy were more likely to participate. AYAs diagnosed with stage III cancer were more likely to participate than AYAs diagnosed with stage I cancer. AYAs treated with chemotherapy were also more likely to participate compared with AYAs who did not receive chemotherapy.

Table 2. Odds ratios (OR) of respondents versus non-respondents, multivariable logistic regression.

		Respondents		Non-Respondents		Odds of Respondents vs. Non-Respondents			
		N = 4010		N = 7286		OR	95% CI	p-value
Gender	Male	1549	39	3082	42	1.00 (ref)		
	Females	2461	61	4204	58	1.246	1.108–1.400	**0.0002**
Age (at diagnosis)	18–24 years	613	15	1168	16	1.00 (ref)		
	25–34 years	1786	45	3328	46	1.074	0.953–1.210	0.2420
	35–39 years	1611	40	2790	38	1.123	0.989–1.275	0.0734
Years since diagnosis	5–10 years	1386	35	2990	41	1.00 (ref)		
	≥11–15 years	1397	35	2496	34	1.210	1.103–1.328	**0.0001**
	≥16–20 years	1231	31	1806	25	1.489	1.348–1.645	**0.0001**
Social economic status	Low	544	14	1510	21	1.00 (ref)		
	Intermediate	1236	31	2354	32	1.406	1.245–1.587	**0.0001**
	High	2220	56	3417	47	1.763	1.575–1.974	**0.0001**
Type of cancer	Head and neck	124	3	305	4	0.933	0.711–1.224	0.6153
	Colon and rectal	82	2	151	2	1.080	0.793–1.472	0.6246
	Digestive tract, other	31	1	63	1	1.146	0.719–1.827	0.5673
	Respiratory tract	30	1	71	1	0.991	0.626–1.570	0.9696
	Melanoma	290	7	617	8	1.069	0.856–1.334	0.5576
	Breast	944	24	1553	21	1.00 (ref)		
	Female genitalia	445	11	878	12	1.042	0.864–1.257	0.6642
	Male genitalia	6	0	12	0	1.258	0.460–3.439	0.6546
	Urinary tract	46	1	105	1	1.086	0.736–1.604	0.6769
	Thyroid gland	248	6	468	6	1.213	0.976–1.508	0.0816
	Central nervous system	150	4	231	3	1.402	0.998–1.969	0.0515
	Bone or soft tissue sarcoma	172	4	291	4	1.289	1008–1.648	**0.0430**
	Germ cell tumors	692	17	1394	19	1.124	0.920–1.374	0.2532
	Lymphoid hematological malignancies	591	15	903	12	1.381	1.048–1.820	**0.0220**
	Myeloid hematological malignancies	148	4	226	3	1.294	0.877–1.908	0.1939
	Other	11	0	18	0	1.318	0.596–2.912	0.4951

Table 2. Cont.

		Respondents		Non-Respondents		Odds of Respondents vs. Non-Respondents		
		N = 4010		N = 7286		OR	95% CI	p-value
Tumor stage	I	1726	43	3480	48	1.00 (ref)		
	II	1063	27	1850	25	1.026	0.916–1.149	0.6579
	III	573	14	923	13	1.174	1.022–1.348	**0.0231**
	IV	179	4	298	4	1.139	0.916–1.417	0.2412
	Missing	469	12	735	10	1.121	0.892–1.409	0.3278
Primary treatment modality	Surgery	3126	78	5863	81	1.121	0.901–1.395	0.3059
	Chemotherapy	2239	56	3632	50	1.262	1.118–1.425	**0.0002**
	Radiotherapy	1902	47	3293	45	1.030	0.935–1.135	0.5475
	Hormone therapy	484	12	786	11	0.991	0.841–1.168	0.9156
	Targeted therapy	308	8	514	7	1.013	0.862–1.191	0.8762
	Stem cell therapy	142	4	207	3	0.996	0.772–1.284	0.9738

3.2. Methods of Invitation

The overall response rate was 36%. To be more specific, 25% of the AYAs responded to the initial invitation, 11% after a reminder was sent (Figure 2). Of the total invited AYA cancer patients in the paper-optional group, 3041 (36%) responded, whereof the reminder still yielded 13% of the response rate. The highest response rate ($n = 544$, 41%) was achieved in the paper-included group (32% after initial invitation and the remaining 9% after the reminder). The lowest response rate ($n = 429$, 26%) was shown in the group to which no reminder was sent.

3.3. Reasons of Non-Participation

Of the non-respondents, 765 (11%) AYAs returned the postcard upon which they indicated (multiple) reason(s) for why they did not participate in the SURVAYA study. Nearly half of the AYAs (49%) who completed the postcard were not interested in participating in the study (Table 3). Furthermore, AYAs did not want to participate because they did not want to think about cancer (32%), were too busy (19%), considered the questionnaire as too long, personal or difficult (13%), and/or had never considered themselves as a young adult cancer patient (13%). The open answer category revealed additional reasons, such as privacy aspects, study participation invitation mail was not appreciated by AYAs, or AYAs were not capable to participate due to sickness or language problems.

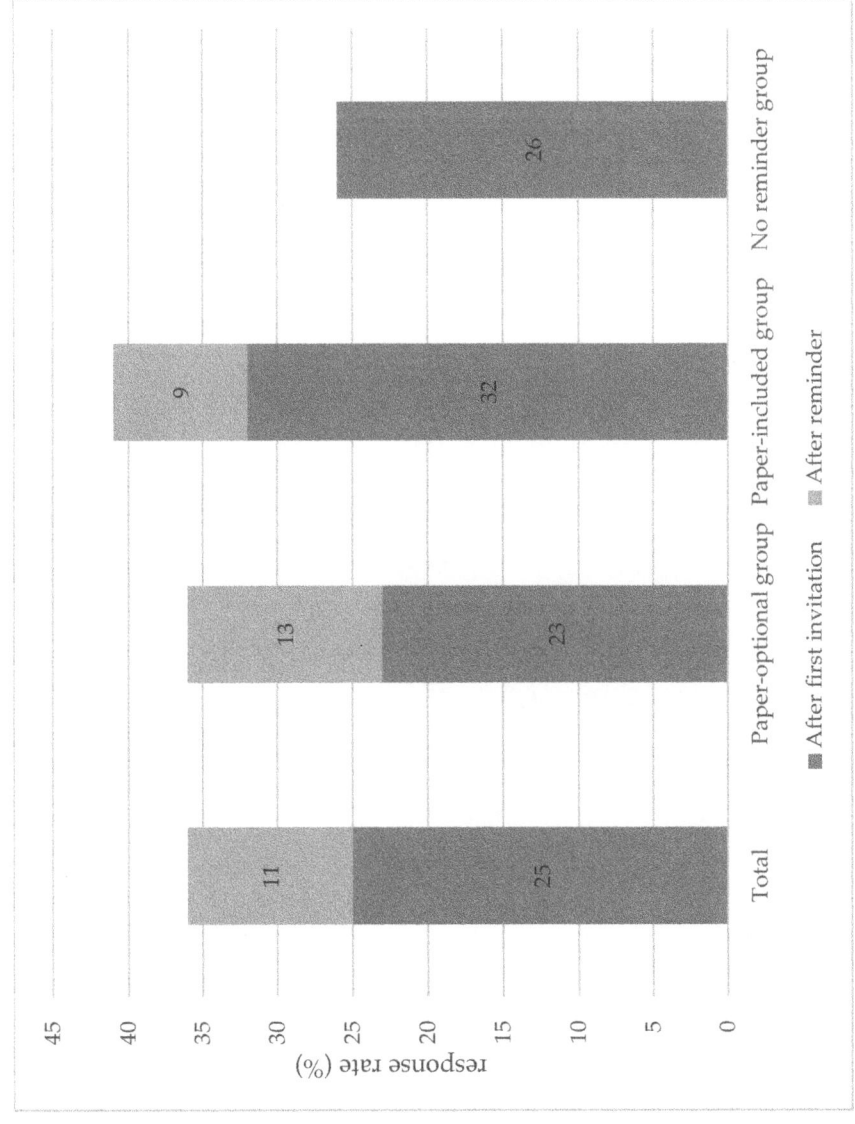

Figure 2. Response rates of the paper-optional group, paper-included group, and no reminder group.

Table 3. Self-reported reasons of AYA (n = 765) who did not want to participate in PRO research.

	N	%
Not interested in the research	379	49
Don't want to think about cancer	243	32
Too busy	148	19
Questionnaire is too long/too personal/difficult	97	13
Don't consider themself a young adult cancer patient	97	13
Have participated in research too many times	58	8
No personal incentive or benefit	32	4
Not capable to participate *	20	3
Don't see the added value of this research	21	3
Worried about privacy aspects	16	2
Practical problems in participating **	16	2
Other ***	16	2
Unclear what causes symptoms because of comorbidities	14	2
Prefer an in person invitation	9	1

Multiple answers could be given

* Too sick/tired/no energy, language problems, ** Log-in problems or want to participate online or just on paper, *** Felt that their situation do not contribute, didn't appreciate study participation invitation.

4. Discussion

This large observational population-based, cross-sectional cohort study, addressing (sub)groups that are less inclined to participate, possible reasons for this and different ways of recruiting patients, recruited more than 4000 long-term AYA cancer survivors. Males and patients with a lower SES, diagnosed less than 10 years ago, having a lower disease stage, and not treated with chemotherapy were less likely to participate, as well as patients with specific tumor types. Paper questionnaires and reminders both had a positive impact on response rates. Reasons for non-participating in the study mainly included not being interested in the study or not wanting to be reminded of cancer.

In terms of the characteristics and representativeness of the SURVAYA study sample, similar to our findings, in previous studies among AYAs, males were less likely to participate in research [14,19,25,30]. In general, in health (behaviour) research, males are less likely to participate [31]. Reasons for lower participation among males are that they were generally less interested in participating than females, and that they were more likely to decline research participation due to time constraints [32]. Ryan et al. found that response rate among males improved substantially through the use of targeted Facebook advertising, incorporating features such as using images of men that appealed to leadership themes and using concise text [33]. In addition, male enrolments increased by asking female participants to invite males.

AYAs who were diagnosed with cancer more than 10 years ago were more likely to participate. AYAs who are more than 10 years diagnosed with cancer are more often older adults. We hypothesize that their willingness to take part could have to do with life stage. It is probably harder to be closer to diagnosis and treatment and juggling with competing demands.

Contrary to our findings, AYAs diagnosed with melanoma were underrepresented in previous research [14,25]. AYAs diagnosed with cancer in the central nervous system, bone and soft tissues, and with a lymphoid hematological malignancy were more likely to participate compared with AYAs with breast cancer. A possible explanation for this difference could be that patients diagnosed with less common cancer types probably are less often invited for participation in research. In addition, they might experience more consequences from their cancer diagnosis and treatment and might be more willing to tell their story, which could result in higher response rates among these patients.

Patients with a low SES have shown to be largely underrepresented in research [34]. Barriers for participation of low SES patients could be language barriers, low health literacy, and distrust of the healthcare system [35]. Adults with a low health literacy were less interested in participating in research, probably because of the difficulties associated with understanding and skills needed to complete questionnaires [36]. Unfortunately, we did not have data on ethnicity, as these data are not collected by the NCR or in electronic patient files. We know from literature that Hispanic black and Hispanic patients were less likely to participate than non-Hispanic white patients as well [19,26].

In contrast to what was found in an older cancer population, we found that AYAs who were treated with chemotherapy were more likely to participate in the study [34,37]. Possibly, because AYAs who received chemotherapy experience daily long-term health consequences from their cancer diagnosis and treatment and were therefore more willing to participate.

Our observed participation rate is, on average, similar compared with studies among AYA populations using similar recruitment strategies [21–24]. Given the younger age of this study population compared with the general cancer population, it is expected that they experience less problems or barriers with completing questionnaires online. However, the response rate improved by including a paper version of the questionnaire. Researchers from the AYA HOPE study found the same and explained this by the fact that unless thrown away, a questionnaire on paper is a constant reminder, whereas a computer/telephone can be turned off [38]. Sending a reminder resulted in a higher response rate and this is consistent with previous studies [39–41]. Among adolescents, in a study of Richards et al., personal contact seems to be effective. The initial response rate of 20% was improved by adding follow-up mailing (31%) and after conducting the consent process and questionnaire by phone (61%) [39].

To the best of our knowledge, no previous studies have assessed self-reported reasons for non-participation in PRO research among AYAs. Studies among the general population identified absence of interest and time constraints as reasons for non-participation in research, which was also found in our study [42–44]. Although patients did not want to participate in our study, they took the effort and time to return the postcard with reason(s) for non-participating. Remarkably, in our study, 13% of the AYAs did not consider themselves as a young cancer patient. A possible explanation could be that a significant part of the participants outgrew the AYA age and mistakenly did not consider themselves as an AYA. When approaching AYAs for future studies regarding long-term outcomes,' it is important that participants feel connected and can identify with the target population of the study. In recent decades, the oncology community became aware of the gap in the care needs and outcomes of AYA patients [45]. Globally, but also in the Netherlands, development of AYA programs has flourished. This evolution in the field of AYA oncology could increase awareness and knowledge among future AYAs about age-specific care and research, and could thereby increase their willingness to participate in AYA research.

This study was limited by the cross-sectional design, limiting the determination of attrition rates. Study participants were diagnosed with cancer 5-20 years ago, which might have led to feeling less connected and attracted to participate in this study. Differentiating reasons of non-participation by different SES groups was not possible since patients had not given permission for this. It also remains unknown what the impact of COVID-19 is on the SURVAYA study. We could imagine that COVID-19 has had an impact on some of the outcomes of the SURVAYA study. We will examine this in a separate manuscript.

The NCR allowed us to identify more than 17,000 cases of cancer among AYA aged 18–39 years between 1998 and 2015 in the participating hospitals. The NCR did not only act as a sampling frame, but also made it possible to perform a non-responder analysis, which gave insight into certain subgroups who are less likely to participate in observational research. In a previous study among the general cancer population, older patients with poorer Health-related Quality of Life (HRQoL) were less likely to participate, whereas younger patients with poorer HRQoL were more likely to participate [27,30]. To obtain more representative data, future studies should focus on personalized recruitment strategies to reach those who are less likely to participate, such as males and AYAs with lower SES. By performing qualitative research via focus groups and interviews, we could gain more insight into attitude towards participation in research, preferences in research type and invitation methods in specific subgroups of AYAs.

AYAs themselves might play an important role to stimulate and encourage fellow AYAs to participate in research. AYAs are widely acknowledged as key stakeholders in oncology and being used by research committees and advisory boards [44]. Involvement of AYA patient experts could bridge the gap between patient and research(ers). AYA patient experts could align research as closely as possible with the target group and help enhance recruitment, especially those who are less likely to participate (e.g., males, AYAs with low SES, ethnic minorities) [44]. Another option to get more PRO data of AYAs is better alignment between research and clinical care. PROs are more and more integrated in clinical practice. Moreover, PROs are more and more integrated in clinical studies, which reported high participation rates [46]. Ideally, PROs are used and aligned between research, health care and policy initiative, and adapted based on purpose. It is important that age-specific themes (e.g., fertility, body image, sexual health, financial security, life plans (educational and employment goals), and independence) are identified and described in a core outcome set and implemented in care and research [47,48].

5. Conclusions

In summary, the SURVAYA study recruited a large sample of AYA cancer survivors, however several differences were found between respondents and non-respondents based on registry data. Future studies should put effort into recruitment strategies, such as involving AYA patient experts as research partners to reach and encourage AYAs who are less likely to participate, such as males and AYAs with a low SES.

Supplementary Materials: The following supporting information can be downloaded at: https://www.mdpi.com/article/10.3390/curroncol29080428/s1, Table S1: Detailed information on tumor types of the total population-based population, and divided in respondents, non-respondents and excluded.

Author Contributions: Conceptualization, C.V., L.V.v.d.P.-F., W.T.A.v.d.G. and O.H.; data curation, C.V.; formal analysis, C.V.; funding acquisition, L.V.v.d.P.-F., W.T.A.v.d.G. and O.H.; investigation, C.V., S.H.M.J., E.D., M.J.P.R., R.B., T.v.d.H., M.C.M.K., S.E.J.K., J.M.K., J.M.T., M.E.M.M.B., R.I.L., J.N., and O.H.; methodology, C.V., L.V.v.d.P.-F., W.T.A.v.d.G. and O.H.; project administration, C.V. and O.H.; resources, C.V., S.H.M.J., E.D. and M.J.P.R.; software, C.V.; supervision, L.V.v.d.P.-F., W.T.A.v.d.G. and O.H.; validation, C.V. and O.H.; visualization, C.V. and O.H.; writing—original draft preparation, C.V. and O.H.; writing—review and editing, C.V., L.V.v.d.P.-F., S.H.M.J., E.D., M.J.P.R., R.B., T.v.d.H., M.C.M.K., S.E.J.K., J.M.K., J.M.T., M.E.M.M.B., R.I.L., J.N., W.T.A.v.d.G. and O.H. All authors have read and agreed to the published version of the manuscript.

Funding: Carla Vlooswijk Msc is supported by the Dutch Cancer Society (#11788 COMPRAYA study). Dr. Olga Husson and Silvie Janssen MSc are supported by the Netherlands Organization for Scientific Research VIDI grant (198.007). Data collection of the SURVAYA study was partly supported by the investment grant (#480-08-009) from the Netherlands Organization for Scientific Research. These funding agencies had no further role in study design; in the collection, analysis and interpretation of data; in the writing of the paper; or in the decision to submit the paper for publication.

Institutional Review Board Statement: The study was conducted in accordance with the Declaration of Helsinki, and approved by the Netherlands Cancer Institute Institutional Review Board (IRB-IRBd18122) on 6 February 2019.

Informed Consent Statement: Informed consent was obtained from all subjects (responders) involved in the study.

Data Availability Statement: The data presented in this study are available on request from the corresponding author. The data are not publicly available due to privacy issues.

Acknowledgments: The authors wish to thank all the patients for their participation in the study and the registration team of the Netherlands Comprehensive Cancer Organisation (IKNL) for the collection of data for The Netherlands Cancer Registry.

Conflicts of Interest: The authors declare no conflict of interest.

References

1. Lewis, D.R.; Seibel, N.L.; Smith, A.W.; Stedman, M.R. Adolescent and young adult cancer survival. *J. Natl. Cancer Inst. Monogr.* **2014**, *2014*, 228–235. [CrossRef]
2. Galán, S.; de la Vega, R.; Miró, J. Needs of adolescents and young adults after cancer treatment: A systematic review. *Eur. J. Cancer Care* **2018**, *27*, e12558. [CrossRef]
3. Meeneghan, M.R.; Wood, W.A. Challenges for cancer care delivery to adolescents and young adults: Present and future. *Acta Haematol.* **2014**, *132*, 414–422. [CrossRef]
4. Smith, A.W.; Seibel, N.L.; Lewis, D.R.; Albritton, K.H.; Blair, D.F.; Blanke, C.D.; Bleyer, W.A.; Freyer, D.R.; Geiger, A.M.; Hayes-Lattin, B.; et al. Next steps for adolescent and young adult oncology workshop: An update on progress and recommendations for the future. *Cancer* **2016**, *122*, 988–999. [CrossRef]
5. Ferrari, A.; Stark, D.; Peccatori, F.A.; Fern, L.; Laurence, V.; Gaspar, N.; Bozovic-Spasojevic, I.; Smith, O.; De Munter, J.; Derwich, K.; et al. Adolescents and young adults (AYA) with cancer: A position paper from the AYA Working Group of the European Society for Medical Oncology (ESMO) and the European Society for Paediatric Oncology (SIOPE). *ESMO Open* **2021**, *6*, 100096. [CrossRef]
6. van der Meer, D.J.; Karim-Kos, H.E.; van der Mark, M.; Aben, K.K.H.; Bijlsma, R.M.; Rijneveld, A.W.; van der Graaf, W.T.A.; Husson, O. Incidence, Survival, and Mortality Trends of Cancers Diagnosed in Adolescents and Young Adults (15–39 Years): A Population-Based Study in The Netherlands 1990–2016. *Cancers* **2020**, *12*, 3421. [CrossRef]
7. Geue, K.; Mehnert-Theuerkauf, A.; Stroske, I.; Brock, H.; Friedrich, M.; Leuteritz, K. Psychosocial Long-Term Effects of Young Adult Cancer Survivors: Study Protocol of the Longitudinal AYA-LE Long-Term Effects Study. *Front. Psychol.* **2021**, *12*, 688142. [CrossRef]
8. National Comprehensive Cancer Network Guidelines for patients. Adolescents and Young adults with Cancer, 2019. Available online: https://www.nccn.org/patients/guidelines/content/PDF/aya-patient.pdf (accessed on 12 July 2022).
9. Adolescent and Young Adult Oncology Progress Review Group. Closing the Gap: Research and Care Imperatives for Adolescents and Young Adults with Cancer, 2006. Available online: https://www.livestrong.org/content/closing-gap-research-and-careimperatives-adolescents-and-young-adults-cancer (accessed on 12 July 2022).
10. Janssen, S.H.M.; van der Graaf, W.T.A.; van der Meer, D.J.; Manten-Horst, E.; Husson, O. Adolescent and Young Adult (AYA) Cancer Survivorship Practices: An Overview. *Cancers* **2021**, *13*, 4847. [CrossRef]
11. Smith, A.W.; Keegan, T.; Hamilton, A.; Lynch, C.; Wu, X.C.; Schwartz, S.M.; Kato, I.; Cress, R.; Harlan, L. Understanding care and outcomes in adolescents and young adult with Cancer: A review of the AYA HOPE study. *Pediatr. Blood Cancer* **2019**, *66*, e27486. [CrossRef] [PubMed]
12. Patterson, P.; McDonald, F.E.J.; Zebrack, B.; Medlow, S. Emerging Issues Among Adolescent and Young Adult Cancer Survivors. *Semin. Oncol. Nurs.* **2015**, *31*, 53–59. [CrossRef]
13. Chao, C.; Bhatia, S.; Xu, L.; Cannavale, K.L.; Wong, F.L.; Huang, P.S.; Cooper, R.; Armenian, S.H. Chronic Comorbidities Among Survivors of Adolescent and Young Adult Cancer. *J. Clin. Oncol.* **2020**, *38*, 3161–3174. [CrossRef]
14. Schulte, F.S.M.; Chalifour, K.; Eaton, G.; Garland, S.N. Quality of life among survivors of adolescent and young adult cancer in Canada: A Young Adults With Cancer in Their Prime (YACPRIME) study. *Cancer* **2021**, *127*, 1325–1333. [CrossRef]
15. Unger, J.M.; Cook, E.; Tai, E.; Bleyer, A. The Role of Clinical Trial Participation in Cancer Research: Barriers, Evidence, and Strategies. *Am. Soc. Clin. Oncol. Educ. Book* **2016**, *35*, 185–198. [CrossRef]
16. Tai, E.; Buchanan, N.; Eliman, D.; Westervelt, L.; Beaupin, L.; Lawvere, S.; Bleyer, A. Understanding and addressing the lack of clinical trial enrollment among adolescents with cancer. *Pediatrics* **2014**, *133* (Suppl. S3), S98–S103. [CrossRef]
17. Shnorhavorian, M.; Doody, D.R.; Chen, V.W.; Hamilton, A.S.; Kato, I.; Cress, R.D.; West, M.; Wu, X.C.; Keegan, T.H.M.; Harlan, L.C.; et al. Knowledge of Clinical Trial Availability and Reasons for Nonparticipation Among Adolescent and Young Adult Cancer Patients: A Population-based Study. *Am. J. Clin. Oncol.* **2018**, *41*, 581–587. [CrossRef]
18. Bleyer, W.A.; Tejeda, H.; Murphy, S.B.; Robison, L.L.; Ross, J.A.; Pollock, B.H.; Severson, R.K.; Brawley, O.W.; Smith, M.A.; Ungerleider, R.S. National cancer clinical trials: Children have equal access; adolescents do not. *J. Adolesc. Health* **1997**, *21*, 366–373. [CrossRef]
19. Harlan, L.C.; Lynch, C.F.; Keegan, T.H.; Hamilton, A.S.; Wu, X.C.; Kato, I.; West, M.M.; Cress, R.D.; Schwartz, S.M.; Smith, A.W.; et al. Recruitment and follow-up of adolescent and young adult cancer survivors: The AYA HOPE Study. *J. Cancer Surviv.* **2011**, *5*, 305–314. [CrossRef] [PubMed]
20. Kaal, S.E.J.; Lidington, E.K.; Prins, J.B.; Jansen, R.; Manten-Horst, E.; Servaes, P.; van der Graaf, W.T.A.; Husson, O. Health-Related Quality of Life Issues in Adolescents and Young Adults with Cancer: Discrepancies with the Perceptions of Health Care Professionals. *J. Clin. Med.* **2021**, *10*, 1833. [CrossRef] [PubMed]
21. Murnane, A.; Gough, K.; Thompson, K.; Holland, L.; Conyers, R. Adolescents and young adult cancer survivors: Exercise habits, quality of life and physical activity preferences. *Support. Care Cancer* **2015**, *23*, 501–510. [CrossRef]
22. Bellizzi, K.M.; Smith, A.; Schmidt, S.; Keegan, T.H.; Zebrack, B.; Lynch, C.F.; Deapen, D.; Shnorhavorian, M.; Tompkins, B.J.; Simon, M. Positive and negative psychosocial impact of being diagnosed with cancer as an adolescent or young adult. *Cancer* **2012**, *118*, 5155–5162. [CrossRef]
23. Michel, G.; François, C.; Harju, E.; Dehler, S.; Roser, K. The long-term impact of cancer: Evaluating psychological distress in adolescent and young adult cancer survivors in Switzerland. *Psychooncology* **2019**, *28*, 577–585. [CrossRef]

24. McCarthy, M.C.; McNeil, R.; Drew, S.; Dunt, D.; Kosola, S.; Orme, L.; Sawyer, S.M. Psychological Distress and Posttraumatic Stress Symptoms in Adolescents and Young Adults with Cancer and Their Parents. *J. Adolesc. Young Adult Oncol.* **2016**, *5*, 322–329. [CrossRef]
25. Leuteritz, K.; Friedrich, M.; Nowe, E.; Sender, A.; Taubenheim, S.; Stoebel-Richter, Y.; Geue, K. Recruiting young adult cancer patients: Experiences and sample characteristics from a 12-month longitudinal study. *Eur. J. Oncol. Nurs.* **2018**, *36*, 26–31. [CrossRef] [PubMed]
26. Nichols, H.B.; Baggett, C.D.; Engel, S.M.; Getahun, D.; Anderson, C.; Cannizzaro, N.T.; Green, L.; Gupta, P.; Laurent, C.A.; Lin, P.C.; et al. The Adolescent and Young Adult (AYA) Horizon Study: An AYA Cancer Survivorship Cohort. *Cancer Epidemiol. Biomark. Prev.* **2021**, *30*, 857–866. [CrossRef]
27. van de Poll-Franse, L.V.; Horevoorts, N.; van Eenbergen, M.; Denollet, J.; Roukema, J.A.; Aaronson, N.K.; Vingerhoets, A.; Coebergh, J.W.; de Vries, J.; Essink-Bot, M.L.; et al. The Patient Reported Outcomes Following Initial treatment and Long term Evaluation of Survivorship registry: Scope, rationale and design of an infrastructure for the study of physical and psychosocial outcomes in cancer survivorship cohorts. *Eur. J. Cancer* **2011**, *47*, 2188–2194. [CrossRef]
28. Fritz, A.; Percy, C.; Jack, A.S.; Shanmugaratnam, K.; Sobin, L.; Parkin, D.M.; Whelan, S. *International Classification of Diseases for Oncology*, 3rd ed.; World Health Organization: Geneva, Switzerland, 2000.
29. Sobin, L.; Gospodarowicz, M.K.; Wittekind, C. *TNM Classification of Malignant Tumours*; Wiley: New York, NY, USA, 2011.
30. Rosenberg, A.R.; Junkins, C.C.; Sherr, N.; Scott, S.; Klein, V.; Barton, K.S.; Yi-Frazier, J.P. Conducting Psychosocial Intervention Research among Adolescents and Young Adults with Cancer: Lessons from the PRISM Randomized Clinical Trial. *Children* **2019**, *6*, 117. [CrossRef]
31. Glass, D.C.; Kelsall, H.L.; Slegers, C.; Forbes, A.B.; Loff, B.; Zion, D.; Fritschi, L. A telephone survey of factors affecting willingness to participate in health research surveys. *BMC Public Health* **2015**, *15*, 1017. [CrossRef]
32. Otufowora, A.; Liu, Y.; Young, H., 2nd; Egan, K.L.; Varma, D.S.; Striley, C.W.; Cottler, L.B. Sex Differences in Willingness to Participate in Research Based on Study Risk Level Among a Community Sample of African Americans in North Central Florida. *J. Immigr. Minor. Health* **2021**, *23*, 19–25. [CrossRef]
33. Ryan, J.; Lopian, L.; Le, B.; Edney, S.; Van Kessel, G.; Plotnikoff, R.; Vandelanotte, C.; Olds, T.; Maher, C. It's not raining men: A mixed-methods study investigating methods of improving male recruitment to health behaviour research. *BMC Public Health* **2019**, *19*, 814. [CrossRef] [PubMed]
34. de Rooij, B.H.; Ezendam, N.P.M.; Mols, F.; Vissers, P.A.J.; Thong, M.S.Y.; Vlooswijk, C.C.P.; Oerlemans, S.; Husson, O.; Horevoorts, N.J.E.; van de Poll-Franse, L.V. Cancer survivors not participating in observational patient-reported outcome studies have a lower survival compared to participants: The population-based PROFILES registry. *Qual. Life Res.* **2018**, *27*, 3313–3324. [CrossRef]
35. Price, K.N.; Lyons, A.B.; Hamzavi, I.H.; Hsiao, J.L.; Shi, V.Y. Facilitating Clinical Trials Participation of Low Socioeconomic Status Patients. *Dermatology* **2021**, *237*, 843–846. [CrossRef] [PubMed]
36. Kripalani, S.; Heerman, W.J.; Patel, N.J.; Jackson, N.; Goggins, K.; Rothman, R.L.; Yeh, V.M.; Wallston, K.A.; Smoot, D.T.; Wilkins, C.H. Association of Health Literacy and Numeracy with Interest in Research Participation. *J. Gen. Intern. Med.* **2019**, *34*, 544–551. [CrossRef] [PubMed]
37. Perneger, T.V.; Chamot, E.; Bovier, P.A. Nonresponse bias in a survey of patient perceptions of hospital care. *Med. Care* **2005**, *43*, 374–380. [CrossRef]
38. Rosenberg, A.R.; Bona, K.; Wharton, C.M.; Bradford, M.; Shaffer, M.L.; Wolfe, J.; Baker, K.S. Adolescent and Young Adult Patient Engagement and Participation in Survey-Based Research: A Report From the "Resilience in Adolescents and Young Adults With Cancer" Study. *Pediatr. Blood Cancer* **2016**, *63*, 734–736. [CrossRef]
39. Richards, J.; Wiese, C.; Katon, W.; Rockhill, C.; McCarty, C.; Grossman, D.; McCauley, E.; Richardson, L.P. Surveying adolescents enrolled in a regional health care delivery organization: Mail and phone follow-up—What works at what cost? *J. Am. Board Fam. Med.* **2010**, *23*, 534–541. [CrossRef] [PubMed]
40. Christensen, A.I.; Ekholm, O.; Kristensen, P.L.; Larsen, F.B.; Vinding, A.L.; Glümer, C.; Juel, K. The effect of multiple reminders on response patterns in a Danish health survey. *Eur. J. Public Health* **2015**, *25*, 156–161. [CrossRef] [PubMed]
41. Edwards, P.J.; Roberts, I.; Clarke, M.J.; Diguiseppi, C.; Wentz, R.; Kwan, I.; Cooper, R.; Felix, L.M.; Pratap, S. Methods to increase response to postal and electronic questionnaires. *Cochrane Database Syst Rev.* **2009**, *2009*, Mr000008. [CrossRef] [PubMed]
42. Akmatov, M.K.; Jentsch, L.; Riese, P.; May, M.; Ahmed, M.W.; Werner, D.; Rösel, A.; Prokein, J.; Bernemann, I.; Klopp, N.; et al. Motivations for (non)participation in population-based health studies among the elderly—Comparison of participants and nonparticipants of a prospective study on influenza vaccination. *BMC Med. Res. Methodol.* **2017**, *17*, 18. [CrossRef] [PubMed]
43. Alkerwi, A.A.; Sauvageot, N.; Couffignal, S.; Albert, A.; Lair, M.-L.; Guillaume, M. Comparison of participants and non-participants to the ORISCAV-LUX population-based study on cardiovascular risk factors in Luxembourg. *BMC Med. Res. Methodol.* **2010**, *10*, 80. [CrossRef] [PubMed]
44. Anampa-Guzmán, A.; Freeman-Daily, J.; Fisch, M.; Lou, E.; Pennell, N.A.; Painter, C.A.; Sparacio, D.; Lewis, M.A.; Karmo, M.; Anderson, P.F.; et al. The Rise of the Expert Patient in Cancer: From Backseat Passenger to Co-navigator. *JCO Oncol. Pract.* **2022**, OP2100763. [CrossRef]
45. Barr, R.D.; Ferrari, A.; Ries, L.; Whelan, J.; Bleyer, W.A. Cancer in Adolescents and Young Adults: A Narrative Review of the Current Status and a View of the Future. *JAMA Pediatr.* **2016**, *170*, 495–501. [CrossRef] [PubMed]

46. Basch, E.; Barbera, L.; Kerrigan, C.L.; Velikova, G. Implementation of Patient-Reported Outcomes in Routine Medical Care. *Am. Soc. Clin. Oncol. Educ. Book* **2018**, *38*, 122–134. [CrossRef] [PubMed]
47. Husson, O.; Reeve, B.B.; Darlington, A.S.; Cheung, C.K.; Sodergren, S.; van der Graaf, W.T.A.; Salsman, J.M. Next Step for Global Adolescent and Young Adult Oncology: A Core Patient-Centered Outcome Set. *J. Natl. Cancer Inst.* **2021**, *114*, 496–502. [CrossRef]
48. Salsman, J.M.; Danhauer, S.C.; Moore, J.B.; Canzona, M.R.; Victorson, D.E.; Zebrack, B.J.; Reeve, B.B. Optimizing the measurement of health-related quality of life in adolescents and young adults with cancer. *Cancer* **2020**, *126*, 4818–4824. [CrossRef] [PubMed]

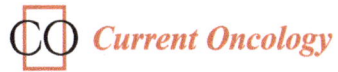

Article

Exploring the Relationship between Self-Rated Health and Unmet Cancer Needs among Sexual and Gender Minority Adolescents and Young Adults with Cancer

Nina Francis-Levin [1], Lauren V. Ghazal [2], Jess Francis-Levin [3], Bradley Zebrack [4], Meiyan Chen [4] and Anao Zhang [4,*]

1 Division of Endocrinology, Metabolism & Diabetes, Michigan Medicine, University of Michigan, Ann Arbor, MI 48109, USA; ninalev@umich.edu
2 School of Nursing, University of Rochester, Rochester, NY 14642, USA; lauren_ghazal@urmc.rochester.edu
3 Institute for Social Research, University of Michigan, Ann Arbor, MI 48104, USA; jessfran@umich.edu
4 School of Social Work, University of Michigan, Ann Arbor, MI 48109, USA; zebrack@umich.edu (B.Z.); myanchen@umich.edu (M.C.)
* Correspondence: zhangan@med.umich.edu; Tel.: +1-734-647-6787

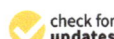

Citation: Francis-Levin, N.; Ghazal, L.V.; Francis-Levin, J.; Zebrack, B.; Chen, M.; Zhang, A. Exploring the Relationship between Self-Rated Health and Unmet Cancer Needs among Sexual and Gender Minority Adolescents and Young Adults with Cancer. *Curr. Oncol.* 2023, *30*, 9291–9303. https://doi.org/10.3390/curroncol30100671

Received: 30 August 2023
Revised: 14 October 2023
Accepted: 19 October 2023
Published: 20 October 2023

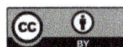

Copyright: © 2023 by the authors. Licensee MDPI, Basel, Switzerland. This article is an open access article distributed under the terms and conditions of the Creative Commons Attribution (CC BY) license (https://creativecommons.org/licenses/by/4.0/).

Abstract: This study evaluates the unmet needs of sexual and gender minority (SGM) adolescent and young adult (AYA) cancer survivors by comparing SGM AYA self-rated health (SRH) scores to their non-SGM (i.e., cisgender/heterosexual) counterparts. The Cancer Needs Questionnaire—Young People (CNQ-YP) and self-rated health measures were used to assess unmet needs in AYAs aged 15–39 who had been diagnosed with cancer in the previous ten years (n = 342). Participants were recruited from a National Cancer Institute (NCI) Comprehensive Cancer Center registry using the modified Dillman's method. Self-reported sexual orientation and gender identity (SO/GI) data were collected. Independent t-tests were used to test between-group differences in unmet needs and Pearson's chi-square test was used to determine the difference in SRH scores between SGM and non-SGM AYA cancer survivors. SGM AYA cancer survivors reported greater mean needs than their non-SGM counterparts across all six domains and reported significantly greater needs in the domains of Feelings and Relationships, $t(314) = -2.111$, $p = 0.036$, Information and Activities, $t(314) = -2.594$, $p = 0.009$, and Education, $t(207) = -3.289$, $p < 0.001$. SGM versus non-SGM SRH scores were significantly different, indicating that a higher percentage of SGM AYAs reported poor/fair health compared to those who were non-SGM. Unmet life and activities needs were negatively associated with AYA cancer survivors' SRH, whereas unmet work needs were positively associated with AYA cancer survivors' SRH. An AYA's gender identity (SGM versus non-SGM) was not a moderator. SGM AYAs are an understudied group within an already vulnerable patient population. Unmet psychosocial needs related to one's feelings and relationships, and information and activity needs merit further research to develop tailored interventions that reflect the experiences of SGM AYAs.

Keywords: sexual and gender minority; adolescent and young adult cancer; self-rated health

1. Introduction

Adolescent and young adult (AYA) cancer patients and survivors (15 to 39 years old) are a vulnerable population who face distinct age-related challenges throughout their disease trajectory [1,2]. Based on data from the National Cancer Institute (NCI), approximately 4.5% (over 89,500) of new cancer cases are among the AYA population in 2022, and nearly 633,000 of survivors in the United States are below the age of 39 [2–4]. On top of the many common challenges confronting cancer survivors across the age spectrum (e.g., treatment-related side- and late-effects), AYA cancer survivors face additional life-stage-driven concerns, including but not limited to occupational disruptions, financial burden, compromised infertility, intimate relationship delays and challenges, sexual dysfunction, and substance misuse, among others [5–10]. Accordingly, AYAs face unmet psychosocial needs in the domains of health and healthcare, informational needs, communication and relationships, sexual and reproductive health, emotional wellbeing and coping skills, vocational disruptions and financial burden [11–13].

Sexual and gender minorities (SGM)—i.e., those who identify as lesbian, gay, bisexual, transgender, nonbinary, queer, and/or other non-cis-heteronormative identities—are an underserved population of cancer survivors [14–16]. AYAs who sit at the intersection of multiple marginalized identities (i.e., AYA and SGM) may face compounded challenges [17]. Including the above-mentioned challenges for all AYAs, SGM AYAs also experience a higher risk for certain cancers, lower rates of prophylactic screening, fear of discrimination or denial of care by healthcare providers, internalized homophobia, increased substance use, and increased psychological distress [15,18–23]. Beyond the unmet needs facing cisgender/heterosexual AYAs, SGM AYAs face further unmet needs related to identity development, including disclosing SGM identities to providers, navigating stigmatization, and accessing safe and relevant care for sexual-, reproductive-, and gender-health before, during and after active treatment [24–26].

In 2021, about 20.8% of emerging adults, born 1997–2003, also referred to as "Gen Z", and 10.5% of young adults, born 1981–1996, also known as "Millennials", identified as SGM. These data represent a major increase in self-identification and identity disclosure when compared to the rate of US adults born before 1980 who self-identified with/disclosed SGM identities (7.6%) [27]. Therefore, it is reasonable to believe that SGM AYAs are likely to comprise a sizable fraction of the AYA survivor population, highlighting the epidemiological significance of attending to the SGM AYA population. The SGM population as a vulnerable group, compounded by the AYA age-range (another risk factor), have been consistently connected with a broad domain of compromised physical and behavioral health outcomes, including, but not limited to, psychological distress, psychosocial functioning, cancer-related quality of life, and general wellness [20–30]. One salient patient-reported outcome (PRO), however, that has not been comprehensively studied among SGM AYA cancer survivors is self-rated health (SRH) [31].

SRH is a patient-centered measure of an individual's general health status, which integrates the biopsychosocial and functional aspects of their health, including cultural beliefs and health behaviors [32,33]. Despite the brevity of SRH as a single-question measure of global health, studies have documented the predictive power of SRH in relation to individuals' morbidity and mortality rates across diverse populations [34,35]. Notably, specifically for the cancer population, SRH has been extensively validated across the sexes, age spectrum, racial/ethnic groups, and cancer stages, endorsing the broad psychometric applicability of SRH [36–38]. Several studies have utilized the SRH measure among the AYA cancer population, suggesting its validity for this population [39,40]. Yet, limited investigations into risk factors impacting AYA cancer survivors' SRH exist, with insufficient examination specifically among SGM AYA.

As such, in this study, our goal was to use the multi-dimensional unmet needs measure for AYAs with cancer, the Cancer Needs Questionnaire—Young People (CNQ-YP) to evaluate the unmet needs of SGM AYA cancer survivors by comparing between-group SRH score differences to those of their non-SGM (i.e., cisgender/heterosexual) counterparts [41,42]. We hypothesized that SGM AYAs would have significantly higher unmet needs across all domains and lower SRH compared to their non-SGM counterparts.

2. Materials and Methods

2.1. Study Design

We used a cross-sectional survey design and evaluated the unmet psychosocial needs of AYAs living with a cancer diagnosis who are receiving or have received care at an NCI-Designated Comprehensive Cancer Center (Unversity of Michigan Rogel Cancer Center at Michigan Medicine). Specifically in this project, we had the following main objectives:

(1) to describe the unmet psychosocial needs of AYA cancer survivors; (2) to evaluate the difference between SGM and non-SGM AYA cancer survivors' SRH and unmet psychosocial needs; and (3) to preliminarily explore the unmet cancer care needs of AYAs with cancer in relation to their SRH, especially considering SGM status as a potential moderator. The study was approved by the University of Michigan IRBMED (HUM00180540).

2.2. Participant Recruitment and Study Procedure

Figure 1 describes the recruitment process. For a participant to be considered eligible for the study, a respondent must have been between the ages of 15 and 39 years old, with a current diagnosis of cancer, or a survivor of cancer diagnosed within the previous 10 years, with at least one appointment for cancer care at the study institution. In accordance with the definition of the NCI, an individual is considered as a cancer survivor from the time of diagnosis [43]. Therefore, we included participants in both active treatment and post-treatment survivorship stages in the current project. Upon approval from the institutional medical IRB, our team used convenience sampling within the cancer registry at Michigan Medicine to identify potential participants. The registry query yielded medical record number (MRN), class of case (role of the institution in patient's case), current age (date of birth), date of first and last contact with Michigan Medicine first and last name, primary cancer site, ICD-O-3 Histology and Behavior code, current address, and vital status. A total of $n = 3823$ potential participants were identified in this manner and were contacted via postal mail.

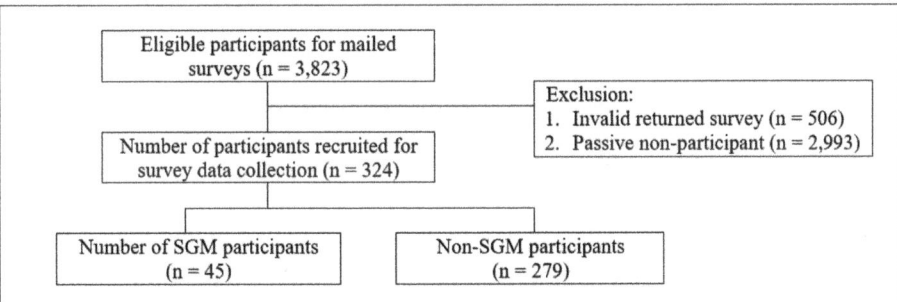

Figure 1. Flow chart for the recruitment of adolescent and young adult cancer survivors.

As a first step, we mailed surveys and consent forms ($n = 3823$) to participants between August 2021 and February 2022 using the modified Dillman's method [44] Participants opted to complete the survey by paper or online via Qualtrics. As a result of the survey dissemination, we received a total of $n = 830$ returned mailers, including $n = 506$ invalid returns (e.g., address no longer active) and $n = 324$ valid returns ($n = 318$ by paper, $n = 6$ by Qualtrics). Participants self-reported sexual orientation and gender identity (SO/GI) using a 'select all that apply' format informed by methodological considerations for SO/GI self-reported data [45]. Participants who selected SO/GI items other than cisgender and/or heterosexual were categorized as SGM ($n = 45$).

As a final step, the first author (N.F.-L.) and a research assistant tracked and documented all returned surveys and extracted data to a database internally stored in a University of Michigan firewall-protected server. The study's principal investigator (A.Z.) randomly selected and double-checked the data input of 25% of all valid surveys, revealing a 99.9% inter-extractor reliability rate. All enrolled study participants were tracked and reported in the clinical and translational oncology research platform—OnCore. Participants were mailed a $15 USD incentive to thank them for participating.

2.3. Measurement

2.3.1. Demographic and Clinical Variables

Demographic and clinical variables were collected as potential covariates. We obtained participants' age (in years), current cancer treatment status (1 = active treatment, 2 = within 1 year post-treatment, 3 = 1–3 years post-treatment, 4 = 3–5 years post-treatment, and 5 = 5 or more years post-treatment), and race/ethnicity (which was recoded into non-Hispanic White versus others given the distribution of this variable). SO/GI items included gender identity (1 = Women/Girl, 2 = Man/Boy, and 3 = Transfeminine, 4 = Transmasculine, 5 = Nonbinary, 6 = Two-spirit, 7 = Cisgender, 8 = Open-response/free-text, and 9 = Prefer not to say), and sexual orientation (1 = Lesbian, 2 = Gay, 3 = Bisexual, 4 = Pansexual, 5 = Straight/heterosexual, 6 = Queer, 7 = Open-response/free-text, 8 = prefer not to say). For race/ethnicity and SO/GI items, participants were instructed to select all that apply and are reported as such. Individuals who selected "Prefer not to say" were included as SGM.

2.3.2. The Unmet Needs of AYAs with Cancer

The unmet cancer care needs of the participants were measured using the Cancer Needs Questionnaire—Young People (CNQ-YP). The CNQ-YP was developed to evaluate the unmet psychosocial and supportive care needs of AYA cancer survivors using a comprehensive process of literature review, focus groups with AYAs, and feedback from health care providers, researchers, and other professionals [41,42]. The CNQ-YP contains a total of 112 questions and covers 6 main areas of (unmet) needs: (1) Treatment Environment and Care, (2) Feelings and Relationships, (3) Daily Life, (4) Information and Activities, (5) Education and (6) Work. Notably, the CNQ-YP has been well-validated by published literature, indicating strong psychometric properties [41,42]. All six dimensions of the CNQ-YP in this study reported satisfactory internal consistency, with Cronbach's alphas ranging from 76% to 82%.

2.3.3. Self-Rated Health (SRH)

SRH was measured by a single question asking the participant, "In general, would you say your health is?" A participant responded to a 5-point Likert scale of "5 = Excellent", "4 = Very Good", "3 = Good", "3 = Fair", or "1 = Poor" to indicate their perceived health status. Given the distribution of this variable, SRH was regrouped into "Excellent or Very Good", "Good", or "Poor or Fair".

2.4. Statistical Analysis Plan

Data analysis was conducted in R statistical software (version 4.2.1). Two research assistants first conducted descriptive statistics for the entire sample, reporting means and standard deviations for continuous variables; frequency and percentage for nominal variables. Then, descriptive statistics were reported separately using participants' SO/GI combined as the group variable. Finally, we evaluated the between-group difference (SGM versus non-SGM groups) for unmet needs and SRH to determine if there were any significant differences. We conducted the independent sample's t-test for continuous outcomes (using the Levene's Test for Equality of Variances to determine the p value) and the chi-square test for nominal variables. Given the distribution of the SRH variable, we used multinomial logistic regression to evaluate the relationship between unmet cancer care needs and SRH (recoded into: 0 = poor or fair health, 1 = good health, or 2 = very good or excellent health). Important covariates were controlled for, including age, race/ethnicity, SO/GI (SGM versus non-SGM), and cancer treatment stage. We explored the possible mediation role of sexual orientation/gender identity by creating a series of interaction terms between significant factors correlated with SRH.

3. Results

3.1. Descriptive Statistics of the Study Population

Key findings indicate that SGM participants reported greater mean unmet needs across all dimensions overall, and significantly greater unmet needs in areas of Feelings and Relationships, Information and Activities, and Education. Findings also reveal a statistically significant difference in SRH between SGM versus non-SGM participants, with SGM participants reporting poorer SRH.

Table 1 displays the descriptive statistics of the study population. A total of $n = 324$ eligible AYAs with cancer completed and returned valid surveys. Participants reported an average age of 30.22 years old (SD = 6.50) and ranged from 16 to 39 years old. Most participants (28.4%) were long-term survivors who, at the time of the study, were more than 5 years post-treatment. The second largest treatment group were AYAs who were 1–3 years post-treatment (26.2%), followed by those who were 3–5 years post-treatment (17.3%). The two smaller treatment groups were AYAs within 1 year post-treatment (14.2%) and about 13.9% were in active treatment at the time of the study.

Most participants identified as non-Hispanic White ($n = 289$, 89.2%), with the remaining participants identifying as Black/African American ($n = 8$; 2.5%), Asian ($n = 8$; 2.5%), Native Hawaiian or other Pacific Islander ($n = 8$; 2.5%), American Indian or Alaska Native ($n = 1$; 0.3%), Hispanic/Latino ($n = 5$; 1.6%), Bi/Multi-racial ($n = 3$; 0.9%), or Another race/ethnicity not listed ($n = 2$; 0.6%). SGM participants (i.e., those who selected SO/GI items other than cisgender and/or heterosexual) comprised $n = 45$. Nearly 8.95% ($n = 29$) participants identified as both non-cisgender and non-heterosexual.

For gender, most participants ($n = 215$; 66.4%) identified as Woman/Girl (participants who selected Woman/Girl, or Woman/Girl AND Cisgender). Ninety-four (29%) identified as Man/Boy (participants who selected Man/Boy, or Man/Boy AND cisgender). One (0.3%) identified as Transmasculine, one (0.3%) identified as a Man/Boy AND Transmasculine, and several participants identified as Nonbinary ($n = 7$; 2.2%).

Regarding sexual orientation, most participants identified as Straight/heterosexual ($n = 279$; 86.4%), followed by seventeen (5.3%) who identified as Bisexual, five (1.6%) as Pansexual, six (1.5%) as Gay, three (0.9%) as Queer, and one (0.3%) as Lesbian, and the remainder are outlined in Table 1.

For SRH, over one-third of the study participants reported Good overall health ($n = 120$, 37%) or Very Good overall health ($n = 106$, 32.7%), while sixty-three participants (19.4%) reported Fair overall health, whereas twenty-eight participants (8.6%) reported Excellent overall health and seven participants (2.2%) reported Poor overall health.

3.2. Between-Group Differences in Self-Rated Health (SRH) and Unmet Cancer Needs

Table 2 shows the between-group differences in SRH and unmet cancer needs between SGM and non-SGM participants. Overall, the difference in SRH between SGM and non-SGM AYA participants was statistically significant, with $\chi^2(4) = 15.95$, $p = 0.031$. The result of the chi-square test revealed that SGM AYA cancer survivors reported significantly lower SRH when compared to their counterparts who are non SGM AYAs with cancer.

In addition, in terms of unmet cancer needs, SGM participants reported higher needs across all dimensions as shown by the higher means of all dimensions compared to non-SGM participants. Furthermore, SGM participants reported significantly greater needs than their non-SGM counterparts in areas of Feelings and Relationships, $t(314) = -2.111$, $p = 0.036$, Information and Activities, $t(314) = -2.594$, $p = 0.009$, and Education, $t(207) = -3.289$, $p < 0.001$. Between-group differences were statistically non-significant in areas of Treatment Environment and Care, Daily Life, and Work.

Table 1. Descriptive Statistics of Adolescents and Young Adults with Cancer (n = 324) *.

Name of Variable	Mean/SD OR Frequency (%)
Dimensions of Unmet Needs	
Treatment Environment and Care	3.99/0.61
Feelings and Relationships	2.13/0.89
Daily Life	2.19/0.94
Information and Activity	2.98/0.91
Education	2.97/1.26
Work	3.14/1.44
Age (Years)	30.22/6.50
Cancer Status	
Active treatment	45 (13.9%)
Within 1 year survivor	46 (14.2%)
1–3 years survivor	85 (26.2%)
3–5 years survivor	56 (17.3%)
>5 years survivor	92 (28.4%)
Race/ethnicity	
Black/African American	8 (2.5%)
Hispanic/Latino	5 (1.5%)
Non-Hispanic White only	289 (89.2%)
American Indian or Alaska Native	1 (0.3%)
Another race/ethnicity not listed	2 (0.6%)
Hispanic/Latino and Bi/Multi-racial or ethnicity	1 (0.3%)
Non-Hispanic White and American Indian or Alaska Native	1 (0.3%)
Bi/Multi-racial or ethnicity	1 (0.3%)
Asian American	8 (2.5%)
Native Hawaiian or Other Pacific Islander	8 (2.5%)
Gender	
Woman/Girl	215 (66.4%)
Man/Boy	94 (29%)
Transmasculine	1 (0.3%)
Nonbinary	7 (2.2%)
Woman/Girl and Nonbinary	1 (0.3%)
Woman/Girl and Cisgender	2 (0.6%)
Man/Boy and Transmasculine	1 (0.3%)
Man/Boy and Cisgender	3 (0.9%)
Sexual Orientation	
Lesbian	1 (0.3%)
Gay	6 (1.5%)
Bisexual	17 (5.2%)
Pansexual	5 (1.5%)
Straight/Heterosexual	279 (86.4%)
Queer	3 (0.9%)
Another sexual orientation not listed	1 (0.3%)
Prefer not to say	5 (1.6%)
Lesbian and Queer	1 (0.3%)
Gay and Queer	1 (0.3%)
Bisexual and Pansexual	2 (0.6%)
Bisexual and Straight/Heterosexual	1 (0.3%)
Bisexual and Queer	1 (0.3%)
Pansexual and Queer	1 (0.3%)
Self-Rated Health	
Poor	7 (2.2%)
Fair	63 (19.4%)
Good	120 (37.0%)
Very good	106 (32.7%)
Excellent	28 (8.6%)

* mean/SD for continuous variables, and n (%) for categorical variables.

Table 2. Between Group Differences of Self-Rated Health *.

Name of Variable	SGM ** (n = 45)	Non-SGM ** (n = 279)	Difference
Dimensions of Unmet Needs			
Treatment Environment and Care	4.027/0.640	3.990/0.610	$t(309) = -0.376, p = 0.707$
Feelings and Relationships	2.460/0.940	2.144/0.928	$t(314) = -2.111, p = 0.036$
Daily Life	2.327/0.892	2.109/0.889	$t(229) = -1.116, p = 0.276$
Information and Activities	3.307/0.928	2.931/0.895	$t(314) = -2.594, p = 0.009$
Education	3.634/1.086	2.849/1.249	$t(207) = -3.289, p < 0.001$
Work	3.250/1.240	3.121/1.466	$t(278) = -0.527, p = 0.599$
Age (years)	28.568/6.460	30.491/6.479	$t(317) = 1.846, p = 0.066$
Cancer Status			
Active treatment	6 (13.3%)	39 (14%)	
Within 1 year survivor	6 (13.3%)	40 (14.3%)	
1–3 years survivor	13 (28.9%)	72 (25.8%)	--
3–5 years survivor	9 (20.0%)	47 (16.8%)	
>5 years survivor	11 (24.4%)	81 (29%)	
Race/ethnicity			
Black/African American	2 (4.4%)	6 (2.2%)	
Hispanic/Latino	0 (0.0%)	5 (1.8%)	
Non-Hispanic White only	40 (88.9%)	249 (89.2%)	
American Indian or Alaska Native	0 (0.0%)	1 (0.4%)	
Asian American	1 (2.2%)	7 (2.5%)	--
Native Hawaiian or Other Pacific Islander	2 (4.4%)	6 (2.2%)	
Another race/ethnicity not listed	0 (0.0%)	2 (0.7%)	
Hispanic/Latino and Bi/Multi-racial or ethnicity	0 (0.0%)	1 (0.4%)	
Non-Hispanic White and American Indian or Alaska Native	0 (0.0%)	1 (0.4%)	
Non-Hispanic Asian or Bi/Multi-racial or ethnicity	0 (0.0%)	1 (0.4%)	
Self-Rated Health			
Poor	4 (8.9%)	3 (1.1%)	
Fair	12 (26.7%)	51 (18.6%)	
Good	17 (37.8%)	103 (36.9%)	$\chi^2(4) = 15.95, p = 0.031$
Very good	11 (24.4%)	95 (33.9%)	
Excellent	1 (2.2%)	27 (9.5%)	

* mean/SD for continuous variables, and n (%) for categorical variables. ** SGM = Sexual and gender minority.

3.3. The Relationship between Unmet Cancer Needs and SRH

Table 3 demonstrates the relationship between unmet cancer care needs and SRH. For both SGM and non-SGM AYAs with cancer, an AYA cancer survivor's daily life needs were significantly associated with their SRH. Specifically, for each unit increase in an AYA cancer survivor's unmet daily life needs, they are 9.5% less likely to report good health versus fair or poor health, OR = 0.905, 95% CI [0.839, 0.977], $p < 0.01$. For each unit increase in their unmet daily life needs, an AYA is 11.5% less likely to report very good or excellent health versus fair or poor health, OR = 0.885, 95% CI [0.816, 0.961], $p < 0.001$. In addition, the unmet work needs are significantly associated with SRH. Interestingly, for each unit increase in their unmet work needs, an AYA is 1.21 times more likely to report good health versus fair or poor health, OR = 1.210, 95% CI [1.009, 1.451]. Similarly, for each unit increase in their unmet work needs, an AYA is 1.225 times more likely to report excellent or very good health versus fair or poor health, OR = 1.225, 95% CI [1.016, 1.476], $p < 0.05$. Moderator analysis evaluating the moderating role of SGM identities on the relationship between the unmet daily life needs and SRH, and between the unmet work needs and SRH, did not indicate SGM status being a significant moderator.

Table 3. Multinomial Logistic Regression [†,1].

	Reference Group: Fair or Poor Health			
	Good Health		Excellent or Very Good Health	
	OR	95% CI	OR	95% CI
Non-SGM (versus SGM)	0.709	[0.097, 5.175]	4.056	[0.347, 47.415]
Unmet cancer care needs				
Treatment environment and care	0.989	[0.955, 1.025]	1.008	[0.971, 1.045]
Daily life	0.905 **	[0.839, 0.977]	0.885 **	[0.816, 0.961]
Feelings and relationships	1.025	[0.957, 1.097]	0.958	[0.886, 1.036]
Information and activities	0.938	[0.794, 1.109]	0.937	[0.785, 1.118]
Education	1.033	[0.870, 1.226]	1.058	[0.885, 1.265]
Work	1.210 *	[1.009, 1.451]	1.225 *	[1.016, 1.476]

[1] Other variables controlled in the model included age, cancer treatment stage, and race/ethnicity. We also evaluated the potential moderating role of SGM versus non-SGM for significant predictors in the model, none were statistically significant, thus not presented in the model. [†] $p < 0.06$, * $p < 0.05$, ** $p < 0.01$.

4. Discussion

The current study provides novel insights into the relationship between unmet needs and self-rated health among SGM AYA cancer survivors. Additionally, our study sheds light on the experiences of a population of cancer survivors about whom little is known: SGM AYAs. We hypothesized that SGM AYAs would have significantly greater unmet needs across all six domains and lower SRH compared to their non-SGM counterparts.

Our finding that SGM AYAs have greater mean unmet needs across all domains builds on the literature which shows that SGM populations are more likely to report unmet medical needs [46]. SGM populations as a whole report a lack of knowledge on the part of health care providers about their health care needs [47]. Specifically, in oncology, most provider knowledge is centered on cancer screening and prevention. Further, transgender and gender-diverse patients have additional distinct needs [48]. In terms of health care delivery, distinct needs for transgender and gender-diverse AYAs include specialized counsel for fertility preservation decision making in light of emergent gender-diverse identities [49]; guidance regarding the contra indications of gender-affirming hormone use before, during, or after chemotherapy [17]; and therapeutic counsel about gender dysphoria arising from disruption to gender-affirming hormones if indicated by therapeutic or supportive treatments [50–52]. Future research into transgender and gender-diverse AYAs' unmet health care needs is urgently needed.

The finding that SGM AYAs have significantly greater unmet needs regarding Feelings and Relationships, Information and Activities, and Education aligns with the literature that has shown that SGM cancer survivors across all ages are more likely to experience psychosocial distress than non-SGM cancer survivors [22]. In another study of adult SGM cancer survivors, the majority reported unmet needs regarding feelings and relationships, and indicated a significant need for mental health resources [53]. In terms of supportive relationships, SGM young people frequently face family-of-origin rejection after coming out. As such, SGM AYAs may lack supportive familial networks [14]. Therefore, family-of-origin support for SGM AYAs must not be presumed by the health care team. Targeted screenings and interventions for mental health, financial, and other instrumental resource needs (e.g., health care navigation; housing) are advised for SGM AYAs. Furthermore, family rejection is predictive of self-harm and suicide for SGM AYAs, especially transgender and gender-diverse individuals [54]. Cancer patients are an at-risk group for self-harm and suicidal behaviors [55]. Therefore, SGM AYAs may be a high-risk group for self-harm, and future research is advised to evaluate this potential risk.

The timing of our data collection is notable in terms of our findings that SGM AYAs expressed greater unmet educational needs. Past research has highlighted that the timing of a cancer diagnosis during adolescence and young adulthood disrupts the achievement of typical educational milestones [56,57]. Recent research published from data collected during the COVID-19 pandemic has also shown that AYAs in general are also more likely to experience educational disruptions than older adults [58,59]. This may be partly explained by the social/physical distancing that resulted from the pandemic, and educational institution closures, which have been shown to have disproportionately affected SGM AYAs who endorsed greater distress and isolation, with fewer coping resources than non-SGM AYAs in one study [60]. Currently, there are no interventions among SGM AYAs with cancer to improve educational or employment outcomes [61]. Among AYA cancer survivors in general, and SGM AYAs in particular, educational support is critically needed.

The finding that SGM AYAs have significantly lower SRH compared to non-SGM AYAs is a notable finding and supports past work reporting that SGM adults endorse worse SRH than non-SGM adults [62,63]. Poor SRH has been shown to be related to minority stress components including discrimination, victimization, concealment of SGM status, and structural stigma [64]. In one study, disclosure of SGM status to oncology providers was associated with better self-reported health among SGM adults [65]. Our past work has highlighted that current AYAs live in a society with fluid sexual attractions and gender expressions, where one cannot make assumptions about goals for relationships and children, and when navigating illnesses such as cancer, SGM AYAs often seek refuge in a "chosen family" [66,67]. These intersecting identities brought forth by both illness, AYA and SGM status warrant further research on addressing discrimination in the healthcare setting where there is a need for recognition and support of non-heteronormative supportive care models. That is, cultivating SGM-competent cancer research may be connected to addressing unmet needs among SGM AYAs [68].

Finally, we found that for both SGM and non-SGM AYA's with cancer there is a significant association between unmet daily life needs and SRH, such that those reporting higher unmet daily life needs were more likely to report poorer health. This is of particular importance as SRH has been extensively shown to be predictive of overall mortality [69,70]. Moreover, as SGM AYAs with cancer are posited to have a greater prevalence of unmet needs than their non-SGM counterparts, this finding could indicate the potential for disparity in survival rates. The findings also suggest a significant association between unmet work needs and SRH such that those AYAs with cancer who reported higher unmet work needs were more likely to report better health. This finding—although seemingly counterintuitive—may indicate that AYAs with unmet work needs are well enough to return to work following completion of active treatment and may be struggling to transition back to the workplace for numerous reasons (e.g., "chemo brain"; disrupted work schedule due to surveillance appointments). By the same logic, those reporting poorer health may, in turn, not be primarily focused on work, may be on hiatus from work (i.e., temporarily receiving Social Security Disability Insurance), and/or may be at a point in their cancer trajectory where determining needs surrounding work proves difficult or impossible [71]. Nevertheless, this association should be explored further. Furthermore, researchers are advised to explore how employers may best empower AYA cancer survivors during their transition back into the workplace. Particularly following the COVID-19 pandemic, there has been a surge in the popularity and prevalence of "remote work," or working from home [72]. We call upon researchers to explore the impact of remote work on the needs of this population to determine what resources will be necessary for successful, supportive, and sustainable reintegration into the workplace.

The current study was limited by a low response rate. Such a limitation may be explained by the timing of data collection in terms of research fatigue following the onset of the COVID-19 pandemic. People affected by disasters—especially vulnerable and marginalized groups—often receive multiple requests for study participation which may lead to participant fatigue and divestment [73]. Accordingly, the representativeness of the sample may have been mitigated by self-selection bias (i.e., those who participated suffered less research fatigue). Recruitment methods may also explain a low response rate. We used postal mail to reach eligible participants because it was the most consistent and reliable form of contact information made available through the cancer registry. However,

AYA is a population that relocates residences frequently. Furthermore, this age cohort is more likely to participate in research activity via text message, email, social media, or other interactive digital methods [74]. Future studies are advised to continue innovating toward age-tailored recruitment and retention strategies. Furthermore, cancer registries are also advised to consistently and regularly collect and update phone number and email contact information so that researchers may identify and engage the population through channels that are meaningful to AYAs.

Secondly, while we included respondents from both active treatment and post-active treatment phases, we did not analyze time since diagnosis as a factor in evaluating unmet needs. Future research is advised to explore changes in unmet needs over time, especially given our group's previous findings which indicated cancer survivors' mental health needs (e.g., worry) increased over time following the completion of treatment [75].

Finally, given the cross-sectional nature of the data, we were only able to evaluate association but not causality, and future research should consider a longitudinal design to strengthen the implication for causality.

Overall, the findings of the current study underscore how vital it is to understand the unique needs of SGM populations and to work toward highlighting potential targets for future intervention.

Author Contributions: Conceptualization, N.F.-L., B.Z. and A.Z.; Methodology, M.C. and A.Z.; Validation, N.F.-L.; Formal analysis, N.F.-L. and A.Z.; Investigation, N.F.-L., L.V.G. and A.Z.; Writing—original draft, N.F.-L., A.Z., L.V.G. and J.F.-L.; Writing—review and editing, N.F.-L., J.F.-L., B.Z., M.C. and A.Z.; Supervision, B.Z. and A.Z.; Project administration, N.F.-L., B.Z. and A.Z. All authors have read and agreed to the published version of the manuscript.

Funding: N. Francis-Levin and L.V. Ghazal received research support from the National Cancer Institute institutional training grant T32-CA-236621. N. Francis-Levin also received support from T32-DK-007245. J. Francis-Levin received support from R01AG067506. The content is solely the responsibility of the authors and does not necessarily represent the official views of the National Institutes of Health or the National Cancer Institute. A. Zhang and N. Francis-Levin received research support from the University of Michigan Vivian A. and James L. Curtis School of Social Work Center for Health Equity Research and Training, Signature Programs Initiatives U070401.

Institutional Review Board Statement: This study was approved by the institutional review board at the University of Michigan Medical School (HUM00180540).

Informed Consent Statement: Written informed consent has been obtained from the patient(s) to publish this paper.

Data Availability Statement: Raw data can be made available upon reasonable request.

Acknowledgments: The authors thank our research assistants, Dalton Meister and Joseph Delly, and project administrator Lisa Kelley for their contributions toward the study.

Conflicts of Interest: The authors declare no conflict of interest.

References

1. Miller, K.D.; Fidler-Benaoudia, M.; Keegan, T.H.; Hipp, H.S.; Jemal, A.; Siegel, R.L. Cancer Statistics for Adolescents and Young Adults, 2020. *CA Cancer J. Clin.* **2020**, *70*, 443–459. [CrossRef]
2. Janssen, S.H.M.; van der Graaf, W.T.A.; van der Meer, D.J.; Manten-Horst, E.; Husson, O. Adolescent and Young Adult (AYA) Cancer Survivorship Practices: An Overview. *Cancers* **2021**, *13*, 4847. [CrossRef] [PubMed]
3. Yarbrough, D.N.P.A.; Yarbrough, A. Survivorship in Adolescents and Young Adults With Cancer. *JNCI Monogr.* **2021**, *2021*, 15–17. [CrossRef]
4. Cancer among Adolescents and Young Adults (AYAs)—Cancer Stat Facts. Available online: https://seer.cancer.gov/statfacts/html/aya.html (accessed on 3 October 2023).
5. Ji, X.; Cummings, J.R.; Mertens, A.C.; Wen, H.; Effinger, K.E. Substance Use, Substance Use Disorders, and Treatment in Adolescent and Young Adult Cancer Survivors-Results from a National Survey. *Cancer* **2021**, *127*, 3223–3231. [CrossRef] [PubMed]
6. Cherven, B.; Sampson, A.; Bober, S.L.; Bingen, K.; Frederick, N.; Freyer, D.R.; Quinn, G.P. Sexual Health among Adolescent and Young Adult Cancer Survivors: A Scoping Review from the Children's Oncology Group Adolescent and Young Adult Oncology Discipline Committee. *CA Cancer J. Clin.* **2021**, *71*, 250–263. [CrossRef] [PubMed]

7. Perez, G.K.; Salsman, J.M.; Fladeboe, K.; Kirchhoff, A.C.; Park, E.R.; Rosenberg, A.R. Taboo Topics in Adolescent and Young Adult Oncology: Strategies for Managing Challenging but Important Conversations Central to Adolescent and Young Adult Cancer Survivorship. *Am. Soc. Clin. Oncol. Educ. Book* **2020**, *40*, e171–e185. [CrossRef] [PubMed]
8. Levin, N.J.; Zebrack, B.; Cole, S.W. Psychosocial Issues for Adolescent and Young Adult Cancer Patients in a Global Context: A Forward-Looking Approach. *Pediatr. Blood Cancer* **2019**, *66*, e27789. [CrossRef] [PubMed]
9. Zebrack, B.; Isaacson, S. Psychosocial Care of Adolescent and Young Adult Patients with Cancer and Survivors. *J. Clin. Oncol.* **2012**, *30*, 1221–1226. [CrossRef]
10. Oberoi-Jassal, R.; Chang, Y.D.; Smith, J.; Rajasekhara, S.; Desai, V.; Fenech, A.L.; Reed, D.R.; Portman, D.; Donovan, K.A. Illicit Substance Use and Opioid Misuse in Adolescent and Young Adult (AYA) Patients with Cancer. *J. Clin. Oncol.* **2017**, *35*, 205. [CrossRef]
11. Okamura, M.; Fujimori, M.; Sato, A.; Uchitomi, Y. Unmet Supportive Care Needs and Associated Factors among Young Adult Cancer Patients in Japan. *BMC Cancer* **2021**, *21*, 17. [CrossRef]
12. Sender, A.; Friedrich, M.; Leuteritz, K.; Nowe, E.; Stöbel-Richter, Y.; Mehnert, A.; Geue, K. Unmet Supportive Care Needs in Young Adult Cancer Patients: Associations and Changes over Time. Results from the AYA-Leipzig Study. *J. Cancer Surviv.* **2019**, *13*, 611–619. [CrossRef] [PubMed]
13. Wong, A.W.K.; Chang, T.-T.; Christopher, K.; Lau, S.C.L.; Beaupin, L.K.; Love, B.; Lipsey, K.L.; Feuerstein, M. Patterns of Unmet Needs in Adolescent and Young Adult (AYA) Cancer Survivors: In Their Own Words. *J. Cancer Surviv.* **2017**, *11*, 751–764. [CrossRef]
14. Power, R.; Ussher, J.M.; Perz, J.; Allison, K.; Hawkey, A.J. "Surviving Discrimination by Pulling Together": LGBTQI Cancer Patient and Carer Experiences of Minority Stress and Social Support. *Front. Oncol.* **2022**, *12*, 918016. [CrossRef] [PubMed]
15. Quinn, G.P.; Sanchez, J.A.; Sutton, S.K.; Vadaparampil, S.T.; Nguyen, G.T.; Green, B.L.; Kanetsky, P.A.; Schabath, M.B. Cancer and Lesbian, Gay, Bisexual, Transgender/Transsexual, and Queer/Questioning Populations (LGBTQ). *CA Cancer J. Clin.* **2015**, *65*, 384–400. [CrossRef] [PubMed]
16. Pratt-Chapman, M.L.; Alpert, A.B.; Castillo, D.A. Health Outcomes of Sexual and Gender Minorities after Cancer: A Systematic Review. *Syst. Rev.* **2021**, *10*, 183. [CrossRef] [PubMed]
17. Francis-Levin, N. Meta/Static Ethnography of Adolescent and Young Adult Oncofertility Research and Practice at a United States Hospital: Implications for Sexual and Gender Minorities. Ph.D. Dissertation, University of Michigan, Ann Arbor, MI, USA, 2023.
18. Williams, S.L.; Mann, A.K. Sexual and Gender Minority Health Disparities as a Social Issue: How Stigma and Intergroup Relations Can Explain and Reduce Health Disparities. *J. Soc. Issues* **2017**, *73*, 450–461. [CrossRef]
19. Mattocks, K.M.; Kauth, M.R.; Sandfort, T.; Matza, A.R.; Sullivan, J.C.; Shipherd, J.C. Understanding Health-Care Needs of Sexual and Gender Minority Veterans: How Targeted Research and Policy Can Improve Health. *LGBT Health* **2014**, *1*, 50–57. [CrossRef]
20. Griggs, J.; Maingi, S.; Blinder, V.; Denduluri, N.; Khorana, A.A.; Norton, L.; Francisco, M.; Wollins, D.S.; Rowland, J.H. American Society of Clinical Oncology Position Statement: Strategies for Reducing Cancer Health Disparities among Sexual and Gender Minority Populations. *J. Clin. Oncol.* **2017**, *35*, 2203–2208. [CrossRef]
21. Kamen, C.; Palesh, O.; Gerry, A.A.; Andrykowski, M.A.; Heckler, C.; Mohile, S.; Morrow, G.R.; Bowen, D.; Mustian, K. Disparities in Health Risk Behavior and Psychological Distress among Gay versus Heterosexual Male Cancer Survivors. *LGBT Health* **2014**, *1*, 86. [CrossRef]
22. Kamen, C.; Mustian, K.M.; Dozier, A.; Bowen, D.J.; Li, Y. Disparities in Psychological Distress Impacting Lesbian, Gay, Bisexual and Transgender Cancer Survivors. *Psychooncology* **2015**, *24*, 1384. [CrossRef]
23. Obedin-Maliver, J. Time to Change: Supporting Sexual and Gender Minority People—An Underserved Understudied Cancer Risk Population. *J. Natl. Compr. Cancer Netw.* **2017**, *15*, 1305. [CrossRef] [PubMed]
24. Wheldon, C.W.; Schabath, M.B.; Hudson, J.; Bowman Curci, M.; Kanetsky, P.A.; Vadaparampil, S.T.; Simmons, V.N.; Sanchez, J.A.; Sutton, S.K.; Quinn, G.P. Culturally Competent Care for Sexual and Gender Minority Patients at National Cancer Institute-Designated Comprehensive Cancer Centers. *LGBT Health* **2018**, *5*, 203–211. [CrossRef] [PubMed]
25. Kent, E.E.; Wheldon, C.W.; Smith, A.W.; Srinivasan, S.; Geiger, A.M. Care Delivery, Patient Experiences, and Health Outcomes among Sexual and Gender Minority Patients with Cancer and Survivors: A Scoping Review. *Cancer* **2019**, *125*, 4371–4379. [CrossRef] [PubMed]
26. Kattari, S.K.; Bakko, M.; Hecht, H.K.; Kattari, L. Correlations between Healthcare Provider Interactions and Mental Health among Transgender and Nonbinary Adults. *SSM Popul. Health* **2019**, *10*, 100525. [CrossRef] [PubMed]
27. LGBT Identification in U.S. Ticks Up to 7.1%. Available online: https://news.gallup.com/poll/389792/lgbt-identification-ticks-up.aspx (accessed on 3 October 2023).
28. Saab, R. Burden of Cancer in Adolescents and Young Adults. *Lancet Oncol.* **2022**, *23*, 2–3. [CrossRef] [PubMed]
29. Duan, Y.; Wang, L.; Sun, Q.; Liu, X.; DIng, S.; Cheng, Q.; Xie, J.; Cheng, A. Prevalence and Determinants of Psychological Distress in Adolescent and Young Adult Patients with Cancer: A Multicenter Survey. *Asia Pac. J. Oncol. Nurs.* **2021**, *8*, 314–321. [CrossRef] [PubMed]
30. Kaal, S.E.J.; Lidington, E.K.; Prins, J.B.; Jansen, R.; Manten-Horst, E.; Servaes, P.; van der Graaf, W.T.A.; Husson, O. Health-Related Quality of Life Issues in Adolescents and Young Adults with Cancer: Discrepancies with the Perceptions of Health Care Professionals. *J. Clin. Med.* **2021**, *10*, 1833. [CrossRef]

31. Idler, E.L.; Kasl, S. Health Perceptions and Survival: Do Global Evaluations of Health Status Really Predict Mortality? *J. Gerontol.* **1991**, *46*, S55–S65. [CrossRef]
32. Bombak, A.E. Self-Rated Health and Public Health: A Critical Perspective. *Front. Public Health* **2013**, *1*, 47799. [CrossRef]
33. Wuorela, M.; Lavonius, S.; Salminen, M.; Vahlberg, T.; Viitanen, M.; Viikari, L. Self-Rated Health and Objective Health Status as Predictors of All-Cause Mortality among Older People: A Prospective Study with a 5-, 10-, and 27-Year Follow-Up. *BMC Geriatr.* **2020**, *20*, 120. [CrossRef]
34. Lorem, G.; Cook, S.; Leon, D.A.; Emaus, N.; Schirmer, H. Self-Reported Health as a Predictor of Mortality: A Cohort Study of Its Relation to Other Health Measurements and Observation Time. *Sci. Rep.* **2020**, *10*, 4886. [CrossRef] [PubMed]
35. Erving, C.L.; Zajdel, R. Assessing the Validity of Self-Rated Health across Ethnic Groups: Implications for Health Disparities Research. *J. Racial Ethn. Health Disparities* **2022**, *9*, 462–477. [CrossRef] [PubMed]
36. Shadbolt, B.; Barresi, J.; Craft, P. Self-Rated Health as a Predictor of Survival among Patients with Advanced Cancer. *J. Clin. Oncol.* **2002**, *20*, 2514–2519. [CrossRef] [PubMed]
37. Kananen, L.; Enroth, L.; Raitanen, J.; Jylhävä, J.; Bürkle, A.; Moreno-Villanueva, M.; Bernhardt, J.; Toussaint, O.; Grubeck-Loebenstein, B.; Malavolta, M.; et al. Self-Rated Health in Individuals with and without Disease Is Associated with Multiple Biomarkers Representing Multiple Biological Domains. *Sci. Rep.* **2021**, *11*, 6139. [CrossRef] [PubMed]
38. Giri, S.; Mir, N.; Al-Obaidi, M.; Clark, D.; Kenzik, K.M.; McDonald, A.; Young-Smith, C.; Paluri, R.; Nandagopal, L.; Gbolahan, O.; et al. Use of Single-Item Self-Rated Health Measure to Identify Frailty and Geriatric Assessment-Identified Impairments Among Older Adults with Cancer. *Oncologist* **2022**, *27*, e45. [CrossRef] [PubMed]
39. Zhang, A.; Delly, J.; Meister, D.; Jackson Levin, N.; Blumenstein, K.; Stuchell, B.; Walling, E. The Relationship between Unmet Cancer Care Needs and Self-Rated Health among Adolescents and Young Adults with Cancer. *Support. Care Cancer* **2023**, *31*, 332. [CrossRef]
40. Tai, E.; Buchanan, N.; Townsend, J.; Fairley, T.; Moore, A.; Richardson, L.C. Health Status of Adolescent and Young Adult Cancer Survivors. *Cancer* **2012**, *118*, 4884–4891. [CrossRef] [PubMed]
41. Clinton-McHarg, T.; Carey, M.; Sanson-Fisher, R.; D'Este, C.; Shakeshaft, A. Preliminary Development and Psychometric Evaluation of an Unmet Needs Measure for Adolescents and Young Adults with Cancer: The Cancer Needs Questionnaire—Young People (CNQ-YP). *Health Qual. Life Outcomes* **2012**, *10*, 13. [CrossRef]
42. Carey, M.L.; Clinton-McHarg, T.; Sanson-Fisher, R.W.; Shakeshaft, A. Development of Cancer Needs Questionnaire for Parents and Carers of Adolescents and Young Adults with Cancer. *Support Care Cancer* **2012**, *20*, 991–1010. [CrossRef]
43. Denlinger, C.S.; Carlson, R.W.; Are, M.; Baker, K.S.; Davis, E.; Edge, S.B.; Friedman, D.L.; Goldman, M.; Jones, L.; King, A.; et al. Survivorship: Introduction and Definition. Clinical Practice Guidelines in Oncology. *J. Natl. Compr. Cancer Netw.* **2014**, *12*, 34–45. [CrossRef]
44. Hoddinott, S.N.; Bass, M.J.; Hoddinott, S. The Dillman Total Design Survey Method. *Can. Fam. Physician* **1986**, *32*, 2366. [PubMed]
45. Levin, N.J.; Zhang, A.; Kattari, S.; Moravek, M.; Zebrack, B. "Queer Insights": Considerations and Challenges for Assessing Sex, Gender Identity, and Sexual Orientation in Oncofertility Research. *Ann. LGBTQ Public Popul. Health* **2022**, *3*, 111–128. [CrossRef]
46. Cathcart-Rake, E.J. Cancer in Sexual and Gender Minority Patients: Are We Addressing Their Needs? *Curr. Oncol. Rep.* **2018**, *20*, 85. [CrossRef] [PubMed]
47. Pratt-Chapman, M.L.; Murphy, J.; Hines, D.; Brazinskaite, R.; Warren, A.R.; Radix, A. "When the Pain Is so Acute or If I Think That I'm Going to Die": Health Care Seeking Behaviors and Experiences of Transgender and Gender Diverse People in an Urban Area. *PLoS ONE* **2021**, *16*, e0246883. [CrossRef]
48. Kamen, C.S.; Pratt-Chapman, M.L.; Meersman, S.C.; Quinn, G.P.; Schabath, M.B.; Maingi, S.; Merrill, J.K.; Garrett-Mayer, E.; Kaltenbaugh, M.; Schenkel, C.; et al. Sexual Orientation and Gender Identity Data Collection in Oncology Practice: Findings of an ASCO Survey. *JCO Oncol. Pract.* **2022**, *18*, e1297–e1305. [CrossRef] [PubMed]
49. Persky, R.W.; Gruschow, S.M.; Sinaii, N.; Carlson, C.; Ginsberg, J.P.; Dowshen, N.L. Attitudes toward Fertility Preservation Among Transgender Youth and Their Parents. *J. Adolesc. Health* **2020**, *67*, 583–589. [CrossRef] [PubMed]
50. Sterling, J.; Garcia, M.M. Fertility Preservation Options for Transgender Individuals. *Transl. Androl. Urol.* **2020**, *9*, S215. [CrossRef] [PubMed]
51. Vyas, N.; Douglas, C.R.; Mann, C.; Weimer, A.K.; Quinn, M.M. Access, Barriers, and Decisional Regret in Pursuit of Fertility Preservation among Transgender and Gender-Diverse Individuals. *Fertil. Steril.* **2021**, *115*, 1029–1034. [CrossRef]
52. Defreyne, J.; Van Schuylenbergh, J.; Motmans, J.; Tilleman, K.L.; Rik T'Sjoen, G.G. Parental Desire and Fertility Preservation in Assigned Female at Birth Transgender People Living in Belgium. *Fertil. Steril.* **2020**, *113*, 149–157.e2. [CrossRef]
53. Seay, J.; Mitteldorf, D.; Yankie, A.; Pirl, W.F.; Kobetz, E.; Schlumbrecht, M. Survivorship Care Needs among LGBT Cancer Survivors. *J. Psychosoc. Oncol.* **2018**, *36*, 393–405. [CrossRef]
54. Marquez-Velarde, G.; Miller, G.H.; Shircliff, J.E.; Suárez, M.I. The Impact of Family Support and Rejection on Suicide Ideation and Attempt among Transgender Adults in the U.S. *LGBTQ+ Fam. Interdiscip. J.* **2023**, *19*, 275–287. [CrossRef]
55. Heynemann, S.; Thompson, K.; Moncur, D.; Silva, S.; Jayawardana, M.; Lewin, J. Risk Factors Associated with Suicide in Adolescents and Young Adults (AYA) with Cancer. *Cancer Med.* **2021**, *10*, 7339–7346. [CrossRef] [PubMed]
56. Ghazal, L.V.; Merriman, J.; Santacroce, S.J.; Dickson, V.V. Survivors' Dilemma: Young Adult Cancer Survivors' Perspectives of Work-Related Goals. *Workplace Health Saf.* **2021**, *69*, 506–516. [CrossRef] [PubMed]

57. Vetsch, J.; Wakefield, C.E.; McGill, B.C.; Cohn, R.J.; Ellis, S.J.; Stefanic, N.; Sawyer, S.M.; Zebrack, B.; Sansom-Daly, U.M. Educational and Vocational Goal Disruption in Adolescent and Young Adult Cancer Survivors. *Psychooncology* **2018**, *27*, 532–538. [CrossRef] [PubMed]
58. Shanahan, L.; Steinhoff, A.; Bechtiger, L.; Murray, A.L.; Nivette, A.; Hepp, U.; Ribeaud, D.; Eisner, M. Emotional Distress in Young Adults during the COVID-19 Pandemic: Evidence of Risk and Resilience from a Longitudinal Cohort Study. *Psychol. Med.* **2022**, *52*, 824–833. [CrossRef] [PubMed]
59. Bécares, L.; Kneale, D. Inequalities in Mental Health, Self-Rated Health, and Social Support among Sexual Minority Young Adults during the COVID-19 Pandemic: Analyses from the UK Millennium Cohort Study. *Soc. Psychiatry Psychiatr. Epidemiol.* **2022**, *57*, 1979–1986. [CrossRef]
60. Salerno, J.P.; Devadas, J.; Pease, M.; Nketia, B.; Fish, J.N. Sexual and Gender Minority Stress Amid the COVID-19 Pandemic: Implications for LGBTQ Young Persons' Mental Health and Well-Being. *Public Health Rep.* **2020**, *135*, 721–727. [CrossRef] [PubMed]
61. Devine, K.A.; Christen, S.; Mulder, R.L.; Brown, M.C.; Ingerski, L.M.; Mader, L.; Potter, E.J.; Sleurs, C.; Viola, A.S.; Waern, S.; et al. Recommendations for the Surveillance of Education and Employment Outcomes in Survivors of Childhood, Adolescent, and Young Adult Cancer: A Report from the International Late Effects of Childhood Cancer Guideline Harmonization Group. *Cancer* **2022**, *128*, 2405–2419. [CrossRef]
62. Streed, C.G.; McCarthy, E.P.; Haas, J.S. Association between Gender Minority Status and Self-Reported Physical and Mental Health in the United States. *JAMA Intern. Med.* **2017**, *177*, 1210–1212. [CrossRef]
63. Gonzales, G.; Ehrenfeld, J.M. The Association between State Policy Environments and Self-Rated Health Disparities for Sexual Minorities in the United States. *Int. J. Environ. Res. Public Health* **2018**, *15*, 1136. [CrossRef]
64. Flentje, A.; Clark, K.D.; Cicero, E.; Capriotti, M.R.; Lubensky, M.E.; Sauceda, J.; Neilands, T.B.; Lunn, M.R.; Obedin-Maliver, J. Minority Stress, Structural Stigma, and Physical Health Among Sexual and Gender Minority Individuals: Examining the Relative Strength of the Relationships. *Ann. Behav. Med.* **2022**, *56*, 573–591. [CrossRef] [PubMed]
65. Kamen, C.S.; Smith-Stoner, M.; Heckler, C.E.; Flannery, M.; Margolies, L. Social Support, Self-Rated Health, and Lesbian, Gay, Bisexual, and Transgender Identity Disclosure to Cancer Care Providers. *Oncol. Nurs. Forum.* **2015**, *42*, 44–51. [CrossRef] [PubMed]
66. Levin, N.J.; Kattari, S.K.; Piellusch, E.K.; Watson, E. "We Just Take Care of Each Other": Navigating 'Chosen Family' in the Context of Health, Illness, and the Mutual Provision of Care amongst Queer and Transgender Young Adults. *Int. J. Environ. Res. Public Health* **2020**, *17*, 7346. [CrossRef] [PubMed]
67. Weston, K. Five: Families We Choose. In *Families We Choose: Lesbians, Gays, Kinship*; Columbia Unversity Press: New York, NY, USA, 1997; pp. 103–136.
68. Waters, A.R.; Tennant, K.; Cloyes, K.G. Cultivating LGBTQ+ Competent Cancer Research: Recommendations from LGBTQ+ Cancer Survivors, Care Partners, and Community Advocates. *Semin. Oncol. Nurs.* **2021**, *37*, 151227. [CrossRef] [PubMed]
69. Schwartz, L.A.; Mao, J.J.; DeRosa, B.W.; Ginsberg, J.P.; Hobbie, W.L.; Carlson, C.A.; Mougianis, I.D.; Ogle, S.K.; Kazak, A.E. Self-Reported Health Problems of Young Adults in Clinical Settings: Survivors of Childhood Cancer and Healthy Controls. *J. Am. Board Fam. Med.* **2010**, *23*, 306–314. [CrossRef] [PubMed]
70. Vie, T.L.; Hufthammer, K.O.; Meland, E.; Breidablik, H.J. Self-Rated Health (SRH) in Young People and Causes of Death and Mortality in Young Adulthood. A Prospective Registry-Based Norwegian HUNT-Study. *SSM Popul. Health* **2019**, *7*, 100364. [CrossRef] [PubMed]
71. Godono, A.; Felicetti, F.; Conti, A.; Clari, M.; Dionisi-Vici, M.; Gatti, F.; Ciocan, C.; Pinto, T.; Arvat, E.; Brignardello, E.; et al. Employment among Childhood Cancer Survivors: A Systematic Review and Meta-Analysis. *Cancers* **2022**, *14*, 4586. [CrossRef] [PubMed]
72. COVID-19 Pandemic Continues to Reshape Work in America | Pew Research Center. Available online: https://www.pewresearch.org/social-trends/2022/02/16/covid-19-pandemic-continues-to-reshape-work-in-america/ (accessed on 3 October 2023).
73. Ashley, F. Accounting for Research Fatigue in Research Ethics. *Bioethics* **2021**, *35*, 270–276. [CrossRef]
74. Katz, R.R.; Ogilvie, S.; Shaw, J.; Woodhead, L. *Gen Z, Explained: The Art of Living in a Digital Age*; The University of Chicago Press: Chicago, IL, USA, 2022; p. 266.
75. Jackson Levin, N.; Zhang, A.; Reyes-Gastelum, D.; Chen, D.W.; Hamilton, A.S.; Zebrack, B.; Haymart, M.R. Change in Worry over Time among Hispanic Women with Thyroid Cancer. *J. Cancer Surviv.* **2022**, *16*, 844. [CrossRef]

Disclaimer/Publisher's Note: The statements, opinions and data contained in all publications are solely those of the individual author(s) and contributor(s) and not of MDPI and/or the editor(s). MDPI and/or the editor(s) disclaim responsibility for any injury to people or property resulting from any ideas, methods, instructions or products referred to in the content.

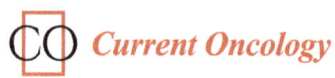

Systematic Review

Education, Employment, and Financial Outcomes in Adolescent and Young Adult Cancer Survivors—A Systematic Review

Aurelia Altherr [1], Céline Bolliger [1], Michaela Kaufmann [1], Daniela Dyntar [1,2], Katrin Scheinemann [1,3,4], Gisela Michel [1], Luzius Mader [5,6] and Katharina Roser [1,*]

1. Faculty of Health Sciences and Medicine, University of Lucerne, Alpenquai 4, 6005 Lucerne, Switzerland; aurelia.altherr@gmail.com (A.A.); celine.bolliger@unilu.ch (C.B.); daniela.dyntar@unibe.ch (D.D.); katrin.scheinemann@kispisg.ch (K.S.); gisela.michel@unilu.ch (G.M.)
2. Cancer Registry of Central Switzerland, 6000 Lucerne, Switzerland
3. Division of Hematology & Oncology, Children's Hospital of Eastern Switzerland, 9006 St. Gallen, Switzerland
4. Department of Pediatrics, McMaster Children's Hospital and McMaster University, Hamilton, ON L8N 3Z5, Canada
5. Institute of Social and Preventive Medicine, University of Bern, 3012 Bern, Switzerland; luzius.mader@unibe.ch
6. Cancer Registry Bern-Solothurn, University of Bern, 3008 Bern, Switzerland
* Correspondence: katharina.roser@unilu.ch

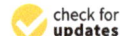

Citation: Altherr, A.; Bolliger, C.; Kaufmann, M.; Dyntar, D.; Scheinemann, K.; Michel, G.; Mader, L.; Roser, K. Education, Employment, and Financial Outcomes in Adolescent and Young Adult Cancer Survivors—A Systematic Review. *Curr. Oncol.* **2023**, *30*, 8720–8762. https://doi.org/10.3390/curroncol30100631

Received: 7 July 2023
Revised: 11 August 2023
Accepted: 2 September 2023
Published: 25 September 2023

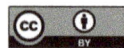

Copyright: © 2023 by the authors. Licensee MDPI, Basel, Switzerland. This article is an open access article distributed under the terms and conditions of the Creative Commons Attribution (CC BY) license (https:// creativecommons.org/licenses/by/ 4.0/).

Abstract: Adolescents and young adults (AYAs) with cancer face unique challenges. We aimed to describe (i) education, employment, and financial outcomes and (ii) determinants for adverse outcomes in AYA cancer survivors. We performed a systematic literature search. We included original research articles on AYA (15–39 years of age) cancer survivors (≥2 years after diagnosis) and our outcomes of interest. We narratively synthesized the results of the included articles. We included 35 articles (24 quantitative and 11 qualitative studies). Patients in education had to interrupt their education during cancer treatment, and re-entry after treatment was challenging. After treatment, most survivors were employed but started their employment at an older age than the general population. Overall, no disadvantages in income were found. Survivors reported more absent workdays than comparisons. We identified chemotherapy, radiotherapy, late effects or health problems, female sex, migration background, and lower education associated with adverse outcomes. Although most AYA cancer survivors were able to re-enter education and employment, they reported difficulties with re-entry and delays in their employment pathway. To facilitate successful re-entry, age-tailored support services should be developed and implemented.

Keywords: adolescent and young adult; cancer; survivors; education; employment; financial outcomes; psychosocial health

1. Introduction

AYAs are diagnosed with cancer during a unique and challenging period of their life [1,2]. The transitional time between childhood and adulthood is characterized by psychosocial milestones related to completing education, starting their employment pathway, and gaining social and financial independence from parents [1,3–8]. The cancer diagnosis may interfere with these psychosocial achievements. It has been shown that psychosocial problems after cancer are more prevalent in AYAs than in older adults [9]. This indicates that cancer might be especially disruptive in AYAs and emphasizes the importance of psychosocial health in AYA cancer survivors.

Cancer in young people is different from cancer in children or cancer in older adults: The epidemiology, the biology of the tumors, and the psychosocial needs of AYA cancer survivors and late outcomes after the cure of the cancer are unique in this specific age group [10–14]. In Europe, about 112'000 AYAs were diagnosed with cancer in 2020 [15]. Survival nowadays exceeds 80% in Europe [16].

The majority of AYA cancer survivors returned to school or work after the end of treatment [17]. However, many AYA cancer survivors reported that cancer had a negative impact on their plans for work or school [17] and that returning to work was challenging [18]. Regarding survivors' educational achievements, some studies indicate different educational pathways for survivors compared to the general population [19,20]. Other studies did not find any differences in educational attainment between survivors and comparisons [21]. However, survivors reported disruptions in their education due to the cancer diagnosis [21]. Regarding employment, some studies did not report an increased risk of unemployment in survivors [19,20]. They started being engaged in paid employment at an older age compared to the general population [20]. In other studies, survivors were less likely to be employed compared to the general population [21,22], and this difference was especially pronounced for health-related unemployment [21].

Cancer and its treatment and disruptions or delays in employment might lead to financial hardship. Different pathways have been suggested for this adverse outcome. Many survivors experience chronic conditions, which are associated with significant increases in medical expenditures and health care use [23]. Furthermore, different educational pathways and a higher risk of unemployment might also increase financial hardship [24–26].

A comprehensive overview of education, employment, and financial outcomes in survivors of AYA cancer is lacking. This systematic review aimed to describe (i) education, employment, and financial outcomes and (ii) determinants for adverse educational, employment, and financial outcomes in AYA cancer survivors.

2. Methods

This systematic review was registered in PROSPERO (number: CRD42021262353) and complies with the PRISMA statement regarding reporting systematic reviews and meta-analyses [27].

2.1. Search Strategy

The literature search was conducted in August 2020 and updated on 15 February 2022. We searched the databases PubMed, Scopus, and PsychINFO. Included publications were hand-searched for additional references. No restrictions on geographical region or publication language were applied. The search was restricted to studies on humans that were published up to 15 February 2022. The search terms included four blocks with search terms referring to the outcomes (education, work, financial outcomes), adolescent and young adult, cancer, and survivorship (Tables S3 and S4 in Supplementary Material).

2.2. Study Selection

The study selection consisted of two steps: title and abstract screening and full text screening.

To select eligible articles, the following inclusion criteria were hierarchically applied: peer-reviewed original research, a sample size of at least 20 for quantitative studies (no sample size restrictions for qualitative and mixed methods studies), study participants having been diagnosed with cancer, AYA cancer (i.e., at least 75% of participants in the age range of 15–39 years at diagnosis), survivors (i.e., at least 75% of participants at least two years after diagnosis), and one of the three outcomes of interest being the primary outcome presented in the article (education, employment, financial outcomes). Review articles, editorials, commentaries, and conference abstracts were excluded. During the full-text screening, articles from which no full text could be obtained were excluded.

We included quantitative, qualitative, and mixed methods studies and any study designs. Studies with and without comparisons (e.g., general population, siblings) were included. Two reviewers each independently assessed eligibility by first screening titles and abstracts followed by the full texts of the remaining articles (involved authors: A.A., C.B., M.K., K.R.). Discrepancies between reviewers were resolved by discussion and consensus or by consulting a third reviewer (L.M.). Reference lists of relevant review articles were screened for potentially eligible articles.

2.3. Data Extraction

The first author, publication year, country, study design, data source, data collection method, sample size, response rate, and population characteristics, including gender, age at time of study, age at diagnosis, time since diagnosis, cancer types, and education, employment, and financial information (which were mentioned additionally to the primary outcomes of the articles), were extracted. If a comparison group was available, the provided information was extracted as well (Table 1 and Table S1 in Supplementary Material for quantitative studies and Table 2 and Table S2 in Supplementary Material for qualitative studies).

2.4. Quality Assessment

The quality of each study was independently assessed by two reviewers each using the JBI critical appraisal tool [28] (involved authors: A.A., M.K., K.R.). Discrepancies between reviewers were resolved by discussion and consensus. Inter-rater reliability, assessed by Kendall's tau, was tau = 0.74 for quantitative studies and tau = 0.71 for qualitative studies. The JBI critical appraisal tool was designed to assess methodological validity and determine the extent to which a study considered possible biases in its design, conduct, and analysis. It is suitable for cross-sectional, cohort, and qualitative studies, which are common in this research area [27]. To assess study quality, 8 questions were asked for cross-sectional studies and 10 questions for qualitative studies. These items could be answered with "yes," "no," "unclear," or "not applicable." To enable a comparable assessment across cross-sectional studies and qualitative studies, the total number of questions answered with "yes" was summed up, and the percentage of "yes" answers was calculated. For cross-sectional studies, a maximum of 8 "yes" and for qualitative studies, a maximum of 10 "yes" answers could be reached (Tables S5 and S6 in Supplementary Material).

2.5. Data Synthesis

Outcomes related to the psychosocial situation of AYA cancer survivors were narratively synthesized. A priori, we did not consider a meta-analytic approach because of the expected heterogeneity in study design, study period, outcome definition across studies, and differences in educational, labor, and financial contexts across geographic regions. The narrative synthesis focused on the educational, employment, and financial outcomes and the determinants for adverse educational, employment, and financial outcomes. Further, the quality of the included studies was evaluated to determine how it may have influenced the synthesis.

Table 1. Characteristics of included quantitative studies.

First Author, Publication Year	Country	Study Design	Sample Size	Response Rate	Gender: Percentage Male	Age at Time of Study	Age at Diagnosis	Time Since Diagnosis	Cancer Types	Comparisons	Study Quality
Abdelhadi et al., 2021 [23]	USA	Retrospective cohort study	n = 2326	MEPS (2011–2016): 53.5–59.3% for the different years	AYA cancer survivors with chronic conditions: 23.90% male, AYA cancer survivors without chronic conditions: 21.85% male	(Weighted proportions) AYA cancer survivors with chronic conditions: 18–29 years old: 6.14%, 30–39 years old: 15.52%, 40–49 years old: 24.36%, 50–64 years old: 36.10%, ≥65 years old: 17.88% AYA cancer survivors without chronic conditions: 18–29 years old: 18.14%, 30–39 years old: 37.52%, 40–49 years old: 27.82%, 50–64 years old: 13.90%, ≥65 years old: 2.70%	range: 15–39 years	AYA cancer survivors with chronic conditions: 0–4 years: 10.86%, 5–9 years: 12.73%, 10–19 years: 26.31%, ≥20 years: 50.09% AYA cancer survivors without chronic conditions: 0–4 years: 31.85%, 5–9 years: 22.96%, 10–19 years: 29.43%, ≥20 years: 15.76%	(Weighted proportions) AYA cancer survivors with chronic conditions: bladder: 0.70%, brain: 1.69%, breast: 12.57%, cervix: 32.90%, colon: 2.94%, leukemia: 1.72%, lung: 2.07%, lymphoma: 4.42%, melanoma: 9.26%, other: 28.26%, prostate: 1.70%, throat: n/a, thyroid: 3.90% AYA cancer survivors without chronic conditions: bladder: n/a, brain: n/a, breast: 11.15%, cervix: 21.86%, colon: 1.76%, leukemia: 1.52%, lung: n/a, lymphoma: 5.45%, melanoma: 10.94%, other: 26.55%, prostate: n/a, throat: n/a, thyroid: 8.50%	None	88%

Table 1. *Cont.*

First Author, Publication Year	Country	Study Design	Sample Size	Response Rate	Gender: Percentage Male	Age at Time of Study	Age at Diagnosis	Time Since Diagnosis	Cancer Types	Comparisons	Study Quality
Abdelhadi et al., 2022 [29]	USA	Retrospective cohort study	n = 2081 (n = 1757 for matched analyses)	MEPS (2011–2016): 53.5–59.3% for the different years	20.0% male	18–29 years old: 10.2%, 30–39 years old: 22.9%, 40–49 years old: 27.3%, 50–64 years old: 26.6%, ≥65 years old: 13.0%	Range: 15–39 years	Not reported	Not reported	Adults without cancer history (n = 5227)	88%
Bhatt et al., 2021 [30]	USA	Retrospective cohort study	n = 1365	Not applicable	56% male	Not reported	Mean age at treatment = 30.8 years old, range: 18–39 years old, 18–24 years old: 19%, 25–29 years old: 26%, 30–34 years old: 27%, 35–39 years old: 28%	Median time since treatment = 60.6 months, range: 12–121 months	Leukemia: 68%, lymphoma: 11%, other malignant diseases: 10%, non-malignant disorders: 11%	None	100%
Dahl et al., 2019 [31]	Norway	Cross-sectional study	n = 1189	42%	27% male	Mean (SD) = 49.7 (7.8), median = 49 years, range: 27–65 years old	Mean (SD) = 33.0 (5.3), median = 35 years old, range: 19–39 years old	Median = 16 years, range: 6–31 years	Breast: 41%, colorectal: 12%, lymphoma: 19%, leukemia: 11%, melanoma: 17%	None	100%

Table 1. *Cont.*

First Author, Publication Year	Country	Study Design	Sample Size	Response Rate	Gender: Percentage Male	Age at Time of Study	Age at Diagnosis	Time Since Diagnosis	Cancer Types	Comparisons	Study Quality
Dieluweit et al., 2011 [20]	Germany	Cross-sectional study	n = 820	43.70%	49% male	Mean (SD) = 29.9 (6) years old	Mean (SD) = 15.8 (0.9) years old, range: 15–18 years old	Mean (SD) = 13.7 (6) years	Lymphoma: 30.5%, malignant bone tumor: 21.2%, leukemia: 19.3%, CNS tumors: 9.5%, soft tissue and other extraosseous sarcomas: 9.2%, germ cell tumors: 6.6%, other malignant epithelial neoplasms and malignant melanomas: 2.4%, renal tumors: 0.9%, neuroblastoma: 0.5%	Age-matched sample from the general population (German Socio-Economic Panel, n = 820)	100%
Ekwueme et al., 2016 [32]	USA	Cross-sectional study	n = 244	Not reported	All female	Mean (SD) = 39.42 (5.29) years old	Mean (SD) = 34.42 (6.95) years old, range: 18–44 years old	<2 years: 30.74%, 2–4 years: 28.69%, 5–10 years: 29.1%, ≥11 years: 11.48%	All breast	Women aged 18–44 without breast cancer (n = 82694), women aged 45–64 at diagnosis with breast cancer (n = 1508), women aged 45–64 without breast cancer (n = 52,586)	88%

Table 1. Cont.

First Author, Publication Year	Country	Study Design	Sample Size	Response Rate	Gender: Percentage Male	Age at Time of Study	Age at Diagnosis	Time Since Diagnosis	Cancer Types	Comparisons	Study Quality
Ghaderi et al., 2013 [33]	Norway	Retrospective cohort study	n = 2561	Not applicable	55.4% male (childhood and AYA cancer survivors)	Not reported	15–19 years old: 1019, 20–24 years old: 1542	Survivors were followed for mean = 13.2 years beginning 5 years after diagnosis (range: 0–39.3 years) (childhood and AYA cancer survivors)	Brain/CNS tumors: 18.2%, testis: 15.4%, lymphatic system: 14.4%, hematopoietic system: 12.9%, melanoma: 10.6%, other: 7.4%, thyroid gland and other endocrine glands: 7.3%, bone and connective tissue: 5.6%, kidney: 2.7%, eye: 2.2%, ovary: 2%, cervix uteri: 1.2% (childhood and AYA cancer survivors)	Childhood cancer survivors (0–14 years of age at diagnosis; n = 1470)	100%
Guy et al., 2014 [34]	USA	Retrospective cohort study	n = 1464	MEPS (2008–2011): 53.5–59.3%	22.2% male	18–29 years old: 11%, 30–39 years old: 21%, 40–49 years old: 26.7%, 50–64 years old: 29.3%, ≥65 years old: 12%	range: 15–39 years	0–9 years: 30.5%, 10–19 years: 27.7%, ≥20 years: 41.9%	Not reported	Adults without cancer in the pooled sample of 2008–2011 MEPS data (n = 86,865)	88%

Table 1. Cont.

First Author, Publication Year	Country	Study Design	Sample Size	Response Rate	Gender: Percentage Male	Age at Time of Study	Age at Diagnosis	Time Since Diagnosis	Cancer Types	Comparisons	Study Quality
Hamzah et al., 2021 [35]	Malaysia	Cross-sectional study	$n = 400$	Not reported	43.3% male	Mean (SD) = 29.1 (7.16) years old, range: 18–40, 18–20 years old: 12.5%, 21–25 years old: 27%, 26–30 years old: 17.8%, 31–35 years old: 12.8%, 36–40 years old: 30%	Not reported	>5 years	Leukemia: 32.25%, Hodgkin lymphoma: 10.0%, ovarian: 8.0%, ependymoma: 7.25%, breast: 6.25%, Wilms' tumor: 5.75%, Ewing's sarcoma: 5.75%, testicular: 3.5%, medulloblastoma: 3.5%, brain tumor: 3.25%, yolk sac tumor: 3%, liver cancer: 2.75%, papillary thyroid: 1.5%, nasopharyngeal cancer: 1.5%, neuroblastoma: 1.5%, intestinal: 1.25%, lung: 1%, germinoma: 1%, embryonal rhabdomyosarcoma: 1%	None	63%

Table 1. Cont.

First Author, Publication Year	Country	Study Design	Sample Size	Response Rate	Gender: Percentage Male	Age at Time of Study	Age at Diagnosis	Time Since Diagnosis	Cancer Types	Comparisons	Study Quality
Ketterl et al., 2019 [24]	USA	Cross-sectional study	n = 872	67%	27.2% male	Not reported	Females: mean (SD) = 32.3 (5.62) years old, males: mean (SD) = 29.8 (6.09) years old	Females: mean (SD) = 3.53 (1.49) years, males: mean (SD) = 3.40 (1.29) years	Breast: 27.6%, leukemia and lymphoma: 18.7%, endocrine system: 14.7%, skin: 9.3%, genital system: 10.9%, brain and other CNS tumors: 4.7%, bones and soft tissue: 4.1%, digestive system: 4.0%, oral cavity and pharynx: 2.9%, urinary system: 1.6%, others: 1.5%	None	100%
Landwehr et al., 2016 [36]	USA	Retrospective cohort study	n = 334	33.60%	20.4% male	Age at time of application submission: mean = 29.3 years old, median = 30.2 years old, 95% CI: 28.7–29.8, SD = 4.4 years old, range: 19–39 years old	Mean (SD) = 24.5 (6.7) years old, median = 26 years old, 95% CI: [23.7–25.2]	Time of treatment completion prior application submission: mean (SD) = 3.5 (4.6) years, median = 1.8 years, 95% CI: 3.0–4.0	Not reported	US census data from 2011 and 2013 using the groups "under age 35" and "25–34 years of age", n = 16,513,000, and MEPS using the group "18–44 years of age", n = 21,877,000	88%
Lim et al., 2020 [37]	Switzerland	Retrospective cohort study	n = 176	Not applicable	43.2% male	Not reported	Median (SD) age at treatment = 30.3 (±7.6) years old, range: 15.1–39.5 years old	Median time since treatment = 66 months, range: 12–236 months	All brain and skull base tumors	None	50%

Table 1. Cont.

First Author, Publication Year	Country	Study Design	Sample Size	Response Rate	Gender: Percentage Male	Age at Time of Study	Age at Diagnosis	Time Since Diagnosis	Cancer Types	Comparisons	Study Quality
Lu et al., 2021 [38]	USA	Cross-sectional study	$n = 2588$	NHIS (2010–2018) 64.2–82.0% for the different years	32.8% male	18–29 years old: 8.3%, 30–39 years old: 23.0%, 40–49 years old: 26.1%, 50–64 years old: 27.4%, 65–80 years old: 12.2%, 81+ years old: 2.9%	Median (IQR) = 31 (26–35) years old	(Categories are not mutually exclusive) <2 years: 8.4%, ≥2 years: 91.6%, >6 years: 75%, >16 years: 50%, >31 years: 25.0%	Lymphoma: 7.8%, melanoma: 12.3%, testicular cancer: 5.5%, thyroid cancer: 9.1%, ovarian cancer: 7.3%, uterine cancer: 10.8%, leukemia: 1.9%, breast cancer: 15.7%	Adults without cancer history ($n = 256,964$)	88%
Mader et al., 2017 [19]	Switzerland	Cross-sectional study	$n = 160$	41.10%	61.3% male	Mean (SD) = 33.5 (5.9) years old, 20–29 years old: 26.9%, 30–39 years old: 53.1%, ≥40 years old: 20%	Mean (SD) = 21.1 (2.9) years old, range: 16–25 years old, 16–20 years old: 43.8%, 21–25 years old: 56.3%	Mean (SD) = 11.9 (4.7) years	Lymphoma: 37.5%, germ cell tumor: 28.8%, CNS tumor: 9.4%, soft tissue sarcoma: 9.4%, leukemia: 8.1%, bone tumor: 3.8%, renal tumor: 1.9%, neuroblastoma: 1.3%	Swiss Health Survey (SHS), participants aged 20–50 years old, residents in the Canton of Zurich ($n = 999$)	100%
Meernik et al., 2020 [25]	USA	Cross-sectional study (restricted to working (full/part-time) at time of diagnosis)	$n = 1328$	12.80%	All female	Median (SD) = 41.0 (6.2) years old	Median (SD) = 34.0 (5.1) years old, range: 16–39 years old	Median (SD) = 7.0 (3.6) years, range: 3–15 years	Breast: 41.7%, thyroid: 22.3%, melanoma: 14.4%, lymphoma: 10.4%, gynaecologic (cervical, uterine, ovarian): 11.2%	None	100%
Nord et al., 2015 [39]	Sweden	Retrospective cohort study	$n = 2146$	Not reported	All male	Not reported,	Median = 32 years old, range: 18–60 years old	Follow-up for study: median = 10 years, range: 2–19 years	All testicular	General population without a cancer history ($n = 8448$)	100%

Table 1. Cont.

First Author, Publication Year	Country	Study Design	Sample Size	Response Rate	Gender: Percentage Male	Age at Time of Study	Age at Diagnosis	Time Since Diagnosis	Cancer Types	Comparisons	Study Quality
Nugent et al., 2018 [40]	USA	Cross-sectional study	$n = 23$	Not reported	69.9% male	Mean (SD) = 23.8 (4.0) years old, median (IQR) = 22.6 (5.0) years old	Mean = 17.4 years old, range: 15–21 years old, length of treatment: mean = *1.2 years	≥2 years since active cancer treatment	Hodgkin lymphoma: 43.4%, acute lymphoblastic leukemia:17.4%, Ewing's sarcoma: 8.7%, osteosarcoma: 8.7%, germ cell tumor: 8.7%, acute myelocytic leukemia: 4.3%, chondrosarcoma: 4.3%, non-Hodgkin lymphoma: 4.3%	Controls were matched to the cancer survivors, being of the same gender and within 2 years of the survivor's age ($n = 14$)	88%
Parsons et al., 2012 [17]	USA	Cohort study	$n = 463$ (all AYA cancer survivors)	Initial survey: 43.4%, follow-up survey: 88.7%	AYA cancer survivors working or in school full-time before diagnosis ($n = 388$): 64% male	Not reported	AYA cancer survivors working or in school full-time before diagnosis ($n = 388$): 15–19 years old: 13.1%, 20–24 years old: 17.8%, 25–29 years old: 24.7%, 30–34 years old: 23.2%, 35–39 years old: 21.1%	AYA cancer survivors working or in school full-time before diagnosis ($n = 388$): 15–19 months: 13.1%, 20–24 months: 42.5%, 25–29 months: 34%, 30–35 months: 10.1%, range: 25–35 months	Germ cell: 40.5%, Hodgkin's lymphoma: 26%, non-Hodgkin's lymphoma: 24.2%, sarcoma: 4.6%, acute lymphoblastic leukemia: 3.9%	AYA cancer survivors 15–24 months after diagnosis and working or in school full-time before diagnosis ($n = 216$)	100%

Table 1. Cont.

First Author, Publication Year	Country	Study Design	Sample Size	Response Rate	Gender: Percentage Male	Age at Time of Study	Age at Diagnosis	Time Since Diagnosis	Cancer Types	Comparisons	Study Quality
Strauser et al., 2010 [41]	USA	Longitudinal study (restricted to AYACS who were unemployed at time of application for vocational services)	n = 368	Not reported	57% male	Mean (SD) = 21.46 (2.39) years old, range: 18–25 years old	Not reported	>2 years	Not reported	None	63%
Sylvest et al., 2022 [42]	Denmark	Register-based cohort study	n = 4222	Not applicable	100% male	≥ 35 years	Range: 0–29 years,	CNS cancer: mean (SD) = 14.59 (9.30) years, hematological cancer: mean (SD) = 16.68 (10.67) years, solid cancer: mean (SD) = 9.37 (8.47) years	CNS tumors: 5.0%, hematological tumors: 6.5%, solid tumors: 88.5%	Age-matched comparison group of the general population (n = 794,589)	100%
Tangka et al., 2020 [43]	USA	Cross-sectional study	n = 830	28.40%	All female	Not reported	18–34 years old: 39.5%, 35–39 years old: 60.5%	Not reported	All breast cancer	None	100%
Tebbi et al., 1989 [44]	USA	Cross-sectional study	n = 40	30%	40% male	Mean (SD) = 26.4 (4.2) years old, range: 18–35 years old	Mean = 16.15 years old, range: 13–19 years old	Mean (SD) = 10.1 (3.2) years	Hodgkin's/non-Hodgkin's lymphoma: 47.5%, soft tissue sarcoma/melanomas: 20.0%, leukemia: 7.5%, bone tumors: 20.0%, ovarian/testicular: 5.0%	15 male and 25 female controls without a cancer history and with age range from 18 to 35 years old (n = 40)	88%

Table 1. *Cont.*

First Author, Publication Year	Country	Study Design	Sample Size	Response Rate	Gender: Percentage Male	Age at Time of Study	Age at Diagnosis	Time Since Diagnosis	Cancer Types	Comparisons	Study Quality
Thom et al., 2021 [45]	USA	Cross-sectional study	n = 212	65%	8.9% male	Mean (SD) = 35.3 (5.25) years old	Mean (SD) = 27.4 (7.17) years old	Mean (SD) time since treatment = 6.2 (5.89) years	Breast: 27.8%, lymphoma: 16.5%, colorectal: 11.3%, leukemia: 9.4%, brain: 7.1%, gynecological: 6.1%, sarcoma: 6.1%, thyroid: 4.7%, other: 8.0%, prefer not to respond: 0.5%	None	88%
Yanez et al., 2013 [46]	USA	Cross-sectional study	n = 106	66.50%	31.6% male	Mean (SD) = 32.2 (5.1) years old	Not reported	Range: 25–60 months, 3 years after treatment completion: 41%, 4 years after treatment completion: 31%, 5 years after treatment completion: 28%	Breast: 24.8%, cervical: 11.5%, melanoma: 9.7%, lung: 8.0%, colorectal: 3.5%, thyroid: 9.7%, testicular: 4.4%	AYA cancer survivors 0–24 months after diagnosis (n = 216)	88%

Abbreviations: d, diagnosis; s, study; t, treatment; fu, follow-up; CI, confidence interval; IQR, interquartile range; SD, standard deviation; NHIS, National Health Interview Surveys; MEPS, Medical Expenditure Panel Survey; CNS, central nervous system; RM, Malaysian ringgit.

Table 2. Characteristics of included qualitative studies.

First Author, Publication Year	Country	Study Design or Approach, Analysis Method	Sample Size	Gender: Percentage Male	Age at Time of Study	Age at Diagnosis	Time Since Diagnosis	Cancer Types	Study Quality
An et al., 2019 [47]	South Korea	Grounded theory/thematic analysis	n = 14	21.43% male	Range: 14–22 years old	Not reported	Not reported; adolescents who visited a hospital for follow-up care following treatment for leukemia	Acute lymphoid leukemia: 42.9%, acute myeloid leukaemia: 50%, chronic myeloid leukemia: 7.1%	80%
Brauer et al., 2017 [48]	USA	Grounded theory; systematic yet flexible coding process	n = 18	61.1% male	Mean = 26 years old, range: 19.8–34.6 years old	Age at treatment: mean = 23.3 years old, range: 18.5–29.7 years old	Time since treatment: mean = 32.8 months, range: 8–60 months	Acute myeloid leukemia: 56%, acute lymphoblastic leukemia: 28%, Hodgkin's lymphoma: 11%, non-Hodgkin's lymphoma: 5%	70%
Drake et al., 2019 [49]	Canada	Phenomenology; thematic analysis	n = 5	40% male	Mean (SD) = 32 (6.78) years old, range: 25–40 years old	Range: 18–39 years old	Not reported	5 participants with Hodgkin's lymphoma, multiple myeloma, malignant neoplasm of the pineal region, thyroid cancer, and appendix cancer	80%
Elsbernd et al., 2018 [50]	Denmark	Thematic analysis	n = 9	22.2% male	Mean = 24.2 years old, median = 25 years old, range: 19–27 years old	Range: 17–24 years old	Time since last treatment: range: < 1–> 10 years	9 participants with lymphoma (2), breast (2), leukemia, cervical, testicular, pancreatic, and brain tumor	50%
Ghazal et al., 2021 [51]	USA	Cross-sectional study	n = 40	36.5% male	Not reported	Median (SD) = 28 (5.26) years old, range: 20–38 years old	Range: 1–5 years	Lymphoma: 82.5%, leukemia: 17.5%	90%
Gupta et al., 2020 [52]	USA	Thematic analysis combined with an abductive approach	n = 52	59.6% male	Mean (SD) = 25.29 (2.88) years old, range: 18–29 years old	Not reported	Mean (SD) = 31.25 (17.12) months	Hematologic: 61.5%, testicular: 38.5%	70%

Table 2. Cont.

First Author, Publication Year	Country	Study Design or Approach, Analysis Method	Sample Size	Gender: Percentage Male	Age at Time of Study	Age at Diagnosis	Time Since Diagnosis	Cancer Types	Study Quality
Kent et al., 2012 [53]	USA	Hermeneutic phenomenology (interpretative method); grounded theory; narrative analysis	n = 19	52.6% male	15–19 years old: 5.3%, 20–23 years old: 10.5%, 24–26 years old: 15.8%, 27–29 years old: 15.8%, 30–33 years old: 26.3%, 34–36 years old: 21.1%, 37–39 years old: 5.3%	15–19 years old: 15.8%, 20–23 years old: 21.1%, 24–26 years old: 21.1%, 27–29 years old: 21.1%, 30–33 years old: 21.1%, 34–36 years old: 10.5%	Range: 6 months–6 years	Non-Hodgkin's lymphoma: 21.1%, Hodgkin's: 10.5%, brain tumor: 10.5%, acute lymphoblastic leukemia: 10.5%, ovarian: 10.5%, melanoma: 5.3%, Wilm's tumor: 5.3%, testicular: 5.3%, ovarian: 5.3%, acute lymphoblastic leukemia: 5.3%, multiple myeloma: 5.3%, aplastic anemia: 5.3%	60%
Magrath et al., 2021 [54]	United Kingdom	Phenomenological analysis, analysis was performed iteratively	n = 8	50% male	Mean = 21.8 years old, median = 2. years old, range: 18–27 years old	Mean = 17.6 years old, median = 17.5 years old, range: 16–19 years old	Not reported	Brain tumor: 12.5%, lymphoma: 75%, leukemia: 12.5%	90%
Parsons et al., 2008 [55]	Canada	Postmodern narrative approach; data analysis occurred in conjunction with data collection	n = 14	57.1% male	Mean = 27.4 years old, median = 26.5 years old, range: 18–38 years old	Mean = 24.2 years old, median = 23 years old, range: 16–35 years old	Range: 1–6 years	All osteosarcoma	70%
Raque-Bogdan et al., 2015 [56]	USA	Consensual method	n = 13	All female	Range: 2.–43 years old	Mean (SD) = 30 (5) years old, median = 27 years old, range: 21–38 years old	Mean = 3.54 years	All breast	80%
Stone et al., 2019 [57]	USA	Constructivist grounded theory; analytic techniques including initial, focused, axial, and theoretical coding procedures	n = 12	25% male	Mean = 43.9 years old, range: 25–59 years old	Mean = 29 years old, 18–29 years old: 50%, 30–39 years old: 50%	Mean = 14.8 years, range: 8–35 years	Breast: 33%, leukemia or lymphoma: 33%, melanoma: 8%, testicular: 317%, thyroid: 8%	90%

Abbreviations: d, diagnosis; s, study; t, treatment.

3. Results

Literature Search and Study Characteristics

While searching the three databases, 6651 articles were identified, and finally, 35 articles were included [17,19,20,23–25,29–57] (Figure 1). We included 24 quantitative (Table 1) and 11 qualitative (Table 2) studies. The majority of the studies were conducted in North America (24, 69%), nine in Europe (26%), and two in Asia (6%). Fourteen of the quantitative studies (58%) studies included a comparison group. The majority of the studies (29, 83%) included different types of cancer. Variations in sample size (quantitative studies: 23–4'222, qualitative studies: 5–52), age at diagnosis or study, and time since diagnosis were observed. Three articles reported only on education outcomes, nine only on employment outcomes, and eight only on financial outcomes. Another six articles described both education and employment outcomes, and nine studies addressed both employment and financial outcomes.

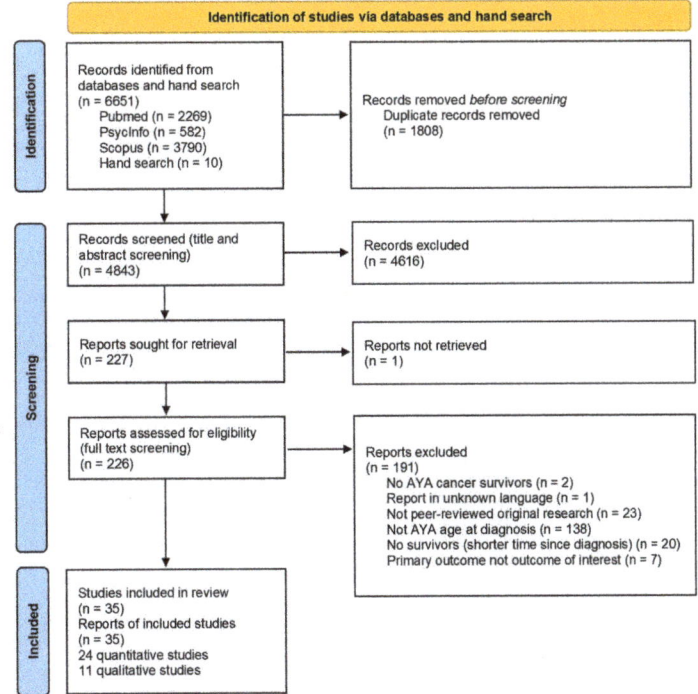

Figure 1. PRISMA flow diagram of included studies.

4. Impact of Cancer

4.1. Education

After being diagnosed with cancer, many AYA cancer survivors experienced a disruption in education [46,48,50] (Table 3). In one study, AYA cancer survivors reported having kept up with school via the Internet while being treated for cancer [47]. Those who left school for cancer treatment wanted to return to school as quickly as possible to keep up with peers but also for a sense of normalcy [47,48,50]. In doing so, they experienced enormous hurdles and challenges, some related to experiencing late effects such as fatigue [54]. Problems arose, especially in re-entry, which could only occur at the beginning of a school year [48,50]. AYA cancer survivors reported different educational pathways compared to the general population: More had completed upper secondary school and fewer university education in Switzerland [19]. In Germany, survivors were more likely to have attended high school, whereas rates of college and university graduation were similar [20]. Survivors of CNS cancer were less progressed in their education compared to age-matched comparisons [42]. On the other hand, survivors of hematological and solid cancers reached higher educational levels [42].

A stay in the intensive care unit (ICU) during treatment, experiencing visual or hearing late effects, and having a migration background were identified as characteristics associated with lower education [19,20].

4.2. Employment

In most studies investigating employment, the majority of AYA cancer survivors were employed at the time of the study [17,19,20,24,25,31,32,34,35,37,40–44,46] (Table 4). Some survivors reported reduced ability to work and were consequently uncertain whether cancer had long-term effects on their ability [31,49]. Compared to before their cancer diagnosis, more survivors were unemployed after their cancer treatment (19% before treatment, 38% six months after treatment [30]; from 9.5% to 23.8% pre- and post-treatment, respectively [37]), about half of survivors reported paid or unpaid time off, and about 10% of survivors quit or lost their job at diagnosis [43]. In most studies comparing survivors with other populations, there was no difference between the employment rates in survivors and the comparison group [19,20,31,40,44]. One study reported that slightly more AYA cancer survivors were outside the workforce compared to the comparison group [42]. Survivors started being engaged in paid employment at an older age compared to the general population [20]. In one study, AYA cancer survivors were significantly less likely to be employed than the comparison group [34]. In two studies from the USA, AYA cancer survivors reported experiencing employment disruption [25,46]. Breast cancer survivors reported stopping working was impossible due to financial hardship or insurance needs [56]. About half of the survivors preserved employment in the same workplace as before the diagnosis [55,57]. For others, the cancer diagnosis meant a change of perspective, be it that they changed their workplace [50,55,56] or that they reported that the meaning of work had changed [51]. Their cancer diagnosis was seen as a catalyst for a change of career and thus an inspiration for a new beginning [49].

Longer time since first cancer diagnosis [31], younger age at diagnosis [19,20], female gender [19,31], lower education [19,31], and experiencing late effects or impaired health [19,20,31] were identified as characteristics associated with unemployment. In another study, with a longer time since end of treatment, the percentage of AYA cancer survivors being unemployed decreased [30].

Table 3. Impact of cancer on education outcomes in adolescent and young adult (AYA) cancer survivors.

First Author, Publication Year	Measurements for Education Outcomes	Education Outcomes	Determinants for Adverse Education Outcomes (Quantitative Studies) or Selected Citations (Qualitative Studies, Indicated in Italics)
An et al., 2019 [47]	Difficulties in school, difficulties in returning to school	Identified themes: feelings of alienation from friends, difficulty in studying, stuck being different from others, apologetic feelings for family, feelings of having an uncertain future	*"I had a university and major in mind, but after an absence from studying for two years, it was very hard to catch up within one year. I put in a great deal of effort in that respect, but it was very difficult." (Female, 22 years old)*
Brauer et al., 2017 [48]	Resuming work and school after hematopoietic cell transplantation	Identified themes: rushing to resume school/work, motivating factors, barriers to successful and sustainable re-entry	*"I had to withdraw from that whole semester, that whole year that I was there. And pay the fee of attending the school when I didn't even get credit for being there, because I missed finals. […] It was basically, 'Hey, you missed finals. That's how our grading system works. There's no exception about it. And here's your five, ten thousand dollar fee that you owe'."*
Dieluweit et al., 2011 [20]	High school attainment, professional training, college or university degree	AYA cancer survivors vs. comparison group: high school attainment: 52.4% vs. 28.3% (Cramer's V = 0.139, $p < 0.001$), professional training: 85.2% vs. 85.9% (Cramer's V = 0.009, not significant), college/university degree: 24.7% vs. 17% (Cramer's V = 0.093, $p = 0.001$)	High school degree: stay in an intensive care unit (OR = 0.73, CI = 0.54–0.99, $p = 0.042$), visual or hearing late effects (OR = 0.69, CI = 0.48–0.99, $p = 0.048$) college/university degree: higher age at time of study (OR = 1.08, CI = 1.05–1.11, $p < 0.001$), female gender (OR = 0.67, CI = 0.48–0.95, $p = 0.0025$), CNS tumor (reference: leukemia and lymphoma) (OR = 0.39, CI = 0.17–0.92, $p = 0.0031$), neuropsychological late effects (OR = 0.5, CI = 0.27–0.91, $p = 0.024$)
Elsbernd et al., 2018 [50]	Management of returning to secondary or higher education	Identified themes: symptoms and late effects, navigating the system, lack of understanding from peers, unofficial support, changed perspectives	*"I think you get a little guidance, but then you are on your own." (Female, 24 years old)*
Mader et al., 2017 [19]	Educational achievement	AYA cancer survivors vs. comparison group: basic education: 8.2% vs. 4.8%, vocational training/apprenticeship: 46.5% vs. 47.2%, upper secondary education: 33.3% vs. 26.7%, university education: 11.9% vs. 21.3%, ($p = 0.012$ for educational achievement)	Only basic education: migration background (OR = 10.23, CI = 4.64 to 22.55, $p < 0.001$)

Table 3. *Cont.*

First Author, Publication Year	Measurements for Education Outcomes	Education Outcomes	Determinants for Adverse Education Outcomes (Quantitative Studies) or Selected Citations (Qualitative Studies, Indicated in Italics)
Magrath et al., 2021 [54]	Experiences while returning to education	Identified themes: late effects, systems, adjusting to losses, mechanisms facilitating resilience	*"The difficulty concentrating was the single most difficult aspect of the cancer because I couldn't look at a screen, I couldn't look at my phone, I couldn't look at a laptop, I couldn't do some work, I couldn't even do a powerpoint."* *"They put me in for the exam on a different day, they also gave me longer time, in exams, which was useful"*. (AYA4) *"I guess I was concerned about just not being able to go to uni, umm, it's always been a plan to go and study [..] so I was concerned about the realisation that maybe that wouldn't be a possibility."* *"I had help from the charity CLIC, they helped arrange for me to go back to university so they arranged with my lecturers to skype me into the lectures as opposed to me physically going in."*
Parsons et al., 2012 [17]	Full-time work or school participation, belief of cancer leading to a negative impact	Results for the 388 AYA cancer survivors who had been working or in school full-time before diagnosis: full-time work or school participation: 15–19 months since diagnosis: 74.0% full-time or work at follow-up, 20–24 months since diagnosis: 75.8% full-time or work at follow-up, 25–29 months since diagnosis: 69.9% full-time or work at follow-up, 30–35 months since diagnosis: 66.7% full-time or work at follow-up Belief: 15–19 months since diagnosis: 44.0% negative impact on plans, 20–24 months since diagnosis: 33.9% negative impact on plans, 25–29 months since diagnosis: 30.8% negative impact on plans, 30–35 months since diagnosis: 38.5% negative impact on plans	-

Table 3. Cont.

First Author, Publication Year	Measurements for Education Outcomes	Education Outcomes	Determinants for Adverse Education Outcomes (Quantitative Studies) or Selected Citations (Qualitative Studies, Indicated in Italics)
Sylvest et al., 2022 [42]	Progression in the educational system	Survivors vs. comparison group: Survivors of CNS cancer had lower odds of having progressed in the educational system than those from the age-matched comparison group: high school: aOR = 0.25; 95% CI: 0.11–0.58; vocational training: aOR = 0.58, 95% CI: 0.42–0.80; short-term further education: aOR = 1.17, 95% CI: 0.71–1.93; medium-term further education: aOR = 0.35, 95% CI: 0.19–0.65; long-term further education: aOR = 0.88, 95% CI: 0.57–1.36. Survivors of hematological and solid cancers showed an opposite trend, with higher odds of progressing to higher educational levels compared to the comparison group: high school: aOR = 0.76; 95% CI: 0.41–1.41 and aOR = 1.00, 95% CI: 0.86–1.16; vocational training: aOR = 0.96, 95% CI: 0.70–1.32 and aOR = 1.07, 95% CI: 0.98–1.16; Short-term further education: aOR = 0.98, 95% CI: 0.59–1.61 and aOR = 1.12, 95% CI: 0.98–1.28; medium-term further education: aOR = 1.15, 95% CI: 0.82–1.62 and aOR = 1.17, 95% CI: 1.07–1.29; long-term further education: aOR = 1.17, 95% CI: 0.84–1.63 and aOR = 1.17, 95% CI: 1.07–1.28.	Cancer type: The percentage of men who attained primary school only was higher in survivors of CNS cancer (36%) than in men with hematological cancer, solid cancer, or no cancer diagnosis (19%, 18%, and 20%, respectively). The opposite was true for medium-term and long-term further education. Age at diagnosis: The percentage of primary school as the highest educational attainment was slightly higher in men diagnosed with cancer when they were 0–9 years old (23%) than in men who were older at diagnosis (10–19 years: 20%, 20–29 years: 19%). Diagnosis decade: This percentage for primary school was also higher in men diagnosed with cancer between 1978 and 1989 (24%) than in those diagnosed in later decades (1990–1999: 18%, 2000–2009: 14%). Contrasting associations were observed for long-term further education (1978–1989: 12%, 1990–1999: 13%, 2000–2009: 20%).
Yanez et al., 2013 [46]	Educational attainment, cancer-related education/work interruption	Educational attainment: 41.6% of AYA cancer survivors reported an educational attainment of less than a college degree. Cancer-related education/work interruption: 62.3% of AYA cancer survivors reported an interruption in education or work.	Time since diagnosis: AYA cancer survivors 25–60 months since diagnosis vs. 13–24 months since diagnosis vs. 0–12 months since diagnosis: Educational attainment: 41.6% vs. 34.3% vs. 39.2% Cancer-related education/work interruption: 62.3% vs. 56.1% vs. 66.1%

Abbreviations: OR, odds ratio; CI, confidence interval; p, p-value; UK, United Kingdom; aOR, adjusted odds ratio; CNS, central nervous system; AYA, adolescent and young adult.

Table 4. Impact of cancer on employment outcomes in adolescent and young adult (AYA) cancer survivors.

First Author, Publication Year	Measurements for Employment Outcomes	Employment Outcomes	Determinants for Adverse Employment Outcomes (Quantitative Studies) or Selected Citations (Qualitative Studies, Indicated in Italics)
Bhatt et al., 2021 [30]	Employment status	Employment status: The percentage of full-time employed survivors was lower 6 months after HCT treatment than before treatment, whereas the rates for part-time employment, unemployment, or medical disability were higher 6 months after treatment than before treatment. Before treatment: full-time 43%, part-time 4%, unemployed 9%, medical disability 16%, unknown 17% 6 months after treatment: full-time 18.3%, part-time 6.9%, unemployed 38.2%, medical disability 36.6%, unknown 0%	Time after treatment: The percentages of survivors working full- or part-time increased with time after treatment (full-time: from 18.3% at 6 months to 50.7% at 3 years; part-time: from 6.9% at 6 months to 10.5% at 3 years). The percentages for unemployment and medical disability decreased over time after treatment (unemployment: from 38.2% at 6 months to 18.3% at 3 years; medical disability: from 36.6% at 6 months to 21% at 3 years).
Brauer et al., 2017 [48]	Resuming work and school after hematopoietic cell transplantation	Identified themes: rushing to resume school or work, motivating factors, barriers to successful and sustainable re-entry	-
Dahl et al., 2019 [31]	Employment status, work ability (current work ability compared to the lifetime best)	Employment status: 75.5% of AYA cancer survivors were employed. Work ability: 62% of AYA cancer survivors reported high current work ability. Mean work ability among employed (8.3) vs. unemployed (3.9) AYA cancer survivors AYA cancer survivors vs. comparison group: Employment status: survivors (m = 83%, f = 73%) vs. Norwegian population (m = 81%, f = 76%) Disability pension recipient: AYA cancer survivors (m = 10%, f = 15%) vs. Norwegian population (m = 11%, f = 13%)	Unemployment: longer time since first cancer diagnosis (OR = 1.03, CI = 1.01–1.05, p = 0.002), increased mean number of adverse events (OR = 1.21, CI = 1.16–1.26, p < 0.001), female gender (OR = 1.77, CI = 1.28–2.46, p = 0.001), low basic education (OR = 2.52, CI = 1.92–3.3, p < 0.001), comorbid cardiovascular disease (OR = 1.85, CI = 1.31–2.63, p = 0.001), decreased general health (OR = 0.98, CI = 0.97–0.98, p < 0.001), increased level of depression (OR = 1.18, CI = 1.15–1.22, p < 0.001)
Dieluweit et al., 2011 [20]	Employment status	AYA cancer survivors vs. comparison group: employment rate: 79.6% vs. 74.2% (Cramer's V = 0.064, p = 0.013)	Employment: higher age at time of study (OR = 1.04, CI = 1.01–1.08, p = 0.017), female (OR = 0.59, CI = 0.34–0.89, p = 0.016), having children (OR = 0.36, CI = 0.23–0.56, p < 0.001), having neuropsychological late effects (OR = 0.55, CI = 0.34–0.89, p = 0.0016)

Table 4. Cont.

First Author, Publication Year	Measurements for Employment Outcomes	Employment Outcomes	Determinants for Adverse Employment Outcomes (Quantitative Studies) or Selected Citations (Qualitative Studies, Indicated in Italics)
Drake et al., 2019 [49]	Perspectives on and experiences with return to work following treatment	Identified themes: uncertainty about return to work, cancer as a catalyst for a career change, importance of employment benefits, benefit of YA-specific resources	*"Ahh because my current role in the [company] is meaningless and repetitive I'd be happy to leave that company... people they, they want to do something that's meaningful. To come through this experience and it kind of ahh turns their world upside down, wakes them up in some ways. They have an awakening and ahh *pause* in my case I guess I have to do something. I have to do work that is meaningful, which is why I'm exploring this opportunity with [company]."*
Ekwueme et al., 2016 [32]	Employment status, work days lost, home productivity days lost	Employment status: 75.43% of AYA cancer survivors employed Work days and home productivity days lost: AYA cancer survivors missed 19 work days and 17 home productivity days. AYA cancer survivors vs. women aged 18–44 without breast cancer: Employment status: employed: 75.43% vs. 78.38% Workdays and home productivity days lost: AYA cancer survivors missed more work days (19 days vs. 4 days, $p < 0.01$) and home productivity days (17 days vs. 4 days, $p < 0.01$).	-
Ghazal et al., 2021 [51]	Perspectives of work-related goals	Identified themes: self-identity and work, perceived health and work ability, financial toxicity	*"(...) in order to take care of myself, I had to quit this job that had been my end goal... I had to go back to the job that I had worked all through school... [with diagnosis and treatment] it's taxing for me to do the job that I chose as my career, and then now I can't even afford to do that job... despite everything I've done in my education to get to this point... I'm literally thinking to myself, "What have I been working my whole life for?"*

Table 4. Cont.

First Author, Publication Year	Measurements for Employment Outcomes	Employment Outcomes	Determinants for Adverse Employment Outcomes (Quantitative Studies) or Selected Citations (Qualitative Studies, Indicated in Italics)
Guy et al., 2014 [34]	Functional limitations, employment status	Functional limitations: 17% of AYA cancer survivors experienced limitations at work, with housework, or in school; 11.9% were completely unable to work at a job, do housework, or go to school. Employment status: 33.4% of AYA cancer survivors were not employed; reasons for not being employed were retirement (41%), inability to work because of illness or disability (34.1%), and not being able to find work (20.7%). AYA cancer survivors vs. comparison group: Functional limitations: limitations in work, housework, or school: 17 vs. 10.5%, $p < 0.001$; being completely unable to work at a job, do housework, or go to school: 11.9 vs. 6.7%, $p < 0.001$. Employment status: not employed: 33.4% vs. 27.4%, $p < 0.001$	-
Hamzah et al., 2021 [35]	Employment status, career engagement and quality of working life	Employment status: 67.5% of AYA cancer survivors had permanent employment, 12.5% had temporary employment, 14.8% were self-employed, 5.2% worked part-time. Career engagement and quality of working life: positive correlation of career engagement with meaning of work ($r = 0.578$, $p < 0.001$), perception of the work situation ($r = 0.665$, $p < 0.001$), atmosphere in the work environment ($r = 0.648$, $p < 0.000$), understanding and recognition in the organization ($r = 0.553$, $p < 0.001$), negative correlation of career engagement with problems because of health situation ($r = -0.688$, $p < 0.001$), effect of disease and treatment ($r = -0.656$, $p < 0.000$)	-

Table 4. Cont.

First Author, Publication Year	Measurements for Employment Outcomes	Employment Outcomes	Determinants for Adverse Employment Outcomes (Quantitative Studies) or Selected Citations (Qualitative Studies, Indicated in Italics)
Ketterl et al., 2019 [24]	Employment status, physical and mental impairment of work-related tasks, extended paid or unpaid time off from work	Employment status: 84.4% of AYA cancer survivors were employed. Physical and mental impairment of work-related tasks: Among employed survivors, 70.2% reported a physical component in their job and 58.6% reported that cancer interfered with physical tasks required by their job. A total of 54.2% reported that cancer interfered with their ability to perform mental tasks required by their job.	Treatment: Chemotherapy: inference with job-related physical tasks (OR = 1.97, CI = 1.22 to 3.11, $p < 0.01$), inference with mental tasks required by a job (OR = 3.22, CI, 2.15 to 4.79, $p < 0.01$), time off from work (OR = 3.56, CI = 2.31 to 5.47, $p < 0.01$), borrowing $\geq$ USD 10,000 (OR = 3.05, CI = 1.53 to 6.09, $p < 0.01$) compared with survivors who were not exposed to chemotherapy. Radiation: interference with job-related physical tasks (OR = 1.66, CI = 1.08 to 2.41, $p < 0.05$) compared with survivors who did not receive radiation. Surgery: extended paid time off from work (OR = 0.54, CI = 0.54 to 1.00, $p < 0.05$) compared with survivors who did not receive surgery.
Lim et al., 2020 [37]	Employment status	Employment status: pre- and post-treatment: unemployment: from 9.5% to 23.8%, employment with sick leave: from 14.3% to 0%, employment: from 42.9% to 63.5%, in education: from 33.3% to 12.7%	-
Mader et al., 2017 [19]	Employment status	AYA cancer survivors vs. comparison group: employment status: 91.2% vs. 89.5% ($p = 0.515$)	Unemployment: female gender (OR = 2.52, CI 1.36 to 4.68, $p = 0.004$), having only basic education (OR = 2.78, CI = 1.01 to 7.65, $p = 0.048$), being married (OR = 0.53, CI = 0.29 to 0.98, $p = 0.042$), younger age at diagnosis (OR = 5.29, CI = 1.32 to 30.79, $p = 0.010$), self-reported late effects (OR 4.70, CI = 1.26 to 19.49, $p = 0.009$)

Table 4. Cont.

First Author, Publication Year	Measurements for Employment Outcomes	Employment Outcomes	Determinants for Adverse Employment Outcomes (Quantitative Studies) or Selected Citations (Qualitative Studies, Indicated in Italics)
Meernik et al., 2020 [25]	Employment status, employment disruption	Employment status: 17% part-time employment, 82.6% full-time employment Employment disruption: 32% of AYA cancer survivors reported an employment disruption, categorized as stopping work completely (14%), reducing work hours (12%), taking temporary leave (6%), or both a reduction in hours and temporary leave (5%).	-
Nord et al., 2015 [39]	Mean days of sick leave or disability pension	AYA cancer survivors vs. comparison group: Mean days of sick leave or disability pension: AYA cancer survivors having received no or limited treatment vs. comparisons: 3rd year after diagnosis: 16 vs. 14 days, 5th year after the diagnosis: 15 vs. 12 days AYA cancer survivors having received extensive treatment vs. comparisons: 3rd year after diagnosis: 26 vs. 14 days, 5th year after diagnosis: 23 vs. 12 days	Treatment intensity: Mean days of sick leave or disability pension: AYA cancer survivors having received no or limited treatment: 3rd year after diagnosis: 16 days, 5th year after diagnosis: 15 days AYA cancer survivors having received extensive treatment: 3rd year after diagnosis: 26 days, 5th year after diagnosis: 23 days
Nugent et al., 2018 [40]	Employment status, occupational function	AYA cancer survivors vs. comparisons: Employment status: full-time student, not working (17.4% vs. 21.4%); student and part-time work (21.7% vs. 28.6%); student and full-time work (4.3% vs. 0%); part time work only (13% vs. 0%); full-time work only (43.4% vs. 50%) Occupational function: no significant difference between AYA cancer survivors (mean score = 4.5 ± 5.28 [2.13–6.87]) and comparisons (mean score 4.67 ± 4.34), Cohen's d = −0.034 [−0.73 to 0.72]	-

Table 4. *Cont.*

First Author, Publication Year	Measurements for Employment Outcomes	Employment Outcomes	Determinants for Adverse Employment Outcomes (Quantitative Studies) or Selected Citations (Qualitative Studies, Indicated in Italics)
Parsons et al., 2008 [55]	Lived experiences of resuming vocational work	50% of AYA cancer survivors returned to their pre-illness occupation, whereas the other half were forced to change careers. Regardless of whether their professional status changed, all respondents recounted how their relationship with their vocation had been profoundly altered by the illness. Return to work was interconnected with aspects of life such as support (including financial), possession of disability and unemployment benefits, and entitlements to sick leave from employment/training/educational programs. All AYA cancer survivors expressed a strong desire to resume vocational pursuits but experienced returning to work as hard work. They portrayed themselves as "hard workers" due to drawing heavily on discourses of "work ethics." Concerns were raised regarding financial pressures, but willingness to physically return was also expressed.	*"I'm afraid to apply for jobs, to be rejected. 'Cause I could send my resume in, and I'm sure I'll get an interview, but I go in there with my crutches or a cane, it's like, even my brother-in-law was saying, "How much work can this person do for me?" (31 years old at diagnosis, 35 years old at interview)*
Parsons et al., 2012 [17]	Full-time work or school participation, belief of cancer leading to a negative impact	Results for the 388 AYA cancer survivors who had been working or in school full-time before diagnosis: Full-time work or school participation: 15–19 months since diagnosis: 74.0% full-time or work at follow-up, 20–24 months since diagnosis: 75.8% full-time or work at follow-up, 25–29 months since diagnosis: 69.9% full-time or work at follow-up, 30–35 months since diagnosis: 66.7% full-time or work at follow-up Belief: 15–19 months since diagnosis: 44.0% negative impact on plans, 20–24 months since diagnosis: 33.9% negative impact on plans, 25–29 months since diagnosis: 30.8% negative impact on plans, 30–35 months since diagnosis: 38.5% negative impact on plans	-

Table 4. Cont.

First Author, Publication Year	Measurements for Employment Outcomes	Employment Outcomes	Determinants for Adverse Employment Outcomes (Quantitative Studies) or Selected Citations (Qualitative Studies, Indicated in Italics)
Raque-Bogdan et al., 2015 [56]	Effect of breast cancer on work lives and career development	Identified themes: cancer-related work challenges, coping with cancer-related work challenges, reappraisal of career development after cancer and components of career, components of career and life satisfaction after cancer	*"So the 2 months that I missed, it has slowed down my learning in my career at a time that learning is very important. Part of that is time away from work. But much of that is that I have not had the capacity to work as intensely at the level that is necessary."*
Stone et al., 2019 [57]	Work experiences	Identified themes: process of revealing the survivor-self, process of sustaining work ability, process of accessing support	*"I was back working, you know, full-time, maybe 3 or 4, 5 days later."*
Strauser et al., 2010 [41]	Competitive employment, use of vocational services	Competitive employment: 51.6% of AYA cancer survivors were competitively employed.	AYA cancer survivors using more services and spending more time in services were more likely to be employed. Employment was associated with the use of following services: vocational training (OR = 2.03, CI: 1.03 to 4.00), miscellaneous training (OR = 3.4, CI: 1.47 to 7.96), job search assistance (OR = 4.01, CI: 1.80 to 8.97), job placement assistance (OR = 2.24, CI: 1.11 to 4.52), on-the-job support (OR = 4.2, CI: 1.66 to 10.63), maintenance (OR = 2.85, CI: 1.38 to 5.90)
Sylvest et al., 2022 [42]	Being outside the workforce	AYA cancer survivors vs. comparison group: The percentage of cancer survivors being outside the workforce (retired/receiving transfer income) was higher (9%) than the percentage in the comparison group with no cancer diagnosis (6%).	-

Table 4. *Cont.*

First Author, Publication Year	Measurements for Employment Outcomes	Employment Outcomes	Determinants for Adverse Employment Outcomes (Quantitative Studies) or Selected Citations (Qualitative Studies, Indicated in Italics)
Tangka et al., 2020 [43]	Employment status, work benefits at diagnosis, impact on employment status	Employment status: 73.4% of participants were employed at the time of diagnosis. Out of these, 64.9% worked for a private or non-profit organization; 21.0% for a branch of federal, state, or local government; and 7.5% were self-employed. Work benefits at diagnosis: The respondents reported that the following work benefits at diagnosis were available for them: paid sick leave: 55.1%, flexible scheduling: 49.4%, disability: 40.5%, unpaid sick leave: 36.8%, flexible location: 21.5%, none of the above: 10.9%. For most of the women, their employer was very supportive during treatment (66.8%). For the others, their employer was neutral or somewhat supportive (17.9%), unsupportive (5.5%), or unaware of the diagnosis (3.7%). Impact on employment status: Survivors reported that their diagnosis and treatment impacted their employment as follows: changed jobs within company: 5.4%, avoided changing jobs to keep health insurance: 23.5%, changed jobs to get health insurance: 1.5%, took paid time off: 55.1%, took unpaid time off: 47.3%, quit job: 12.2%, retired early: 1.2%, lost job: 7.5%, job performance suffered: 40.4%, kept job for health insurance: 30.2%, increased work hours to cover medical costs: 5.1%.	-

Table 4. Cont.

First Author, Publication Year	Measurements for Employment Outcomes	Employment Outcomes	Determinants for Adverse Employment Outcomes (Quantitative Studies) or Selected Citations (Qualitative Studies, Indicated in Italics)
Tebbi et al., 1989 [44]	Employment status, job-related questions, experience in the work environment	Employment status: 62.5% of AYA cancer survivors were full-time employed, 10% part-time employed, and 27.5% unemployed. Job-related questions: 5% of AYA cancer survivors changed jobs as part of the adjustment to cancer. Experience in the work environment: 79% of AYA cancer survivors believed that readjustment to the job would be easier for survivors if the attitudes of others were changed, 64% of AYA cancer survivors believed that changes in certain physical features of the workplace were necessary to facilitate such readjustment, and 16% of AYACS believed that no changes in the workplace were necessary. AYA cancer survivors vs. comparison group: Employment status: full-time employed (62.5% vs. 65%), part-time employed (10% vs. 17.5%), unemployed (27.5% vs. 17.5%), $p = 0.425$. Job-related questions: No significant difference in experience of discrimination in hiring or promotion or problems performing their job or using job-related facilities.	-
Yanez et al., 2013 [46]	Employment status, cancer-related education or work interruption	Employment status: employed: 69%, homemaker: 11.5%, unemployed: 10.7%, student: 6.2% Cancer-related education/work interruption: 62.3% of AYA cancer survivors reported an interruption in education or work.	Time since diagnosis: AYA cancer survivors 25–60 months since diagnosis vs. 13–24 months since diagnosis vs. 0–12 months since diagnosis. Employment status: employed (% vs. 77.5 vs. 64.2), homemaker (11.5 vs. 9.8% vs. 9.2%), unemployed (10.7% vs. 3.8% vs. 15.8%), student (6.2% vs. 7.8% vs. 9.2%), cancer-related education/work interruption: 62.3% vs. 56.1% vs. 66.1%

Abbreviations: m, male; f, female; OR, odds ratio; CI, confidence interval; p, p-value; r, correlation coefficient; WAI, work ability index; aOR, adjusted odds ratio; CI, confidence interval; AYA, adolescent and young adult; HCT, allogeneic hematopoietic cell transplantation.

4.3. Financial Outcomes

Two studies addressed the income of AYA cancer survivors and compared it to the general population [34,36,44] (Table 5). In an early study, AYA cancer survivors had a higher income than the general population [44]. This difference may reflect a strong motivation to achieve higher goals among survivors [44]. In a more recent study, more AYA cancer survivors had a low family income and fewer survivors had a high family income [34]. AYA cancer survivors reported a negative net worth, whereas young adults from the general population reported a positive net worth [36]. Indirect medical costs were reported in three studies, with AYA cancer survivors having reported more missed work days than the comparison group in all studies [32,34,39]. AYA cancer survivors were significantly more likely to experience medical financial hardship compared to adults without a cancer history [29,38], and survivors reported a high level of financial toxicity (financial-related hardship) [45]. About half of the women with breast cancer experienced a financial decline due to their cancer diagnosis [43]. Three Scandinavian studies reported on disability pension uptake [31,33,39]. Compared with the general population, AYA cancer survivors received disability pensions at similar rates [31]. Compared with childhood cancer survivors, AYA cancer survivors were less likely to receive disability pensions [33].

Older age at time of study [36], chemotherapy and radiation [24,39], lower education [43,45], psychological distress [29], and more chronic conditions [23] were identified as characteristics associated with a higher financial burden. AYA cancer survivors with more chemotherapy courses were more likely to receive a disability pension [39].

4.4. Study Quality

Although some studies were designed as longitudinal or cohort studies, outcomes were cross-sectionally assessed. The average quality rating for cross-sectional studies (mean = 90%, range: 50–100%; Table 1) was slightly higher than for qualitative studies (mean = 75%; range: 50–90%; Table 2). No conclusive patterns in reported outcomes by study quality were identified.

Table 5. Impact of cancer on financial outcomes in adolescent and young adult (AYA) cancer survivors.

First Author, Publication Year	Measurements for Financial Outcomes	Financial Outcomes	Determinants for Adverse Financial Outcomes (Quantitative Studies) or Selected Citations (Qualitative Studies, Indicated in Italics)
Abdelhadi et al., 2021 [23]	Annual medical expenses	AYA cancer survivors without chronic conditions had an average of USD 5468 (95% CI, USD 3128 to USD 9559) in annual medical expenditures.	Chronic conditions: AYA cancer survivors with at least one chronic condition (74% of all AYA cancer survivors) spent an additional USD 2777 (95% CI: USD 480 to USD 5958) annually compared to survivors without chronic conditions. AYA cancer survivors with four or more chronic conditions (22%) had an increased average annual medical expenditure of USD 11,178 (95% CI: USD 6325 to USD 18,503). Higher annual medical expenses: physically inactive (USD 3558; 95% CI: USD 2200 to USD 4606), having a usual source of care (USD 687; 95% CI: USD 173 to USD 1415), having regular check-ups during the last year (USD 1117; 95% CI: USD 560 to USD 1867), unable to get care when needed (USD 1291; 95% CI: USD 198 to USD 3335).
Abdelhadi et al., 2022 [29]	Annual medical expenditures	AYA cancer survivors vs. comparison group: AYA cancer survivors without psychological distress had an average of USD 5324 (95% CI, USD 3275–USD 8653) in annual medical expenditures; adults with no history of cancer without psychological distress had an average of USD 2527.03 (USD 1837.76–USD 3474.83) in annual medical expenditures.	Psychological distress: AYA cancer survivors with psychological distress had significantly higher medical expenditures than AYA cancer survivors without psychological distress (p for interaction = 0.013) AYA cancer survivors vs. comparison group: In AYA cancer survivors, psychological distress was associated with an additional USD 4415 (95% CI, USD 993–USD 9690) in annual medical expenditures (p = 0.006). In matched adults without a history of cancer, psychological distress was associated with an additional USD 1802 (95% CI, USD 440–USD 3791) in annual medical expenditures (p = 0.005)
Drake et al., 2019 [49]	Perspectives on and experiences with return to work following treatment	Identified themes: uncertainty about return to work, cancer as a catalyst for a career change, importance of employment benefits, benefit of YA-specific resources	*"(…) so, part of the challenge is as much as I want a new job, umm I know that my cancer is now a pre-existing condition. So, if I was to switch to a different employer, some things won't be covered anymore. So, part of me thinks I can't leave my job because I'm covered under my benefits now and if I was to get new benefits then this is a pre-existing condition that won't be covered."*

Table 5. *Cont.*

First Author, Publication Year	Measurements for Financial Outcomes	Financial Outcomes	Determinants for Adverse Financial Outcomes (Quantitative Studies) or Selected Citations (Qualitative Studies, Indicated in Italics)
Ekwueme et al., 2016 [32]	Income, indirect productivity costs	Income: low (< USD 34,999) 30.59%, medium (USD 35,000–USD 74,999) 29.08%, high (> USD 75,000) 28.59% Indirect productivity costs: AYA cancer survivors missed 19 work days and 17 home productivity days. This resulted in indirect productivity costs of USD 2293 for missed work and USD 442 for missed home productivity days per capita per year. AYA cancer survivors vs. women aged 18–44 without breast cancer: Income: Low (< USD 34,999) 30.59% vs. 33.54%, medium (UDS 35,000–USD 74,999) 29.08% vs. 29.69%, high (> USD 75,000) 28.59% vs. 24.11% Indirect productivity costs: AYA cancer survivors had higher indirect productivity costs (from work days lost and home productivity days lost) per capita.	-
Ghaderi et al., 2013 [33]	Attendance benefit, basic benefit, medical rehabilitation benefit, disability pension	Uptake of benefits (childhood (0–14 years old at diagnosis) vs. AYA (15–19 and 20–24 years old at diagnosis) survivors): Attendance benefit: 20.5% vs. 3.3% and 1.9%, basic benefit: 19.12% vs. 8.05% and 5.12%, medical rehabilitation benefit: 9.18% vs. 10.9% and 10.3%, disability pension: 11.36% vs. 6.9% and 6.6%	Age at diagnosis: uptake of benefits (15–19 vs. 20–24 years at diagnosis): attendance benefit: 3.3% vs. 1.9%, basic benefit: 8.05% vs. 5.12%, medical rehabilitation benefit: 10.9% vs. 10.3%, disability pension: 6.9% vs. 6.6%
Ghazal et al., 2021 [51]	Perspectives of work-related goals	Identified themes: self-identity and work, perceived health and work ability, financial toxicity	*"I ended up getting into some credit card debt. I sold a lot of things that I had bought for myself over the years to try to play catch up on bills that I had monthly."* *"I feel like I need to go do these [new WRGs], but there's that whole financial portion."*

Table 5. Cont.

First Author, Publication Year	Measurements for Financial Outcomes	Financial Outcomes	Determinants for Adverse Financial Outcomes (Quantitative Studies) or Selected Citations (Qualitative Studies, Indicated in Italics)
Gupta et al., 2020 [52]	Experience of cancer-related financial stress	Identified themes: managing health care costs with limited funds, limiting future possibilities of employment and education, developing independence while being financially dependent, potential benefit of financial stress, work environment	*"One thing I would advise [...] is to make sure to have health insurance. [...] You know, most young adults don't think [about] having it. "Nothing's going to happen to me. Why do I need health insurance?"* (Male, 24 years old)
Guy et al., 2014 [34]	Family income, direct medical costs, indirect medical costs	Family income: 21.4% of AYA cancer survivors had a low family income, 41.6% had a middle family income, and 12.3% had a high family income. Annual direct medical costs: AYA cancer survivors had annual per person medical expenditures of USD 7417. Private insurance was the largest source of payment for AYA cancer survivors (USD 3083). Ambulatory and inpatient care were the largest type of service for AYA cancer survivors (USD 2409 + USD 1605). Annual indirect medical costs: All types of lost productivity resulted in a total per capita spending of USD 4564. AYA cancer survivors vs. comparison group: family income: low, 21.4% vs. 16.7%; middle, 41.6% vs. 44%; high, 12.3% vs. 16.3% Annual direct medical costs: Annual per person medical expenditures were USD 7417 vs. $4247. Private insurance was the largest source of payment, USD 3083 vs. USD 1825. Ambulatory and inpatient care saw the largest share of medical expenditures, USD 2409 + USD 1605 vs. USD 1376 + USD 1169 Annual indirect medical costs: AYA cancer survivors reported higher productivity costs due to employment disability, more missed work days among employed people, and greater household productivity loss. All types of lost productivity resulted in a higher total per capita spending of USD 4564 vs. USD 2314.	-

Table 5. *Cont.*

First Author, Publication Year	Measurements for Financial Outcomes	Financial Outcomes	Determinants for Adverse Financial Outcomes (Quantitative Studies) or Selected Citations (Qualitative Studies, Indicated in Italics)
Kent et al., 2012 [53]	Perspectives on cancer survivorship	Concerns about being un- or underinsured as an AYA cancer survivor because they could not afford coverage and/or felt they did not need coverage. About 1/3 of survivors reported difficulties with acquiring or maintaining health insurance. Insured patients were worried about future insurability. Many survivors experienced a gap in coverage between high school, college, and full-time employment. As a result, many survivors first sought out the emergency room due to lack of insurance. Eventually, many uninsured survivors were able to obtain government-sponsored insurance, but in all cases, they indicated that this process delayed their treatment.	*"I was going to the doctors. And I was paying cash. We didn't have insurance at that time. And when they found out from the labs that I had cancer, I went to the emergency room because I was almost dying."* (Female, diagnosed with non-Hodgkin lymphoma in her midtwenties)
Ketterl et al., 2019 [24]	Borrowing money or going into debt	14.4% reported that they borrowed ≥ USD 10,000. 1.5% reported that they had filed for bankruptcy because of their cancer.	Treatment: Chemotherapy: inference with job-related physical tasks (OR = 1.97, CI = 1.22 to 3.11, $p < 0.01$), inference with mental tasks required by a job (OR = 3.22, CI, 2.15 to 4.79, $p < 0.01$), time off from work (OR = 3.56, CI = 2.31 to 5.47, $p < 0.01$), borrowing ≥ USD 10,000 (OR = 3.05, CI = 1.53 to 6.09, $p < 0.01$) compared with survivors who were not exposed to chemotherapy. Radiation: interference with job-related physical tasks (OR = 1.66, CI = 1.08 to 2.41, $p < 0.05$) compared with survivors who did not receive radiation. Surgery: extended paid time off from work (OR = 0.54, CI = 0.54 to 1.00, $p < 0.05$) compared with survivors who did not receive surgery.

Table 5. *Cont.*

First Author, Publication Year	Measurements for Financial Outcomes	Financial Outcomes	Determinants for Adverse Financial Outcomes (Quantitative Studies) or Selected Citations (Qualitative Studies, Indicated in Italics)
Landwehr et al., 2016 [36]	Use of a funding grant, net worth (value of all things owned by an individual), out-of-pocket medical expenses, financial indices	Use of a funding grant: medical/insurance (34%), rent/mortgage (25%), health/wellness (20%), continuing education/loans (14%), car-related (12%), computer (10%), family building (7%), other (12%). AYA cancer survivors vs. comparison group: Net worth: AYA cancer survivors had an average negative net worth value of −USD 35,009.41 in debt compared to young adults from the general population who had a mean net worth of USD 68,479 in assets. Out-of-pocket medical expenses: AYA cancer survivors had higher expenses (mean = USD 2528.76 annually) compared to young adults from the general population (median = USD 610.00 annually).	Age at application (19–29 years old vs. 30–39 years old): Financial indices: mean total liabilities: USD 37,760.16 vs. USD 59,012.16 ($p < 0.05$), mean total medical debt: USD 3616.89 vs. USD 4239.34, mean total credit card debt: USD 3025.93 vs. USD 3913.89, mean monthly income: USD 1385.84 vs. USD 1851.14 ($p < 0.05$), mean monthly expenses: USD 1490.94 vs. USD 2135.70 ($p < 0.01$), mean monthly medical expenses: USD 184.25 vs. USD 242.82, mean monthly student loan payment: USD 112.35 vs. USD 68.53, mean income to expenses ratio: 0.87 vs. 0.89
Lu et al., 2021 [38]	Medical financial hardship	The majority of AYA cancer survivors (62.2%) experienced at least one domain of medical financial hardship. Material hardship (reporting problem paying medical bills): 36.7%, psychological hardship (reporting worry about medical costs): 46.6%, behavioral hardship (reporting delaying or forgoing medical care because of worry about cost or being unable to afford prescription medicine or care): 28.4% AYA cancer survivors vs. comparison group: AYA cancer survivors were significantly more likely to experience medical financial hardship compared to adults without a cancer history. Material hardship (36.7% vs. 27.7%, $p < 0.001$), psychological hardship (46.6% vs. 44.7%, $p = 0.210$), behavioral hardship (28.4% vs. 21.2%, $p < 0.001$).	-

Table 5. Cont.

First Author, Publication Year	Measurements for Financial Outcomes	Financial Outcomes	Determinants for Adverse Financial Outcomes (Quantitative Studies) or Selected Citations (Qualitative Studies, Indicated in Italics)
Meernik et al., 2020 [25]	Financial hardship	Financial hardship: 27% of AYA cancer survivors reported financial hardship (borrowing money, going into debt, and/or filing for bankruptcy), 27% had borrowed money or gone into debt, and 3% reported to have filed for bankruptcy.	Employment disruption: Financial hardship differed significantly between AYA cancer survivors with and without employment disruption: 43% vs. 20%, borrowing money or going into debt: 43% vs. 20%, filing for bankruptcy: 4% vs. 2%.
Nord et al., 2015 [39]	Disability pension	AYA cancer survivors vs. comparison group: number of persons with disability pension: 76/2073 (4%) vs. 209/8140 (3%).	Disability pension: Extensive treatment with 4 courses (HR = 1.93, CI = 1.01 to 3.71), extensive treatment with ≥4 courses (HR = 5.16, CI = 2.00 to 10.3)
Tangka et al., 2020 [43]	Treatment and other non-clinical costs, financial decline	Treatment and other non-clinical costs: 27.7% of women spent less than USD 500, 27.9% spent USD 500 to USD 2000, 18.7% spent USD 2001 to USD 5000, and 17.0% spent USD 5001 to USD 10,000 out of pocket for breast cancer treatment (e.g., for hospital bills, deductibles, and medication) during the 12 months prior to the study. For these costs, most women used personal funds (81.5%), informal borrowing from family and friends (22.9%), the method of leaving some medical bills unpaid (22.7%), or increasing credit card debt (21.7%). Financial decline: 47.0% of women experienced a financial decline due to their cancer diagnosis.	Women showing the following characteristics were most vulnerable to financial decline due to their cancer diagnosis: non-Hispanic other: OR = 2.58 (compared to non-Hispanic White women), some college education: OR = 1.58 (compared to women with a college or postgraduate degree), one comorbidity: OR = 1.80 (compared to women with no comorbid conditions), two or more comorbidities: OR = 2.80 (compared to women with no comorbid conditions), late-stage diagnoses (stage III and IV): OR = 1.76 (compared to women diagnosed at earlier stages), self-funded insurance: OR = 2.29 (compared to women with employer-based insurance coverage).

Table 5. *Cont.*

First Author, Publication Year	Measurements for Financial Outcomes	Financial Outcomes	Determinants for Adverse Financial Outcomes (Quantitative Studies) or Selected Citations (Qualitative Studies, Indicated in Italics)
Tebbi et al., 1989 [44]	Income	Income: AYA cancer survivors had a mean income of USD 16,750. AYA cancer survivors vs. comparison group: mean income: USD 16,750 vs. USD 12,250, $p = 0.006$	-
Thom et al., 2021 [45]	Financial toxicity, medical cost-coping	Financial toxicity: The mean score for financial toxicity was 14.0 (±9.33), which indicates severe financial toxicity in AYA cancer survivors. Medical cost-coping: Participants on average reported 3.2 (±1.89) cost-coping behaviors, including postponing mental health care (46% of the sample) and/or preventative care (36%); having a health problem but not seeing a provider (37%); skipping a medical test, treatment, or fo low-up (34%); and not filling a prescription (27%) or taking a smaller dose of a medication than prescribed (18%).	Financial toxicity was associated with: full-time employment (mean difference of the financial toxicity score between people lacking and people having full-time employment: −4.66; 95% CI: −7.18 to −2.13), less education (correlation coefficient $r = 0.31$; $p < 0.001$), lower income ($r = 0.47$; $p = <0.001$), younger age at time of survey completion ($r = 0.16$; $p = 0.05$), more COVID-19 pandemic-related negative economic events (e.g., not having enough money for medical expenses, food or medication) ($r = −0.59$; $p = <0.001$).

Abbreviations: OR, odds ratio; CI, confidence interval; *p*, *p*-value; WRG, work-related goal; AYA, adolescent and young adult; r, correlation coefficient.

5. Discussion

With this systematic review, we showed that a cancer diagnosis in adolescence or young adulthood significantly impacted educational, employment, and financial outcomes. Re-entry to school or work after cancer treatment was challenging. After treatment, most survivors were employed but started their employment at an older age than the general population. Overall, no disadvantages in income were found. Survivors reported more absent work days than the comparisons. The main determinants for adverse outcomes were female gender, younger age at diagnosis, chemotherapy and radiotherapy, and experiencing late effects.

Our systematic review is in line with the findings of a previous review on work-related issues in AYA cancer survivors [58]. For many AYA cancer survivors, the cancer diagnosis interrupted their current engagement at school or work. This interruption delayed the attainment of education and work goals and sometimes forced survivors to rely on social security benefits or file for bankruptcy. This did not mean that AYA cancer survivors could not achieve a successful career compared to healthy controls, but they did start the career later. Many survivors were willing to return to school or work, although cancer treatment and its side effects often imposed hurdles. Our review showed that these long-term consequences forced some AYA cancer survivors to wait a certain amount of time to return to school, or for formerly employed survivors, it meant a change of workplace. Whereas some AYA cancer survivors perceived working as a return to normalcy, others described a change in perspective and redefined their professional careers.

One study found that AYA cancer survivors earned more compared to the general population [44]. One reason could be the change in perspective leading to a job change, possibly resulting in survivors earning more than they did before diagnosis [59,60]. For instance, jobs with less physical effort might be, on average, better paid compared to jobs with more physical effort involved. Within AYA cancer survivors, financial outcomes varied with age at the time of the study. Although older survivors earned more [36], as seen in the general population, the study also found that older survivors reported a more severe financial impact [36]. Whereas older survivors were more likely to be married and thus had a potential additional source of income through their partner, they received less parental support, were more likely to have dependent children, and were more likely to own a home compared to younger survivors, indicating the need for more financial resources for older survivors. AYA cancer survivors diagnosed with breast cancer missed more work days and home productivity days (spending more than half of the day in bed due to illness) compared to women without breast cancer, resulting in higher indirect productivity costs [32].

According to this review, AYA cancer survivors diagnosed at a younger age were found to be particularly vulnerable to adverse outcomes. One explanation for the lower educational attainment might be that they were still pursuing education and could not keep up with fellow students due to the interruption caused by cancer [47]. Unemployment might be higher because they may prioritize their health over their career [56,61]. Health insurance is organized differently in different countries. In countries where health insurance is not mandatory or related to employment, an explanation for the high financial burden might be that AYA cancer survivors were believed to be too young to need health insurance before the cancer diagnosis.

Chemotherapy and radiotherapy and a stay in the ICU during treatment were found to be determinants for adverse outcomes in all domains studied [20,39]. ICU stays are costly and associated with an increased number of potentially life-threatening complications that can negatively impact patient prognosis [62,63]. This could prolong their absence from school and work and affect their financial situation in the long run.

Our three outcomes of interest, i.e., education, employment, and financial outcomes, are linked to the different life stages (Figure 2). Whereas educational attainment is the primary focus in adolescence, transitioning to work and gaining financial independence becomes more important in young adulthood. However, all stages of life have one aspect in common: a reciprocal relationship with the state of health. If the state of health is deteriorating, this affects the current stage of life and is also likely to have long-term consequences for the following stage of life. Therefore, it is important to consider these three outcomes as mutually dependent rather than independent factors, also in the case of a cancer diagnosis in adolescence or young adulthood. Taking a holistic approach and considering the reciprocal relationship between outcomes and state of health can ensure a successful career even after a cancer diagnosis in adolescence or young adulthood.

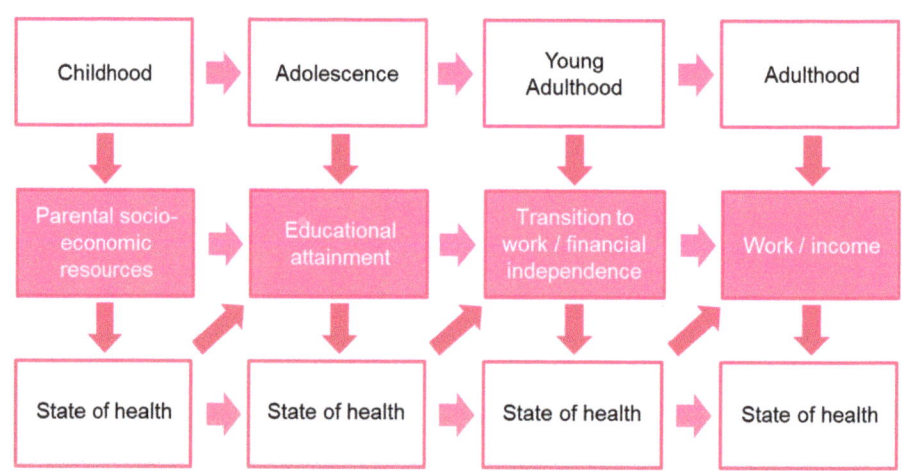

Figure 2. Dynamic interaction between life stages and state of health (own adaptation, based on (Adler et al., 2007 [64]; Fardell et al., 2018 [18]).

6. Limitations and Strengths

Countries have different education, labor, and financial systems. Furthermore, there were significant differences in how the data were collected. This made comparisons across studies challenging. Most of the included studies were based on self-reported data. For these studies, self-report bias might be present. As for other systematic reviews, there is a potential for language and publication bias. We included publications in English and other languages known to the research team (only one publication written in Japanese had to be excluded) and published in the three databases searched.

The comprehensive literature review (search in three relevant databases) is a strength of the study. For this systematic review, over 5000 articles were screened for eligibility. Each article was screened independently by two reviewers, and three reviewers were involved in the decision process. The comprehensive search allowed for the inclusion of studies from different countries with different educational, employment, and financial contexts. The three outcomes were purposely chosen to represent a life course perspective. The carefully selected, mutually exclusive, and collectively exhaustive search terms ensured that we were able to include relevant studies, including a broad range of AYA cancer survivors, different cultural backgrounds, the whole AYA age range at diagnosis, and different time phases after diagnosis. Extensive hand searching and the search update ensured that the most recent articles and articles that would have been missed with the search in the databases were included as well.

7. Implications

Identifying AYA cancer survivors at risk for adverse educational, employment, and financial outcomes is important for developing tailored support strategies for cancer patients and survivors throughout their whole cancer trajectory. We found that most survivors returned to school or work after cancer treatment. However, this re-entry was associated with difficulties and hurdles. To enable a successful return to school or work, AYA cancer survivors should be supported in navigating the system [65] and involve key persons such as peers, teachers, or employers, and employees should be informed and supported as well [66]. Flexible working conditions might help survivors with successfully returning to work [67] and being able to stay in the workforce in the long term. Survivors in their last years of school or their first years of employment might be especially vulnerable to adverse effects on their education and employment. Individual support options focusing on cancer- and treatment-related impairments as well as abilities and potential new directions for their employment should be provided [67]. Furthermore, open conversations about finances should be held with AYA cancer patients and survivors. Such conversations can empower patients and survivors and increase their knowledge about existing financial assistance services. Further research should be done in the area of insurance at a young age. Where health insurance is optional, young people often think they are too young for insurance [68], as chronic illness may affect them less frequently than older people.

Although most AYA cancer survivors experience some degree of negative impact of their diagnosis on education, employment, or financial outcomes, many survivors also do well. It might be worth looking at their strategies to overcome the challenges of a cancer diagnosis during adolescence or young adulthood and to re-enter school or work successfully.

Most of the included studies were of a cross-sectional design. In future research, longitudinal studies in AYA cancer survivors could expand the understanding of the impact of cancer diagnosis and treatment throughout the cancer trajectory. Multiple measurement time points could be used to assess the individual courses of AYA cancer survivors. These results might expand the knowledge on appropriate time points for tailored support to AYA cancer survivors to mitigate their risk for adverse education, employment, and financial outcomes and improve their well-being.

8. Conclusions

Although most AYA cancer survivors were able to re-enter education and employment, they reported difficulties with re-entry and delays in their employment pathway. We found some determinants for adverse outcomes, but the results were heterogeneous. To facilitate successful re-entry, age- and situation-tailored support services along the cancer trajectory should be developed and implemented to prevent future social inequalities and adverse educational, employment, and financial outcomes in the long term.

Supplementary Materials: The following supporting information can be downloaded at: https://www.mdpi.com/article/10.3390/curroncol30100631/s1, Table S1: Characteristics of included quantitative studies (detailed version); Table S2: Characteristics of included qualitative studies (detailed version); Table S3: PICO format for the research questions; Table S4: Search blocks for the search in the literature databases; Table S5: Quality assessment for quantitative cross-sectional studies; Table S6: Quality assessment for qualitative studies.

Author Contributions: Conceptualization, A.A., G.M., L.M. and K.R.; methodology, G.M., L.M. and K.R.; formal analysis, A.A., M.K. and K.R.; investigation, A.A., C.B., M.K., L.M. and K.R.; data curation, K.R.; writing—original draft preparation, A.A. and K.R.; writing—review and editing, C.B., D.D., K.S., G.M. and L.M.; visualization, A.A. and K.R.; supervision, G.M. and K.R.; project administration, K.R.; funding acquisition, K.R. and G.M. All authors have read and agreed to the published version of the manuscript.

Funding: This work was supported by Palatin-Stiftung Switzerland (Nr. 0028/2020 to KR), Krebsliga Zentralschweiz Switzerland (to KR), Avenira Stiftung Switzerland (to KR), and the Swiss National Science Foundation (SNSF, Nr. 10001C_182129/1 to GM).

Conflicts of Interest: The authors declare no conflict of interest.

References

1. Epelman, C.L. The adolescent and young adult with cancer: State of the art—Psychosocial aspects. *Curr. Oncol. Rep.* **2013**, *15*, 325–331. [CrossRef] [PubMed]
2. Soliman, H.; Agresta, S.V. Current issues in adolescent and young adult cancer survivorship. *Cancer Control. J. Moffitt Cancer Cent.* **2008**, *15*, 55–62. [CrossRef] [PubMed]
3. Bellizzi, K.M.; Smith, A.; Schmidt, S.; Keegan, T.H.M.; Zebrack, B.; Lynch, C.F.; Deapen, D.; Shnorhavorian, M.; Tompkins, B.J.; Simon, M.; et al. Positive and negative psychosocial impact of being diagnosed with cancer as an adolescent or young adult. *Cancer* **2012**, *118*, 5155–5162. [CrossRef]
4. Zebrack, B.J. Psychological, social, and behavioral issues for young adults with cancer. *Cancer* **2011**, *117* (Suppl. S10), 2289–2294. [CrossRef] [PubMed]
5. Patterson, P.; McDonald, F.E.; Zebrack, B.; Medlow, S. Emerging issues among adolescent and young adult cancer survivors. *Semin. Oncol. Nurs.* **2015**, *31*, 53–59. [CrossRef]
6. Geue, K.; Schmidt, R.; Sender, A.; Sauter, S.; Friedrich, M. Sexuality and romantic relationships in young adult cancer survivors: Satisfaction and supportive care needs. *Psycho-Oncology* **2015**, *24*, 1368–1376. [CrossRef]
7. Murphy, D.; Klosky, J.L.; Reed, D.R.; Termuhlen, A.M.; Shannon, S.V.; Quinn, G.P. The importance of assessing priorities of reproductive health concerns among adolescent and young adult patients with cancer. *Cancer* **2015**, *121*, 2529–2536. [CrossRef]
8. Barnett, M.; McDonnell, G.; DeRosa, A.; Schuler, T.; Philip, E.; Peterson, L.; Touza, K.; Jhanwar, S.; Atkinson, T.M.; Ford, J.S. Psychosocial outcomes and interventions among cancer survivors diagnosed during adolescence and young adulthood (AYA): A systematic review. *J. Cancer Surviv. Res. Pract.* **2016**, *10*, 814–831. [CrossRef]
9. Lang, M.J.; Giese-Davis, J.; Patton, S.B.; Campbell, D.J.T. Does age matter? Comparing post-treatment psychosocial outcomes in young adult and older adult cancer survivors with their cancer-free peers. *Psycho-Oncology* **2017**, *27*, 1404–1411. [CrossRef]
10. Fidler, M.M.; Gupta, S.; Soerjomataram, I.; Ferlay, J.; Steliarova-Foucher, E.; Bray, F. Cancer incidence and mortality among young adults aged 20–39 years worldwide in 2012: A population-based study. *Lancet Oncol.* **2017**, *18*, 1579–1589. [CrossRef]
11. Bleyer, A.; Ferrari, A.; Whelan, J.; Barr, R.D. Global assessment of cancer incidence and survival in adolescents and young adults. *Pediatr. Blood Cancer* **2017**, *64*, e26497. [CrossRef] [PubMed]
12. Stark, D.; Bielack, S.; Brugieres, L.; Dirksen, U.; Duarte, X.; Dunn, S.; Erdelyi, D.; Grew, T.; Hjorth, L.; Jazbec, J.; et al. Teenagers and young adults with cancer in Europe: From national programmes to a European integrated coordinated project. *Eur. J. Cancer Care* **2016**, *25*, 419–427. [CrossRef] [PubMed]
13. Barr, R.D.; Ries, L.A.G.; Trama, A.; Gatta, G.; Steliarova-Foucher, E.; Stiller, C.A.; Bleyer, W.A. A system for classifying cancers diagnosed in adolescents and young adults. *Cancer* **2020**, *126*, 4634–4659. [CrossRef]
14. Bleyer, A. Increasing Cancer in Adolescents and Young Adults: Cancer Types and Causation Implications. *J. Adolesc. Young Adult Oncol.* **2023**, *12*, 285–296. [CrossRef]
15. Trama, A.; Stark, D.; Bozovic-Spasojevic, I.; Gaspar, N.; Peccatori, F.; Toss, A.; Bernasconi, A.; Quarello, P.; Scheinemann, K.; Jezdic, S.; et al. Cancer burden in adolescents and young adults in Europe. *ESMO Open* **2023**, *8*, 100744. [CrossRef]
16. Trama, A.; Botta, L.; Foschi, R.; Ferrari, A.; Stiller, C.; Desandes, E.; Maule, M.M.; Merletti, F.; Gatta, G. Survival of European adolescents and young adults diagnosed with cancer in 2000–2007: Population-based data from EUROCARE-5. *Lancet Oncol.* **2016**, *17*, 896–906. [CrossRef]
17. Parsons, H.M.; Harlan, L.C.; Lynch, C.F.; Hamilton, A.S.; Wu, X.-C.; Kato, I.; Schwartz, S.M.; Smith, A.W.; Keel, G.; Keegan, T.H. Impact of cancer on work and education among adolescent and young adult cancer survivors. *J. Clin. Oncol. Off. J. Am. Soc. Clin. Oncol.* **2012**, *30*, 2393–2400. [CrossRef]
18. Fardell, J.E.; Wakefield, C.E.; Patterson, P.; Lum, A.; Cohn, R.J.; Pini, S.A.; Sansom-Daly, U.M. Narrative Review of the Educational, Vocational, and Financial Needs of Adolescents and Young Adults with Cancer: Recommendations for Support and Research. *J. Adolesc. Young Adult Oncol.* **2018**, *7*, 143–147. [CrossRef]
19. Mader, L.; Vetsch, J.; Christen, S.; Baenziger, J.; Roser, K.; Dehler, S.; Michel, G. Education, employment and marriage in long-term survivors of teenage and young adult cancer compared with healthy controls. *Swiss Med. Wkly.* **2017**, *147*, w14419. [CrossRef] [PubMed]
20. Dieluweit, U.; Debatin, K.-M.; Grabow, D.; Kaatsch, P.; Peter, R.; Seitz, D.C.; Goldbeck, L. Educational and vocational achievement among long-term survivors of adolescent cancer in Germany. *Pediatr. Blood Cancer* **2011**, *56*, 432–438. [CrossRef]
21. Warner, E.L.; Kent, E.E.; Trevino, K.M.; Parsons, H.M.; Zebrack, B.J.; Kirchhoff, A.C. Social well-being among adolescents and young adults with cancer: A systematic review. *Cancer* **2016**, *122*, 1029–1037. [CrossRef] [PubMed]
22. Kirchhoff, A.C.; Yi, J.; Wright, J.; Warner, E.L.; Smith, K.R. Marriage and divorce among young adult cancer survivors. *J. Cancer Surviv. Res. Pract.* **2012**, *6*, 441–450. [CrossRef] [PubMed]
23. Abdelhadi, O.A.; Joseph, J.; Pollock, B.H.; Keegan, T.H.M. Additional medical costs of chronic conditions among adolescent and young adult cancer survivors. *J. Cancer Surviv. Res. Pract.* **2021**, *16*, 487–496. [CrossRef] [PubMed]
24. Ketterl, T.G.; Syrjala, K.L.; Casillas, J.; Jacobs, L.A.; Palmer, S.C.; McCabe, M.S.; Ganz, P.A.; Overholser, L.; Partridge, A.; Rajotte, E.J.; et al. Lasting effects of cancer and its treatment on employment and finances in adolescent and young adult cancer survivors. *Cancer* **2019**, *125*, 1908–1917. [CrossRef] [PubMed]

25. Meernik, C.; Kirchhoff, A.C.; Anderson, C.; Edwards, T.P.; Deal, A.M.; Baggett, C.D.; Kushi, L.H.; Chao, C.R.; Nichols, H.B. Material and psychological financial hardship related to employment disruption among female adolescent and young adult cancer survivors. *Cancer* **2020**, *127*, 137–148. [CrossRef] [PubMed]
26. Thom, B.; Benedict, C.; Friedman, D.N.; Kelvin, J.F. The intersection of financial toxicity and family building in young adult cancer survivors. *Cancer* **2018**, *124*, 3284–3289. [CrossRef]
27. Page, M.J.; McKenzie, J.E.; Bossuyt, P.M.; Boutron, I.; Hoffmann, T.C.; Mulrow, C.D.; Shamseer, L.; Tetzlaff, J.M.; Akl, E.A.; Brennan, S.E.; et al. The PRISMA 2020 statement: An updated guideline for reporting systematic reviews. *BMJ* **2021**, *372*, n71. [CrossRef]
28. Aromataris, E.; Munn, Z. (Eds.) JBI Manual for Evidence Synthesis. JBI. 2020. Available online: https://synthesismanual.jbi.global (accessed on 1 September 2023). [CrossRef]
29. Abdelhadi, O.A.; Pollock, B.H.; Joseph, J.G.; Keegan, T.H.M. Psychological distress and associated additional medical expenditures in adolescent and young adult cancer survivors. *Cancer* **2022**, *128*, 1523–1531. [CrossRef]
30. Bhatt, N.S.; Brazauskas, R.; Salit, R.B.; Syrjala, K.; Bo-Subait, S.; Tecca, H.; Badawy, S.M.; Baker, K.S.; Beitinjaneh, A.; Bejanyan, N.; et al. Return to Work Among Young Adult Survivors of Allogeneic Hematopoietic Cell Transplantation in the United States. *Transplant. Cell. Ther.* **2021**, *27*, 679.e1–679.e8. [CrossRef]
31. Dahl, A.A.; Fosså, S.D.; Lie, H.C.; Loge, J.H.; Reinertsen, K.V.; Ruud, E.; Kiserud, C.E. Employment Status and Work Ability in Long-Term Young Adult Cancer Survivors. *J. Adolesc. Young Adult Oncol.* **2019**, *8*, 304–311. [CrossRef]
32. Ekwueme, D.U.; Trogdon, J.G.; Khavjou, O.A.; Guy, G.P., Jr. Productivity Costs Associated With Breast Cancer Among Survivors Aged 18–44 Years. *Am. J. Prev. Med.* **2016**, *50*, 286–294. [CrossRef] [PubMed]
33. Ghaderi, S.; Engeland, A.; Moster, D.; Ruud, E.; Syse, A.; Wesenberg, F.; Bjørge, T. Increased uptake of social security benefits among long-term survivors of cancer in childhood, adolescence and young adulthood: A Norwegian population-based cohort study. *Br. J. Cancer* **2013**, *108*, 1525–1533. [CrossRef] [PubMed]
34. Guy, G.P., Jr.; Yabroff, K.R.; Ekwueme, D.U.; Smith, A.W.; Dowling, E.C.; Rechis, R.; Nutt, S.; Richardson, L.C. Estimating the health and economic burden of cancer among those diagnosed as adolescents and young adults. *Health Aff.* **2014**, *33*, 1024–1031. [CrossRef] [PubMed]
35. Hamzah SRa Musa, S.N.S.; Muda, Z.; Ismail, M. Quality of working life and career engagement of cancer survivors: The mediating role of effect of disease and treatment. *Eur. J. Train. Dev.* **2021**, *45*, 181–199. [CrossRef]
36. Landwehr, M.S.; Watson, S.E.; Macpherson, C.F.; Novak, K.A.; Johnson, R.H. The cost of cancer: A retrospective analysis of the financial impact of cancer on young adults. *Cancer Med.* **2016**, *5*, 863–870. [CrossRef]
37. Lim, P.S.; Tran, S.; Kroeze, S.G.; Pica, A.; Hrbacek, J.; Bachtiary, B.; Walser, M.; Leiser, D.; Lomax, A.J.; Weber, D.C. Outcomes of adolescents and young adults treated for brain and skull base tumors with pencil beam scanning proton therapy. *Pediatr. Blood Cancer* **2020**, *67*, e28664. [CrossRef]
38. Lu, A.D.; Zheng, Z.; Han, X.; Qi, R.; Zhao, J.; Yabroff, K.R.; Nathan, P.C. Medical Financial Hardship in Survivors of Adolescent and Young Adult Cancer in the United States. *J. Natl. Cancer Inst.* **2021**, *113*, 997–1004. [CrossRef]
39. Nord, C.; Olofsson, S.-E.; Glimelius, I.; Cedermark, G.C.; Ekberg, S.; Cavallin-Ståhl, E.; Neovius, M.; Jerkeman, M.; Smedby, K.E. Sick leave and disability pension among Swedish testicular cancer survivors according to clinical stage and treatment. *Acta Oncol.* **2015**, *54*, 1770–1780. [CrossRef]
40. Nugent, B.D.; Bender, C.M.; Sereika, S.M.; Tersak, J.M.; Rosenzweig, M. Cognitive and occupational function in survivors of adolescent cancer. *J. Adolesc. Young Adult Oncol.* **2018**, *7*, 79–87. [CrossRef]
41. Strauser, D.; Feuerstein, M.; Chan, F.; Arango, J.; da Silva Cardoso, E.; Chiu, C.-Y. Vocational services associated with competitive employment in 18–25 year old cancer survivors. *J. Cancer Surviv.* **2010**, *4*, 179–186. [CrossRef]
42. Sylvest, R.; Vassard, D.; Schmidt, L.; Schmiegelow, K.; Macklon, K.T.; Forman, J.L.; Pinborg, A. Family Formation and Socio-Economic Status among 35-Year-Old Men Who Have Survived Cancer in Childhood and Early Adulthood: A Register-Based Cohort Study. *Oncol. Res. Treat.* **2021**, *45*, 102–111. [CrossRef]
43. Tangka, F.K.; Subramanian, S.; Jones, M.; Edwards, P.; Flanigan, T.; Kaganova, Y.; Smith, K.W.; Thomas, C.C.; Hawkins, N.A.; Rodriguez, J.; et al. Insurance Coverage, Employment Status, and Financial Well-Being of Young Women Diagnosed with Breast Cancer. *Cancer Epidemiol. Biomark. Prev.* **2020**, *29*, 616–624. [CrossRef]
44. Tebbi, C.K.; Bromberg, C.; Piedmonte, M. Long-term vocational adjustment of cancer patients diagnosed during adolescence. *Cancer* **1989**, *63*, 213–218. [CrossRef]
45. Thom, B.; Benedict, C.; Friedman, D.N.; Watson, S.E.; Zeitler, M.S.; Chino, F. Economic distress, financial toxicity, and medical cost-coping in young adult cancer survivors during the COVID-19 pandemic: Findings from an online sample. *Cancer* **2021**, *127*, 4481–4491. [CrossRef] [PubMed]
46. Yanez, B.; Garcia, S.F.; Victorson, D.; Salsman, J.M. Distress among young adult cancer survivors: A cohort study. *Support. Care Cancer Off. J. Multinatl. Assoc. Support. Care Cancer* **2013**, *21*, 2403–2408. [CrossRef] [PubMed]
47. An, H.; Lee, S. Difficulty in returning to school among adolescent leukemia survivors: A qualitative descriptive study. *Eur. J. Oncol. Nurs.* **2019**, *38*, 70–75. [CrossRef]
48. Brauer, E.R.; Pieters, H.C.; Ganz, P.A.; Landier, W.; Pavlish, C.; Heilemann, M.V. "From Snail Mode to Rocket Ship Mode": Adolescents and Young Adults' Experiences of Returning to Work and School After Hematopoietic Cell Transplantation. *J. Adolesc. Young Adult Oncol.* **2017**, *6*, 551–559. [CrossRef] [PubMed]

49. Drake, E.K.; Urquhart, R. "Figure Out What It Is You Love to Do and Live the Life You Love": The Experiences of Young Adults Returning to Work After Primary Cancer Treatment. *J. Adolesc. Young Adult Oncol.* **2019**, *8*, 368–372. [CrossRef]
50. Elsbernd, A.; Pedersen, K.J.; Boisen, K.A.; Midtgaard, J.; Larsen, H.B. "On Your Own": Adolescent and Young Adult Cancer Survivors' Experience of Managing Return to Secondary or Higher Education in Denmark. *J. Adolesc. Young Adult Oncol.* **2018**, *7*, 618–625. [CrossRef]
51. Ghazal, L.V.; Merriman, J.; Santacroce, S.J.; Dickson, V.V. Survivors' Dilemma: Young Adult Cancer Survivors' Perspectives of Work-Related Goals. *Workplace Health Saf.* **2021**, *69*, 506–516. [CrossRef]
52. Gupta, S.K.; Mazza, M.C.; Hoyt, M.A.; Revenson, T.A. The experience of financial stress among emerging adult cancer survivors. *J. Psychosoc. Oncol.* **2020**, *38*, 435–448. [CrossRef]
53. Kent, E.E.; Parry, C.; Montoya, M.J.; Sender, L.S.; Morris, R.A.; Anton-Culver, H. "You're too young for this": Adolescent and young adults' perspectives on cancer survivorship. *J. Psychosoc. Oncol.* **2012**, *30*, 260–279. [CrossRef] [PubMed]
54. Magrath, C.M.; Critoph, D.J.; Smith, L.A.M.; Hatcher, H.M. "A Different Person Entirely": Adolescent and Young Adults' Experiences Returning to Education after Cancer Treatment. *J. Adolesc. Young Adult Oncol.* **2021**, *10*, 562–572. [CrossRef] [PubMed]
55. Parsons, J.A.; Eakin, J.M.; Bell, R.S.; Franche, R.-L.; Davis, A.M. "So, are you back to work yet"? Re-conceptualizing 'work' and 'return to work' in the context of primary bone cancer. *Soc. Sci. Med.* **2008**, *67*, 1826–1836. [CrossRef] [PubMed]
56. Raque-Bogdan, T.L.; Hoffman, M.A.; Ginter, A.C.; Piontkowski, S.; Schexnayder, K.; White, R. The work life and career development of young breast cancer survivors. *J. Couns. Psychol.* **2015**, *62*, 655–669. [CrossRef] [PubMed]
57. Stone, D.S.; Pavlish, C.L.; Ganz, P.A.; Thomas, E.A.; Casillas, J.N.; Robbins, W.A. Understanding the Workplace Interactions of Young Adult Cancer Survivors With Occupational and Environmental Health Professionals. *Workplace Health Saf.* **2019**, *67*, 179–188. [CrossRef] [PubMed]
58. Stone, D.S.; Ganz, P.A.; Pavlish, C.; Robbins, W.A. Young adult cancer survivors and work: A systematic review. *J. Cancer Surviv.* **2017**, *11*, 765–781. [CrossRef] [PubMed]
59. Dumas, A.; Berger, C.; Auquier, P.; Michel, G.; Fresneau, B.; Allodji, R.S.; Haddy, N.; Rubino, C.; Vassal, G.; Valteau-Couanet, D.; et al. Educational and occupational outcomes of childhood cancer survivors 30 years after diagnosis: A French cohort study. *Br. J. Cancer* **2016**, *114*, 1060–1068. [CrossRef] [PubMed]
60. Dumas, A.; Cailbault, I.; Perrey, C.; Oberlin, O.; De Vathaire, F.; Amiel, P. Educational trajectories after childhood cancer: When illness experience matters. *Soc. Sci. Med.* **2015**, *135*, 67–74. [CrossRef]
61. Caumette, E.; Di Meglio, A.; Vaz-Luis, I.; Charles, C.; Havas, J.; de Azua, G.R.; Martin, E.; Vanlemmens, L.; Delaloge, S.; Everhard, S.; et al. Change in the value of work after breast cancer: Evidence from a prospective cohort. *J. Cancer Surviv. Res. Pract.* **2023**, *17*, 694–705. [CrossRef]
62. Laky, B.; Janda, M.; Kondalsamy-Chennakesavan, S.; Cleghorn, G.; Obermair, A. Pretreatment malnutrition and quality of life—Association with prolonged length of hospital stay among patients with gynecological cancer: A cohort study. *BMC Cancer* **2010**, *10*, 232. [CrossRef] [PubMed]
63. Lilly, C.M. Hospital Mortality, Length of Stay, and Preventable Complications Among Critically Ill Patients Before and After Tele-ICU Reengineering of Critical Care Processes. *JAMA* **2011**, *305*, 2175. [CrossRef] [PubMed]
64. Adler, N. Reaching for a Healthier Life: Facts on Socioeconomic Status and Health in the US. 2007. Available online: https://scholar.harvard.edu/davidrwilliams/reports/reaching-healthier-life (accessed on 1 September 2023).
65. Pedersen, K.J.; Boisen, K.A.; Midtgaard, J.; Elsbernd, A.; Larsen, H.B. Facing the Maze: Young Cancer Survivors' Return to Education and Work-A Professional Expert Key Informant Study. *J. Adolesc. Young Adult Oncol.* **2018**, *7*, 445–452. [CrossRef] [PubMed]
66. Davis, E.L.; Clarke, K.S.; Patterson, P.; Cohen, J. Using Intervention Mapping to Develop an Education and Career Support Service for Adolescents and Young Adults Diagnosed with Cancer: Identification of the Contextual Factors That Influence Participation in Education and Employment. *Cancers* **2022**, *14*, 4590. [CrossRef] [PubMed]
67. Braun, I.; Friedrich, M.; Morgenstern, L.; Sender, A.; Geue, K.; Mehnert-Theuerkauf, A.; Leuteritz, K. Changes, challenges and support in work, education and finances of adolescent and young adult (AYA) cancer survivors: A qualitative study. *Eur. J. Oncol. Nurs. Off. J. Eur. Oncol. Nurs. Soc.* **2023**, *64*, 102329. [CrossRef]
68. Jones, J.M.; Fitch, M.; Bongard, J.; Maganti, M.; Gupta, A.; D'agostino, N.; Korenblum, C. The Needs and Experiences of Post-Treatment Adolescent and Young Adult Cancer Survivors. *J. Clin. Med.* **2020**, *9*, 1444. [CrossRef]

Disclaimer/Publisher's Note: The statements, opinions and data contained in all publications are solely those of the individual author(s) and contributor(s) and not of MDPI and/or the editor(s). MDPI and/or the editor(s) disclaim responsibility for any injury to people or property resulting from any ideas, methods, instructions or products referred to in the content.

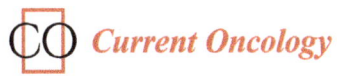

Article

Young Adults' Lived Experiences with Cancer-Related Cognitive Impairment: An Exploratory Qualitative Study

Sitara Sharma [1] and Jennifer Brunet [1,2,3,*]

1. School of Human Kinetics, University of Ottawa, Ottawa, ON K1N 6N5, Canada
2. Cancer Therapeutic Program, Ottawa Hospital Research Institute, The Ottawa Hospital, Ottawa, ON K1H 8L6, Canada
3. Institut du Savoir Montfort, Hôpital Montfort, Ottawa, ON K1N 6N5, Canada
* Correspondence: jennifer.brunet@uottawa.ca

Abstract: Cancer-related cognitive impairment (CRCI; e.g., disrupted memory, executive functioning, and information processing) affects many young adults, causing significant distress, reducing quality of life (QoL), and thwarting their ability to engage in professional, recreational, and social experiences. The purpose of this exploratory qualitative study was to investigate young adults' lived experiences with CRCI, and any strategies (including physical activity) they use to self-manage this burdensome side effect. Sixteen young adults (M_{age} = 30.8 ± 6.0 years; 87.5% female; $M_{years\ since\ diagnosis}$ = 3.2 ± 3) who reported clinically meaningful CRCI whilst completing an online survey were interviewed virtually. Four themes comprising 13 sub-themes were identified through an inductive thematic analysis: (1) *descriptions and interpretations of the CRCI phenomenon*, (2) *effects of CRCI on day-to-day and QoL*, (3) *cognitive–behavioural self-management strategies*, and (4) *recommendations for improving care*. Findings suggest CRCI is detrimental to young adults' QoL and must be addressed more systematically in practice. Results also illuminate the promise of PA in coping with CRCI, but research is needed to confirm this association, test how and why this may occur, and determine optimal PA prescriptions for young adults to self-manage their CRCI.

Keywords: cognition; exercise; oncology; interviews

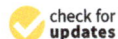

Citation: Sharma, S.; Brunet, J. Young Adults' Lived Experiences with Cancer-Related Cognitive Impairment: An Exploratory Qualitative Study. *Curr. Oncol.* **2023**, *30*, 5593–5614. https://doi.org/10.3390/curroncol30060422

Received: 8 May 2023
Revised: 5 June 2023
Accepted: 8 June 2023
Published: 9 June 2023

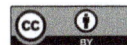

Copyright: © 2023 by the authors. Licensee MDPI, Basel, Switzerland. This article is an open access article distributed under the terms and conditions of the Creative Commons Attribution (CC BY) license (https:// creativecommons.org/licenses/by/ 4.0/).

1. Introduction

Annually, over one million young adults aged 18–39 years are diagnosed with cancer worldwide [1]. As their disease survival rate surpasses 80% [2], young adults are increasingly burdened with a host of physical and psychological sequelae that severely impair their daily functioning and quality of life (QoL) [3]. Cancer-related cognitive impairment (CRCI) is among the most common adverse effects reported by survivors across their lifespan [4], and is characterized by disturbances in mental processes related to thinking, reasoning, remembering, concentrating, learning, and processing information [5]. Since cognitive deficits often persist long after completion of treatment [6–8], many survivors experience significant psychological distress [9] and struggle with several emotional, interpersonal, and economic problems [10]. This is especially important to consider in a young adult population as unmanaged CRCI can disrupt their abilities to achieve major developmental milestones and establish functional roles in society [10]. However, published studies on CRCI have predominantly targeted middle-aged and older breast cancer survivors [5], and consequently, the extent and nature of young adults' CRCI experiences remain poorly understood, resulting in inadequate management of CRCI in practice.

Another limitation of previous studies pertains to the methods used to assess CRCI, which have largely been quantitative in nature and thus provide limited insight into young adults' lived experiences with this adverse effect. Given the clinical relevance of patient-reported outcome measures [11], self-report questionnaires are often used for cognitive assessment; the *European Organization for the Research and Treatment of Cancer Quality of Life*

Questionnaire (EORTC QLQ-C30; [12]), *Functional Assessment of Cancer Therapy—Cognitive Function* (FACT-Cog; [13]), and *Cognitive Failures Questionnaire* [14] are some popular examples. However, whilst most have shown evidence of reliability and validity [15], there are critical conceptual issues related to the content of the self-report measures employed in oncology research. For instance, the EORTC QLQ-C30 is one of the most commonly used self-report instruments for assessing cognition in cancer survivors [16,17]; however, it was designed to measure QoL and only comprises two items related to cognition [12]. Additionally, comparison of extant questionnaires reveals substantial heterogeneity with respect to their cognitive focus (e.g., memory, attention), and measures geared towards young adults are lacking [15]. This not only constitutes a problem for comparing research findings, but using such questionnaires alone fails to yield a rounded understanding of which aspects of/issues with cognitive (dys)function are relevant and important to young adult cancer survivors. Correspondingly, qualitative methods are best suited to uncover their experiences with CRCI. Such methods are attracting increasing interest in oncology (e.g., [18,19]) because they allow for a thick, in-depth description of a phenomenon and the capturing of complex experiences that may not otherwise be explored [20]. Selamat et al. [21] synthesized the sparse corpus of qualitative research on CRCI with breast cancer survivors, concluding that survivors struggle to adjust to/manage cognitive impairments and face hardship on multiple levels (i.e., emotional, psychological, social, occupational). Although these findings *may* translate to young adults, ramifications likely vary according to life stage. Thus, to better understand young adults' lived experiences with CRCI (including its specific burden on this group and potential self-management strategies), it is necessary to make use of qualitative methods.

Therapeutic options to prevent or treat CRCI remain elusive, but physical activity (PA) may help young adults *cope* with CRCI and/or *enhance* their cognition. The cognitive benefits of PA have been observed in several groups including healthy older adults [22], individuals with diseases of cognition (i.e., mild cognitive impairment, dementia) [23–25], and young persons with neurodevelopmental disorders (e.g., attention-deficit hyperactivity disorder) [26–28]. Studies have also shown promising results in cancer survivors. For instance, Galiano-Castillo et al. [29] reported improved performance on two neuropsychological tests assessing memory, executive functioning, and processing speed in middle-aged breast cancer survivors following a resistance PA intervention. Meanwhile, Gokal et al. [30] found improvements in self-reported cognition in middle-aged breast cancer survivors following a home-based aerobic PA intervention. Breast cancer survivors have also spoken in favour of PA as a behavioural strategy in a qualitative study [31], perceiving that it helped them reduce mental fatigue and improve mental clarity. Nevertheless, a major issue remains—evidence to support a link between PA and cognition in cancer survivors is mixed [17,32]. Therefore, qualitative inquiry into young adults' PA beliefs and experiences as they relate to self-management of CRCI may shed light on the causes of such mixed findings and offer suggestions for creating future PA-based CRCI interventions and supports for this population.

Current Study

The objectives of this qualitative study were twofold: (1) understand the lived experiences of young adults who report clinically meaningful CRCI after completing primary treatment for non-metastatic cancer, and (2) explore their use of strategies (including PA) to self-manage CRCI.

2. Materials and Methods
2.1. Design

This qualitative study was undertaken as part of a larger, mixed-methods observational study designed to explore how young adults experience and cope with CRCI after treatment, taking into consideration potential predisposing factors (i.e., medical, psychological), interventional strategies (i.e., PA), and outcomes (i.e., QoL) (quantitative results forthcoming). Both authors identify as women, and at the time of the study, they were a master's student and an Associate Professor in the School of Human Kinetics at the University of Ottawa. The reporting herein complies with the *Consolidated Criteria for Reporting Qualitative Studies (COREQ)* checklist [33] (see Supplementary File S1).

2.2. Participants and Procedures

Following approval from the University of Ottawa Research Ethics Board (H-05-21-6889—REG-6889), young adults were recruited via social media advertisement, online postings on relevant organizations' websites/newsletters, and word of mouth for the larger, mixed-methods study. Eligibility criteria were (1) cancer diagnosis between 15 to 39 years of age and currently aged 16 to 39 years, (2) completed primary treatment for non-metastatic cancer, (3) access to the Internet and audio–visual devices, and (4) ability to read, speak, and provide written informed consent in English. Young adults were ineligible to participate if they (1) had traumatic brain injury or concussion with residual symptoms (e.g., dizziness, headaches, loss of concentration) at the time of screening, (2) were actively taking selective serotonin reuptake inhibitor/serotonin norepinephrine reuptake inhibitor medication to treat a major mood disorder, and/or (3) received a diagnosis of a substance use disorder (e.g., alcohol, narcotics) by a medical professional within the past year. Participants were recruited from August 2021 to May 2022.

An overview of study flow for the larger mixed-methods study is presented in Figure 1. In short, after providing informed consent, participants undertook two quantitative assessments: first, they completed an online survey with multiple questionnaires including the *Functional Assessment of Cancer Therapy—Cognitive Function* (FACT-Cog; [13]), followed by a brief battery of three web-based neuropsychological tests hosted on the *Inquisit 6 Web* platform. For this qualitative study, purposive sampling was used. Specifically, on a rolling basis, participants' responses on the FACT-Cog were compared against clinically meaningful levels of cognitive impairment [34]; those who scored below 54 (out of a possible 72) on the 18-item *Perceived Cognitive Impairments* (PCI) subscale were invited via email to participate in a semi-structured interview. Sixteen of the 46 young adults enrolled in the larger study were invited, and all agreed to be interviewed (see Results for sample characteristics). At cessation of the larger study, participants were entered into a draw to win a CAD $100 gift card, with a total of three possible entries for each study component they began (i.e., survey, neuropsychological tests, interview).

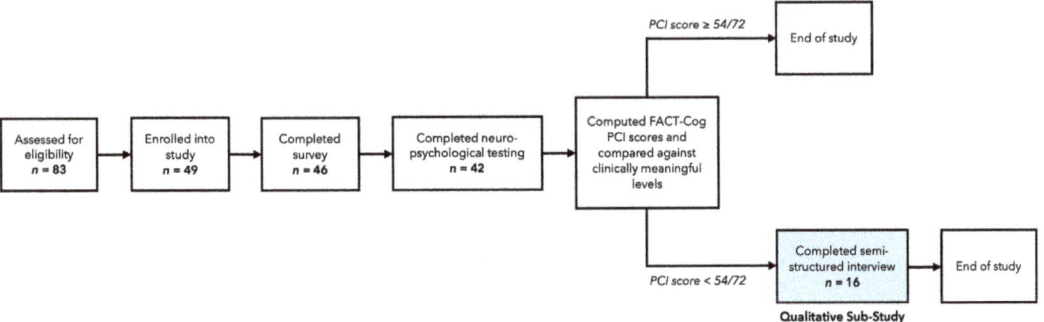

Figure 1. Overview of study flow.

2.3. Measures

2.3.1. Sociodemographic and Medical Characteristics

To describe the sample, participants were asked to self-report their age, sex, gender identity, self-identified ethnicity, civil status, highest level of education attained, household income, employment status, medication, substance-use (if applicable), cancer type and stage, date of cancer diagnosis, and cancer treatment history. Participants also rated their perceived health on a 5-point Likert scale ranging from 1 (*excellent*) to 5 (*poor*) using a single item from the *36-Item Short Form Health Survey* [35].

2.3.2. Self-Reported Cognitive Function

As mentioned above, the FACT-Cog (Version 3) [13] was used to assess self-reported cognitive function and identify participants for this study. The FACT-Cog is a 37-item measure designed specifically to assess cognitive impairment and its impact on QoL in cancer survivors over the past week. This questionnaire comprises four subscales (i.e., *PCI, Comments from Others, Perceived Cognitive Abilities,* and *Impact on QoL*) and responses are given using a 5-point Likert scale ranging from 0 (*never/not at all*) to 4 (*several times a day/very much*). While a total FACT-Cog score can be obtained by reverse-scoring negatively stated items and summing all items, only the 18-item PCI subscale score was used based on recommendations from scale developers (see the scoring document available at www.facit.org/measures/FACT-Cog, accessed on 15 May 2021) to select participants for interviews as described above. This specific subscale asks about difficulties related to forming thoughts, thinking, concentrating, remembering, communicating with others, reacting to situations, and both sustaining and shifting attention. Scores on the FACT-Cog (including PCI subscale scores) have been found to be reliable and valid, and this questionnaire has been used previously with various cancer populations [13,15].

2.3.3. PA

The *Leisure-Time Exercise Questionnaire* (LTEQ; [36]) was used to assess PA levels and describe the sample to provide context for interpreting PA-related data. The first item asks participants how often they engage in mild-, moderate-, and strenuous-intensity PA for a minimum of 15 mins during their leisure time in a typical week. As recommendations for cancer survivors are to accumulate at least 150 mins of moderate-to-vigorous-intensity aerobic training per week for health benefits (e.g., www.cancer.org/healthy/eat-healthy-get-active/get-active/fitting-in-fitness.html, accessed on 30 April 2022), frequency scores for moderate and vigorous PA were multiplied by a corresponding metabolic equivalent for task (MET) value (i.e., moderate ×5; vigorous ×9) and summed to obtain a moderate-to-vigorous-intensity PA (MVPA) Leisure Score Index (LSI). Based on published LSI cut-points [37], participants were classified as either *active* (MVPA LSI $\geq$ 24) or *insufficiently active* (MVPA LSI < 24). LTEQ scores have demonstrated reliability and validity with accelerometer data [38], and this measure has been widely used in studies with adult cancer survivors [39].

2.3.4. Interviews

The first author conducted individual semi-structured interviews with participants using an online platform (i.e., *Zoom*); these were audio-recorded and transcribed verbatim by SS within one week of the interview. On average, interviews lasted 69 mins (range = 42–91). The authors developed an interview guide with questions that focused on participants' lived experiences with, and self-management strategies (including PA) for CRCI. To prompt participants to share their experiences, they were asked questions that centered on: (1) how they viewed their cognitive function and/or impairment, (2) what they perceived as predisposing factors to their CRCI, (3) how they felt these impairments impacted their QoL, (4) how they cope with CRCI, and (5) their thoughts on PA as a self-management strategy. Participants were encouraged to deviate from the interview questions to discuss experiences that had significant meaning to them, and all interviews ended with an opportunity for participants to make final comments and/or add additional pertinent information. Moreover, probes were used when responses lacked sufficient detail, depth, or clarity [40], and follow-up questions were used to further pursue central themes, elaborate on the context of answers, and explore the implications of what was said. Sample questions and probes used during the interview are presented in Table 1. During and immediately after the interviews, the first author took field notes to document any contextual information and observations necessary for conducting a quality analysis.

Table 1. Example questions and probes from the semi-structured interview guide.

Question Categories	Example Questions and Probes
How participants viewed their cognitive function and/or difficulties.	Can you describe your current cognitive function? [Probe] What specific cognitive difficulties or impairments (e.g., impaired memory, attention, ability to process information, etc.) do you experience? Compared to before you were diagnosed, how do you think your cognitive function has changed over the course of your cancer journey? [Probes] After diagnosis? During treatment? Immediately after treatment? What about as time went on after treatment?
What they perceived as predisposing factors to their CRCI.	Do you think that being diagnosed when you were ___ years old and now being where you are in life influence how you experience your cognitive difficulties or impairments? How so? Do you think the cognitive difficulties or impairments you are experiencing are due to your specific cancer (i.e., ___) and/or the medications you have received, namely ___? Why/why not?
How they felt these impairments have impacted their QoL.	Can you tell me how the cognitive difficulties or impairments you mentioned have affected your emotional and/or psychological wellbeing? [Probe] Has this affected the way you see yourself? How?
How they cope with CRCI.	What strategies do you use to manage your cognitive difficulties or impairments? Why these? [Probe] Was/is physical activity one of such strategies? Why so? Why not?
Participants' thoughts on PA as a self-management strategy.	Do you believe PA can improve your cognitive function? Why/why not? [Probes] Do you feel that PA helps improve your memory? Attention? Processing speed? Any other specific cognitive domains? Why or why not? Has anyone ever recommended that you engage in physical activity to improve your cognitive function? If so, who? What did they say?

Notes. CRCI = cancer-related cognitive impairment; QoL = quality of life; PA = physical activity.

2.4. Interviewer

The interviewer (first author) was in her early 20s and had garnered research experience working with cancer survivors (including young adults) in the context of an exercise training/rehabilitation study. She had also received training in qualitative methods from the second author and as part of her graduate education. Her knowledge, skills, and experience made her ideally suited to develop rapport with participants and discuss their experiences with CRCI, as well as PA. Prior to the interviews, she pilot-tested the interview guide with a young adult cancer survivor who was selected purposively to help determine if questions were neutral, clear, flowed, and if it was feasible to conduct the interview in roughly one hour (to minimize participant burden). In doing so, she was also able to practice developing probes and follow-up questions. Data from this pilot interview were not included. However, based on feedback, she deleted one redundant question, re-arranged some for better flow, and made a note to begin each interview by defining "cognitive function" in lay terms to avoid confusion or misinterpretation of questions.

2.5. Sample Size

Given the lack of a definitive recommendation from experts for determining sample size in qualitative research, the criterion of data saturation [41] was used. That is, participants were approached and interviewed for this sub-study until no additional information appeared to be forthcoming; at this point, sampling was discontinued [42]. Saturation was achieved after the fifteenth interview; however, one additional interview was conducted with a participant who had expressed interest before recruitment was terminated, yielding a total sample size of 16.

2.6. Data Analysis

Interviews were transcribed using *NVivo Transcription* (Version 1.7.1). Transcripts were managed and analyzed in *Microsoft Word* (Version 2203) using inductive thematic analysis [43]. Analysis involved six steps: (1) familiarizing oneself with the data and generating initial codes, (2) systematically coding salient features of the raw data across all interviews that were relevant to the research objectives, (3) grouping similar codes to develop sub-themes, (4) reviewing and grouping similar sub-themes into main themes, (5) defining and naming themes and sub-themes to capture their essence, and (6) selecting compelling anonymized quotes from transcripts to illustrate each final theme/sub-theme and communicate participants' experiences in a meaningful way. The first author was responsible for the formal analysis, and the second author provided input at each step; accordingly, codes, themes, and sub-themes were revised following joint reflection. Transcripts were not returned to participants for comments or corrections, and participants did not provide feedback on the findings.

2.7. Study Rigour

Several strategies were undertaken during this study to enhance the rigor and trustworthiness of qualitative data. First, the interview guide was pilot tested with a young adult cancer survivor. Second, open-ended questions were asked to allow participants to express what they felt was important and expand upon/alter responses as they wished. Third, the interviewer developed rapport with participants by being empathetic and attentive throughout, which is key to a constructive qualitative interview [44]. Fourth, an exhaustive, systematic, and reflective analysis of the data was conducted by the first author, and the second author acted as a "critical friend" [45] during the development and reporting of themes/sub-themes to encourage consideration of multiple and alternative interpretations of the data. Importantly, while interpreting data, both authors took time to acknowledge and reflect upon any preconceptions, personal experiences, and prior knowledge of the literature. Finally, detailed descriptions of the research process and analyses have been provided above in accordance with the COREQ checklist [33] to ensure explicit, transparent reporting, along with the quotations below to give participants voice.

3. Results

3.1. Sample

Participants were between 23 to 39 years of age (M = 30.8 ± 6.0) (see Table 2 for characteristics). Most were born female (n = 14; 87.5%;), self-identified as women (n = 14; 87.5%;) and White (n = 12; 75%), single (n = 8; 50%), had completed post-secondary education (n = 15; 93.8%), were either working or transitioning into work (n = 10; 62.5%), and had an annual household income <CAD $100,000 ($n$ = 12; 75%). In terms of medical characteristics, participants were between 15 to 38 years of age at diagnosis (M = 27.6 ± 7.9), and their time since diagnosis ranged from 0 to 10 years (M = 3.2 ± 3). There was diversity in cancer stage, type, and treatments reported, but most were diagnosed with stage II cancer (n = 7; 43.8%), a hematological cancer (25%; n = 4), and received surgery as primary treatment (n = 13; 81.3%). Also, participants largely perceived their overall health as "good to very good" (n = 10; 62.5%). Previous concussion(s) and cannabis use within the past month was reported by two (12.5%) and seven (43.8%) participants, respectively. Also, participants were *insufficiently active* on average, based on their self-reported MVPA (M = 19 ± 12.7; range = 0–46); however, seven (43.8%) had a MVPA LSI score ≥ 24 (i.e., the established cut-point [37] for being classified as "active"). For a better understanding of the sample, the profiles of participants who were interviewed are noted in Table 3.

Table 2. Sociodemographic and medical characteristics for interviewed participants (*n* = 16).

Variables	Values
Sociodemographic Characteristics	
Current Age (M Years ± SD; Range)	30.8 ± 6.0; 23–39
Sex, *n* (% Female)	14 (87.5)
Gender Identity, *n* (% Woman)	14 (87.5)
Ethnicity, *n* (% White)	12 (75.0)
Civil Status, *n* (% Single)	8 (50)
Highest Level of Completed Education, *n* (% Post-secondary)	15 (93.8)
Vocational Status, *n* (% Working/Transitioning to Work)	10 (62.5)
Annual Household Income, *n* (% < CAD $100,000)	12 (75.0)
Medical Characteristics	
Age at Diagnosis (M years ± SD; range)	27.6 ± 7.9; 15–38
Time Since Diagnosis (M years ± SD; range)	3.2 ± 3.0; 0–10
Cancer Stage, *n* (%)	
I	1 (6.3)
II	7 (43.8)
III	3 (18.8)
N/A or "Do Not Know"	5 (31.3)
Cancer Type, *n* (%)	
Hematological	4 (25)
Breast	3 (18.8)
Sarcoma	3 (18.8)
Brain	2 (12.5)
Carcinoma	1 (6.3)
Gynecologic	2 (12.5)
Colorectal	0 (0)
Melanoma	1 (6.3)
Testicular	0 (0)
Treatments Received, *n* (%)	
Surgery	13 (81.3)
Chemotherapy	11 (68.8)
Radiation	9 (56.3)
Hormonal	3 (18.8)
Other	3 (18.8)
Perceived Overall Health, *n* (%)	
Poor to Fair	6 (37.5)
Good to Very Good	10 (62.5)
Excellent	0 (0)
Previous Concussion(s), *n* (%)	2 (12.5)
Cannabis Use in the Past Month, *n* (%)	7 (43.8)

Notes. SD = standard deviation.

Table 3. Profiles of interviewed participants (*n* = 16).

Participant Pseudonym	Sex	Age	Cancer Stage	Cancer Type	Cancer Treatment	PCI Score	MVPA LSI Score/Classification
Cole	M	25	II	Hematological	C + R	8	10/Insufficiently active
Emma	F	39	-[a]	Breast	S + C + R	17	10/Insufficiently active
Erica	F	28	II	Brain	S + C + R	48	25/Active
Eva	F	26	-[a]	Sarcoma	S + C + R	38	0/Insufficiently active
Ivy	F	32	-[a]	Brain	S	39	35/Active
Jack	M	26	II	Sarcoma	C + R	54 [b]	24/Active
Jaime	F	25	-[a]	Hematological	S + C	31	15/Insufficiently active
Lauren	F	25	-[a]	Sarcoma	S + C	51	33/Active
Layla	F	29	II	Hematological	C + R	41	24/Active
Mia	F	38	II	Carcinoma	S	35	25/Insufficiently active
Nina	F	36	I	Gynecologic	S	37	5/Insufficiently active
Peyton	F	27	III	Melanoma	S	29	12.5/Insufficiently active
Priya	F	38	III	Gynecologic	S + C	44	10/Active
Sarah	F	39	III	Breast	S + C + R	33	NR
Sydney	F	37	II	Breast	S + C + R	34	46/Active
Taylor	F	23	II	Hematological	S + C	37	10/Insufficiently active

Notes. C = chemotherapy; F = female; LSI = Leisure Score Index; M = male; MVPA = moderate-to-vigorous-intensity physical activity (LSI scores ≥ 24 = "active"; LSI scores < 24 = "insufficiently active"); NR = not reported; PCI = perceived cognitive impairment (subscale range: 0–72; scores <54/72 indicate clinically meaningful impairment); R = radiation therapy; S = surgery. [a] Reported as "not applicable" or "do not know". [b] Scored on the upper edge of the PCI cut-off value but was invited for an interview to gain male perspective.

3.2. Themes

As displayed in Figure 2, four themes comprising 13 sub-themes were developed based on the data: (1) *descriptions and interpretations of the CRCI phenomenon*, (2) *effects of CRCI on day-to-day and QoL*, (3) *cognitive–behavioural self-management strategies*, and (4) *recommendations for improving care*. Each theme is presented below, supported by quotations from individuals identified by pseudonyms. Of note, in the quotations, [. . .] indicates that text was omitted to enhance clarity.

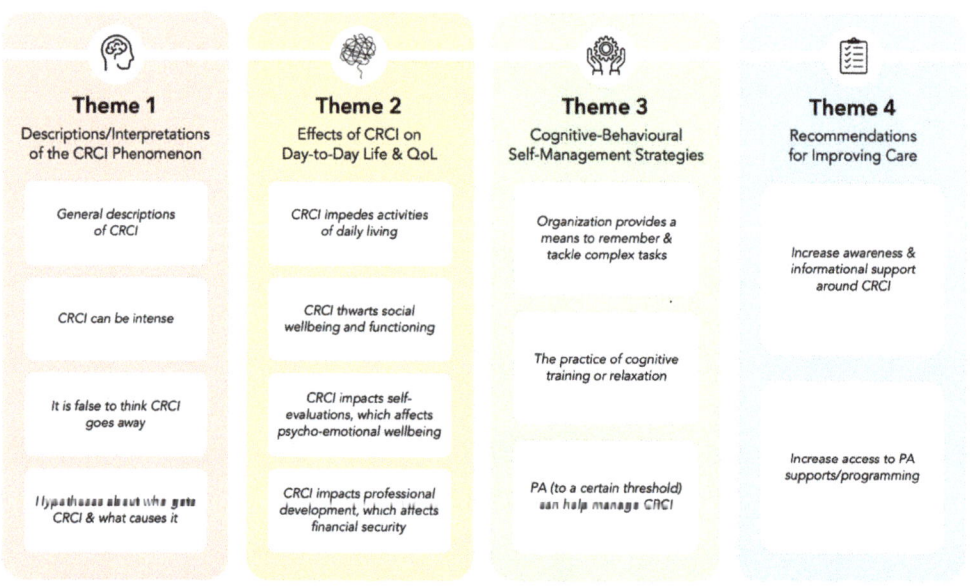

Figure 2. Main themes and sub-themes encompassing young adults' lived experiences with CRCI.

3.2.1. Theme 1: Descriptions and Interpretations of the CRCI Phenomenon

The first theme captures participants' thoughts about the origins, evolution, and meaning of CRCI following cancer treatment. These were organized into four sub-themes: *general descriptions of CRCI, CRCI can be intense, it is false to think CRCI always goes away,* and *hypotheses about who gets CRCI and what causes it*.

The *general descriptions of CRCI* sub-theme illustrates the meanings that participants ascribed to their cognitive impairment, which was painted out to be "fog"-like (Nina), a "constant cloud" (Jaime), and a "black hole" (Priya). According to Sydney, CRCI makes "everything [feel] like it's been muted a bit . . . like . . . when you're sick and your brain's just not moving quite at [the right] speed". She went on to say, "I feel like that all the time, but I'm not sick anymore". Participants illuminated troubles with their memory, word recollection, concentration, and ability to both process and learn information. For Jack and Mia respectively, these deficits added "a layer of difficulty" to everything and made it feel as if she "can't trust [her] brain".

As reflected within the *CRCI can be intense* sub-theme, participants' cognitive impairment often presented frequently and with considerable severity. Lauren remarked, "It's hard to say how frequently I have *actual* issues, but . . . it comes to my attention that I am having this problem . . . at least once or twice a week". Others affirmed struggling with cognitive impairment even more often; that is, either "multiple times a week" (Peyton) or "pretty much every day" (Nina). CRCI was such a constant for Jack that he explained, "I basically build the way that I interact around [CRCI]". When asked to describe their CRCI severity on a scale from 0 to 10, ratings ranged from "two" (Erica) to "severely . . . 10"

(Ivy), although most felt it landed right in the middle of the scale. On average, as Peyton explained, "it bothers me, obviously, but . . . I can still live my life around it". Further, CRCI severity was described to be fluid, such that "some days might be less [severe] than others" (Layla), and that "it's definitely worse [on] the days that [they] do more" (Sarah).

The *it is false to think CRCI goes away* sub-theme encompasses an unfortunate reality. Cognitive impairment was most pronounced during primary treatment and immediately after it had ended. Participants described a "rapid drop" (Jack) in their cognitive function during treatment that was "consuming" (Layla). Indeed, in recalling her experience during this time, Emma said, "I don't think I was functioning at all cognitively". Whilst unsurprising as participants all self-reported clinically meaningful CRCI, cognitive difficulties were typically worse during and immediately after treatment, but many continued to struggle post-treatment. Cole explained that his CRCI got "progressively worse," while others characterized CRCI as dynamic. For instance, Mia explained that her cognitive function changed "in waves," wherein it vacillated between improving and worsening depending on adjustments to medication. Others also noted that their cognitive function continuously changed and that "it's been better than during treatment . . . but it's definitely not a huge improvement" (Emma). Importantly, while slight-to-moderate improvements in cognitive function were discussed, participants largely credited these to "work[ing] really hard" (Layla) to adjust to and self-manage their CRCI because they accepted cognitive impairment as a permanent side effect that they needed to get used to. As Peyton exemplified, "I don't know . . . if [my cognitive function is] getting better, or if I'm just getting . . . used to living with how my brain works".

Finally, the *hypotheses about who gets CRCI and what causes it* sub-theme reflects that participants largely attributed CRCI to treatments received; since individuals diagnosed with different cancers (i.e., type, stage) receive common treatments (e.g., chemotherapy, radiation therapy, surgery, medications), participants felt that CRCI could affect *anybody* receiving treatment. Highlighting this, Emma said, "I think treatment . . . " when speaking to the causes. She then added, "I feel like its [affected] everybody that I've talked to". Likewise, Lauren said, "My guess is that people experience [CRCI] with cancer treatment in general. I don't know if that has to do with the fact that you're given like, so many drugs . . . and all that just messes with your brain . . . I feel like in general, cancer patients . . . have some sort of cognitive issues related to treatment".

3.2.2. Theme 2: Effects of CRCI on Day-to-Day Life and QoL

The second theme demonstrates that participants explicitly linked CRCI to QoL and reveals its tremendous, multidimensional burden. Specifically, participants noted that when cognitive troubles manifested, their physical, social, psycho-emotional, and professional wellbeing and functioning were adversely impacted. Consequences were grouped into four sub-themes: *CRCI impedes activities of daily living, CRCI thwarts social wellbeing and functioning, CRCI impacts self-evaluations which affects psycho-emotional wellbeing*, and *CRCI obstructs professional development which affects financial security*.

The *CRCI impedes activities of daily living* sub-theme captures how CRCI thwarts one's ability to undertake instrumental activities of daily living (IADL); that is, key life tasks needed to live independently and maintain health. Participants described basic tasks such as cooking and housekeeping as challenging because "everything takes more focus, more work" (Sarah) and because they would get easily distracted. For instance, Peyton said, "baking . . . cooking . . . laundry . . . it just takes longer to do stuff and [requires] being more thorough because I have to like, go back and make sure, or like, re-read or that kind of stuff". Due to the extra time and effort required to complete such tasks, participants often had less time for engaging in PA; as Taylor conveyed, "Stuff takes longer for me . . . [so] I don't leave enough time for my walks". Additionally, some neglected basic self-care due to their cognitive struggles, saying "this sounds so gross, but I'd forget to brush my teeth, or I would forget to eat breakfast or something like that" (Erica). Participants also mentioned difficulties with upholding personal values such as being punctual. Sarah said,

"I was never late for anything before . . . Now I'm late for everything and I hate it. It's like there's not enough time in a day for me to get through anything. I just seem like I'm failing a lot". Moreover, driving was discussed as another common IADL affected by CRCI. Particularly due to difficulties with focusing and processing situations, participants limited or stopped driving out of apprehension for threatening the physical safety of oneself and others. Priya remarked, "I've been really nervous about . . . driving just because I feel like my reaction time is kind of slow . . . like if someone ran out in front of my car or turned suddenly, would I be able to react as fast as I could before?" Mirroring this hesitation, Sarah said, "There has been a couple times driving where . . . I just have come home because I know that I shouldn't be out there because I can't focus enough. Or I've had a close call or something, right? Where I'm like, 'Hey . . . I'm not here.' So there ha[ve] been those days where I just shut it down".

The *CRCI thwarts social wellbeing and functioning* sub-theme reflects that CRCI strained relationships with others (e.g., romantic, familial, friendships) as it often caused communication struggles and left individuals feeling misunderstood. For example, Sydney said, "I do need more time to process . . . [than my] very quick-thinking partner . . . that alone is frustrating. I mean, that's basically the crux of like all of our communication problems". Further, Mia mentioned that she "ha[s] a father who . . . doesn't understand being forgetful. He doesn't understand that [CRCI] is something that I'm dealing with so he'll get upset, saying that I don't remember something because I don't want to do it". Lack of understanding and negative comments from others were also discussed by Lauren, who explained, "I would get very hurt when people would tell me . . . 'Oh, you don't remember this?' . . . my memory is not as great . . . it's hard for the people in my life to understand that". Moreover, participants described feeling like a "bad friend" (Taylor) because CRCI made it difficult for them to be as thoughtful or to recall memories and details about loved ones' lives. Collectively, cognitive difficulties created "an internal barrier" (Emma) that inhibited social engagement and led to self-isolation for participants. For instance, Sarah said, "Because I can't articulate how I feel, I just avoid . . . some of my family . . . . They don't understand". Similarly, Nina expressed, "Sometimes when I can't put a sentence together, I feel really ridiculous and then it kind of makes you not want to talk to people because you feel like . . . they're probably thinking, 'Oh my gosh, what's going on with her?' So . . . maybe I am a little bit more isolating myself".

The *CRCI impacts self-evaluations which affects psycho-emotional wellbeing* sub-theme captures the heavy inward struggles and distress that CRCI causes. Participants perceived themselves as "a failure" (Emma), a "damaged version" of themselves (Taylor), and "like a shell of . . . what [they] once thought [they] were" (Peyton) due to their CRCI. Importantly, their damaged self-concept and identity often stemmed from feeling less intelligent than prior to their cancer experience and gave rise to many negative emotions and thoughts. Sarah shared, "It makes you insecure . . . You don't recognize your brain, right? All the things that you grew up learning how to study and knowing how to do . . . they don't work anymore . . . It's very unnerving . . . not being who you were and not being as smart as you were". Correspondingly, Layla expressed, "My memory was quite sharp . . . I always got high grades. So, it was really, really disappointing. I think [CRCI] took a lot of my identity. I lost a lot of my confidence in myself and developed a lot of imposter syndrome . . . Initially, [CRCI] was really, really upsetting . . . I went home and cried every day . . . it was just so hard and frustrating". Paradoxically, negative emotions and thoughts further fueled cognitive troubles, suggesting that the connection between CRCI and psychological distress is bidirectional, or as Taylor put it, a "vicious cycle". Jack explained "I think it happens in both directions. I think if I'm having issues with my cognition, I feel depressed and slow and low. And conversely if I'm having anxiety . . . I'm so hyper-focused on those things that I can't pay attention well, I get distracted, I can't remember what's going on . . . I think they feed all on each other like writhing massive snakes".

Finally, the *CRCI obstructs professional development which affects financial security* sub-theme encapsulates the toll CRCI takes on work/school performance and motivation to pursue vocational opportunities. Nina exemplified this when she said, "I did decide to step back a little bit from work because I felt like I ... couldn't function [cognitively] ... I can't make mistakes in my work ... I've cut down my hours. So yeah, it affected me financially ... And it's frustrating because, like, if I was in my 50s or 60s, I'd probably be retired, and I wouldn't have to work. It wouldn't matter, you know? But it matters right now for me because I'm so young ... I probably have to work another twenty years". As Nina alluded to, young adults bear many financial responsibilities, making this consequence of CRCI especially taxing for them. Moreover, based on the survey data collected, four (25%) participants were currently unemployed or on medical leave, and they described CRCI as a barrier to return to work or school. Cole explained, "It's been very hard to be able to consistently stay with like a full-time job ... There's so much to learn ... There's so many mistakes that you can make in a day ... It just seems that every attempt has been futile for me". Others postponed return to work or ceased their job searches out of fear or discouragement that it would "take [them] longer to finish tasks" (Eva) and ultimately, that they would not "bring value to the team" (Peyton). As Mia said, "It's not fair to a new employer for me to go there and have all of this confusion and everything until I'm all sorted out".

3.2.3. Theme 3: Cognitive–Behavioural Self-Management Strategies

The third theme reflects the cognitive–behavioural self-management strategies participants used to self-manage their CRCI. The strategies described herein were used to help participants cope or to improve their ability to remember, focus, and tackle complex tasks. Of note, none of the strategies were unanimously used, highlighting the personal nature of dealing with CRCI and the potential need for tailored interventions. Despite the diversity in use, strategies are captured within three non-exclusive sub-themes: *organization provides a means to remember and tackle complex tasks, the practice of cognitive training or relaxation, and PA (to a certain threshold) can help self-manage CRCI*.

The *organization provides a means to remember and tackle complex tasks* sub-theme captures the various organizational methods and tools participants used to help them self-manage their CRCI (in some cases), specifically by helping to jog their memory and reserve their cognitive energy. To help manage troubles with memory, participants described "stick[ing] to a routine" (Mia), scheduling "everything in a calendar" with constant reminder alerts (Sarah), "writ[ing] everything down" (Emma), and essentially, as Jaime explained, "putting [stuff] somewhere that's not inside my head". However, for others, "calendars and all that stuff ... just doesn't work" (Cole) because ironically, they were often forgotten or misplaced. For instance, Jack said, "I try and make lists and then a few days later, I forget that I made a list. And then a few months later, I'm going through, like erasing iPhone notes and going, 'Oh, I was supposed to do this or that' ... So, I do make lists, but I'm not successful at using them". Beyond routines, scheduling, and notes/lists, participants mentioned organizing their days intentionally to undertake certain tasks when their cognitive function was at its "best". For example, Layla mentioned, "I know that I have better [cognitive] function in the morning. So, [I try] putting more complex things in the beginning of my day versus trying to do them in the afternoon because I'm exhausted and I ... don't have the capacity as much". Overall, organization was used as a tool to help manage (not improve) poor memory and attention.

The *practice of cognitive training or relaxation* sub-theme captures techniques that participants used to help them better remember and focus. On one hand, some participants integrated different cognitively demanding games/activities into their routines to "get [their] brain[s] working" (Taylor). Erica touched on many of them when saying that "listening to podcasts and that kind of thing... keep[s] my brain working. One thing that I got really into during treatment ... is sudoku puzzles ... just remembering those little things I thought was really good practice ... It made me focus and ... utilize my short-term memory". Similarly, Taylor said, "I started to play a lot of solitaire on my phone ... sometimes I feel like it helps me to like, get my brain working". Other examples Taylor gave included not "turn[ing] on [TV] subtitles so that [she had] to focus more" and "try[ing] to use . . . scientific papers that are in English [when conducting research for university] so that it's harder" (as English is not her first language). Conversely, others wanted to calm their brains through cognitive relaxation techniques which helped them enhance focus and memory while also reducing stress. For instance, Erica cited, "Meditation is like my number one [strategy] . . . it is amazing. It has all these benefits . . . I find my memory is better," and Ivy described that a simple five-minute guided meditation session helped her go "from being, like, very frazzled and fe[eling] like [her] head [is] being pulled in a million different directions to . . . just like, all of a sudden [feeling that things were] manageable . . . it helps put the pieces in order".

Finally, the *PA (to a certain threshold) can help manage CRCI* sub-theme captures that PA was used for various purposes, including allowing participants to better concentrate, remember, and "not be stuck in that . . . weird foggy state as much" (Priya). As shared by Jack and Erica, respectively, "I can [focus] whenever I come back from exercise, I get so much done . . . I'm just more successful," and "I find that the days that I've gone to the gym the day before . . . I feel like my memory is better . . . I feel more alert". Emma found that PA "definitely helped [her] brain" and made it easier for her to tackle tasks that were otherwise difficult. Furthermore, Ivy mentioned that the act of counting strokes and focusing on her breath while swimming (i.e., incorporating mindfulness) helped calm her brain and thus provided some relief from her cognitive struggles, tying into the above sub-theme. She said, "For me, [when I swim laps] . . . the counting of strokes and breath . . . it's just so meditative . . . [I feel] mental effects and benefits". Critically, the key was to engage in PA that was not too intense or undertaken too often to avoid overexertion, as this could lead to cognitive fatigue. For instance, Emma mentioned, "If I push myself too hard [during PA], I'm just done. Like everything—physically, emotionally, cognitively, it's just like total body shutdown . . . I am trying to learn the window where it feels good, when it's not too much". Similarly, Layla explained, "I started working out with a personal trainer in the summer . . . if I worked out too many days . . . the physical fatigue contribute[d] to increased brain fog . . . I tried working out . . . 3–4 times a week, and I had to cut it back to twice a week because . . . it was too much physically, and it really impacted my brain". However, Layla went on to say, "I think other than the overexertion and getting to the fatigue point . . . I feel good in myself . . . [PA] helps with . . . your mental health, and then that translates into having better cognitive function". Although PA was not something used by all to self-manage CRCI, even those *not* using PA as a strategy believed the benefits of PA likely extend to cognitive function. As Sydney conveyed, "PA clears your mind, so I can certainly . . . see the link [between PA and cognitive function]". However, PA was not something that everyone knew how to engage in, which was clear when Sydney went on to say "I don't know exactly . . . which type of PA . . . or if there's kind of a strategy of 'you should be doing *these* five things' and 'you work them in *this* order' or whatever . . . But . . . I can see the reason that they would be linked for sure".

3.2.4. Theme 4: Recommendations for Improving Care

Participants unanimously described feeling ill-informed about CRCI and did not believe they "ha[d] the tools necessary in place that would have helped" (Cole) to navigate this challenging side effect. As such, they provided recommendations for improving care, which are captured within this final theme. Suggestions for successful survivorship were grouped into two sub-themes: *increased informational support around CRCI* and *greater access to PA supports/programming*.

The *increased informational support around CRCI* sub-theme captures participants' desires for more systematic awareness and information around CRCI. Sarah expressed, "I think the more awareness we have that this is a real thing that all cancer patients go through, we won't feel so alienated by it". Likewise, Eva said, "Difficulty focusing . . . memory issues . . . [health professionals] don't tell you about these things and you don't expect it, and then it actually happens to you. You feel like something's wrong with you when it's not.

So, I think it's important to discuss that with you". Many echoed that they felt they were left to understand and heal with cognitive impairment via "trial and error" (Peyton); thus, Mia remarked, "It would have been better if [health professionals] said, '*These* are some of the symptoms that you may have. If you run into these, *these* are some of the coping strategies you can deal with,' instead of leaving it up to me to go onto these Facebook groups". By the same token, Layla remarked "I think preparing people in advance for [CRCI] would be helpful ... Medical professionals need ... to help with cognitive strategies ... To be like, 'Yeah, so you may just have to write things down more.' Like I know ... it should be intuitive, but it wasn't in that moment. So, like ... 'Write things down more,' 'chunk things up in your day' ... 'have [complex] things in the morning.' Like those things would have been really really helpful tips because you're dealing with something that you've never thought about or you never had to do".

The *greater access to PA supports/programming* sub-theme reflects participants' overwhelming desire for PA support during and following cancer treatment (both for CRCI self-management purposes and general health reasons) as it was often not presented as an option or was inaccessible to them. In relation to CRCI, Taylor explained, "[My friend] was prescribed physiotherapy during her treatment ... Her cognitive function, I would say, is better than mine ... She always had to do workouts during treatment, but when I was in treatment, they were like 'Just stay in bed and just rest.' And they told her 'You should move. You should go out of the house at least once every day.' I feel like if my doctors would have told me the same ... that I would definitely have increased my cognitive function or made it less worse". More broadly, participants mentioned that they would have liked more dialogue and information around the benefits of PA and how to engage in it safely and effectively. For instance, Priya said, "It would have been really helpful if the doctor had more of a conversation about PA ... Like providing some kind of tips or even directing people to some resources". In parallel, Layla said, "Some sort of ... graphic info sheet that had either organizations you could access ... as well as information on PA, the importance of it, how much PA cancer patients should be doing, or what activities they should be partaking in versus what's contraindicated ... would be helpful ... I think ... when people are [doing] really, really poorly and they're trying to incorporate exercise, they need to know distance and frequency and timing and that kind of stuff to help". Furthermore, participants believed that help from PA professionals (e.g., kinesiologists) in creating detailed, individualized PA plans would be beneficial in setting them (and future young adults) up for success following cancer treatment. As Sydney mentioned, "An actual recommendation to say, 'We'd like to have you work with somebody to set up what would be a good physical exercise plan for you' ... would go pretty far".

4. Discussion

The purpose of this qualitative study was to better understand young adults' lived experiences with, and self-management strategies for CRCI after completing primary cancer treatment. Overall, results encapsulated by Themes 1 and 2 extend previous research describing the adverse impacts of CRCI on cancer survivors, both in general, and for young adults specifically. Findings captured within Theme 3 support the continued investigation into several cognitive–behavioural strategies (i.e., organization, cognitive training or relaxation, PA) that may help young adults manage this burdensome side effect and suit different preferences. Finally, Theme 4 emphasizes the significance of acknowledging CRCI in research and practice, and the critical need for greater support.

4.1. CRCI Is Consequential for Young Adults

Results revealed the multidimensional consequences that clinically meaningful CRCI has for young adults' QoL, including diminished daily functioning and independence, social and psycho-emotional well-being, professional capabilities, and financial health. This aligns with previous research involving adolescent and young adult cancer survivors [46–49] and breast cancer survivors [50–53]. Additionally, results suggest a bidirectional relationship (or "vicious cycle") between CRCI and psychological outcomes (e.g., depressive symptoms, anxiety, perceived stress). Whilst shown to be associated [8,9,54–58], the lack of longitudinal studies (with repeated measures) that test the two causal directions between CRCI and psychological distress limits confirmation of a bidirectional association, and research exploring underpinning mechanisms (e.g., psychosocial, physiological) is also scarce; these gaps warrant future investigation.

Further, results illuminated that clinically meaningful CRCI affects young adults' views of themselves. This is not surprising as cancer influences young adults' self-evaluations and identify [59]. Current findings add that CRCI can leave young adults feeling less intelligent and threaten their sense of self, which can in turn hinder their vocational aspirations and success [60]. Seeing as young adults constitute a substantial proportion of the workforce [61], such feelings can represent a larger societal issue. Therefore, considering the pressures and difficulties participants described around resuming vocational pursuits after treatment, along with evidence that CRCI can impede occupational re-integration, reduce work capability, and cause job loss [47–50,52,62], it is crucial to help young adult cancer survivors maintain positive views of themselves. Investigating reasons behind such views will aid in identifying risk and protective factors to target when designing supportive care for young adults with clinically meaningful CRCI.

Finally, findings show discordance between young adults' lived experiences and current CRCI measures which lack appraisal of a seemingly important construct—sense of self. This indicates a need to expand CRCI measures designed to capture its impact (e.g., FACT-Cog [13]), and involving young adults in their development/refinement may help increase relevancy. Relatedly, conceptual definitions of CRCI are simplistic and researcher-developed, but results suggest they can be modified to better capture the nuanced meanings young adults ascribe to their cognitive impairment. To do so and escape the limitations of postpositivist epistemologies, qualitative studies are necessary; arguably, these could also be used to build a theoretical framework of CRCI for young adults to support future research and practice.

4.2. Self-Managing CRCI

Similar to research with breast cancer survivors [21], results revealed that young adults with clinically meaningful CRCI struggle to understand, adjust to, and cope with their CRCI given a lack of informational support or resources; this forced many to explore compensatory cognitive–behavioural strategies on their own. As with previous findings [31,50], participants relied heavily on *external* organizational strategies (e.g., to-do lists, scheduling, setting alerts) as memory aids; however, others forgot about or misplaced the very tools they relied on to help them better remember, suggesting such strategies may not suit everyone. Instead, young adults may need to be taught how to use *internal* strategies (e.g., rehearsing/repeating/visualizing information, creating mnemonics/rhymes) to facilitate deeper information association and processing and thus help compensate for memory difficulties, as suggested in research with other populations (e.g., mild cognitive impairment, traumatic brain injury, stroke) [63]. Identifying which strategies work "best" for whom and under what circumstances would help inform decision making.

Also consistent with past studies [50,51,64,65], cognitive training (i.e., "exercising the brain" through mentally challenging games/tasks [e.g., solitaire, sudoku]) was used to manage troubles related to memory and focus. This is unsurprising given that "brain training" has received growing attention in media and research, and several mobile applications claiming to maintain/increase cognitive skills (e.g., *Lumosity, Elevate, CogniFit*) are available [66]. Systematic reviews of CRCI studies with adults [67] and breast cancer survivors [68] have identified cognitive training as an effective *rehabilitation* strategy for strengthening specific cognitive domains. Pilot data from adolescent and young adult cancer survivors [69] suggests it may also be a feasible, possibly beneficial CRCI *prehabilitation* tool; however, evidence is needed to confirm the effectiveness of cognitive training in young adults. Likewise, cognitive relaxation techniques were seen as beneficial to "calm the brain" (and in turn, help improve memory), supporting prior research (e.g., [70]). Whilst meditation was the only technique explicitly mentioned by participants, several others (e.g., mindfulness-based stress reduction [71,72], biofeedback [73], imagery [74]) have been investigated as CRCI interventions in breast and mixed cancer groups and elicited improvements in perceived cognition. As with cognitive training, research is needed to generate evidence on the effectiveness of cognitive relaxation techniques in young adults. Exploring underpinning mechanisms may also help understand how to target specific cognitive domains.

Furthermore, aligning with evidence from adolescent and young adult cancer survivors [75,76] and breast cancer survivors [31], findings emphasize that PA may be an effective CRCI self-management strategy for young adults. Indeed, feeling more focused, alert, and able to remember following bouts of PA were cited as cognitive benefits, and even those who did *not* use PA as an explicit strategy believed it *could* help manage CRCI. This suggests young adults might be willing to engage in PA for their cognitive and mental well-being, and thus, PA-based interventions for ameliorating CRCI should be developed and evaluated. However, not all PA interventions have conferred cognitive benefits (e.g., [77,78]), and some participants herein said not all PA was "good". To inform effective PA intervention design for CRCI, several questions remain, including: *how much PA is needed to induce cognitive benefits, what types/combinations are most beneficial, and how long do the effects of PA last on cognition?* Regarding the latter, as previously suggested [79], the potential cognitive benefits of PA may be more acute than long-lasting. Thus, researchers may wish to investigate the effects of daily PA on young adults' cognition using *Ecological Momentary Assessment* methodology [80] to see if cognitive benefits from PA are indeed acute and/or sustainable.

Interestingly, some participants enjoyed *mindful* PA (i.e., PA involving a heightened sense of attention; e.g., Qigong, yoga), whereas others alluded to benefits following gym-based resistance training; if well-practiced, the latter could be considered a form of *mindless* PA (i.e., PA that allows automaticity to take over). That said, the relative effects of mindful versus mindless PA remain unclear. Diamond and Ling [81] proposed that PA with a cognitive load (i.e., mental effort) may lead to "better" executive functioning than mindless PA; however, this hypothesis has been criticized due to a lack of empirical evidence [82]. Also, the current findings suggest that (a) individuals may prefer one type over the other, and (b) there could be cognitive benefits to both that go beyond executive functioning. Whilst questions on this topic were not asked in this study, findings suggest it may be fruitful to compare the effects of mindful and mindless PA on various cognitive domains in a larger sample of young adult cancer survivors and across different contexts.

While the theory that PA involving a cognitive load is superior to PA with a lesser cognitive component requires substantiation, participants herein used cognitive training or relaxation *and* PA as forms of self-management. This raises the question: *Can additive cognitive effects be experienced by combining these interventions?* Although such work is lacking in oncology, a recent systematic review concluded that PA programs enriched with mental challenges (e.g., exergaming, tai chi, dance) helped improve cognition in older adults with/without mild cognitive impairment [83]. Studies conducted across different groups further support the notion that combining cognitive training with PA may be more beneficial for the brain than PA alone (e.g., [84,85]); it is worth exploring if similar results map onto the young adult cancer population. Conversely, some have examined the effects of mindfulness-based interventions *compared to* PA on CRCI and reported cognitive improvements in both groups (e.g., [86]), but little is known about the impact of combining cognitive relaxation techniques with PA—another area requiring future research.

Nonetheless, certain barriers may stand in the way of young adults' PA participation. This study suggests CRCI can serve as a barrier due to the extra time and effort required to complete essential daily tasks when struggling with this adverse effect. As evidence grows in support of the positive effect(s) of PA on cognition in cancer survivors (e.g., [75,76,87–102]), more messaging is needed to inform young adults about its benefits as a way to help them increase motivation and perhaps overcome barriers. Relatedly, drawing on the *Health Belief Model* [103] for predicting and explaining health behaviours, researchers should aim to identify and understand young adult cancer survivors' perceived benefits, barriers, and self-efficacy in regards to engaging in PA for their brain health; this may help guide the creation of preliminary PA-based CRCI self-management for this group.

Finally, it is worth cautioning young adult cancer survivors that engaging in "too much" PA may compromise their cognition, as participants believed it caused or exacerbated mental fatigue. Drawing on sport psychology models (e.g., *Individual Zones for Optimal Functioning Model* [104,105]) that posit athletic performance is optimal up until/within a certain individualized zone of arousal, there may be an individualized threshold for which PA induces optimal cognitive effects based on one's level of mental fatigue. This may require that healthcare practitioners encourage young adults to actively monitor themselves over time to determine their mental "sweet spot," and engage in PA at this point. Moreover, building off the emerging practice of "personalized medicine" [106] which aims to tailor care based on individual differences (e.g., genes, environment), it would be valuable to study how to match young adults to the right PA parameters (e.g., frequency, intensity) so they may feel cognitive benefits and avoid mental fatigue.

4.3. Limitations and Future Directions

Although this study makes important contributions, it is not without limitations. First, the sample was predominantly comprised of women who were White, had completed post-secondary education, and had an annual household income above CAD $100,000; thus, results from this sample may not be transferable to all cancer survivors. Researchers should aim to adopt more diverse recruitment strategies that allow for maximum sample variation. Second, results predominantly captured the experiences of those who underwent chemotherapy exposure. To better target and understand the CRCI experiences of a wider young adult population, researchers should aim to recruit young adults who undergo anti-cancer treatments other than chemotherapy. Third, this sample had a large range in time since diagnosis (0–10 years); although perspectives were consistent across participants in this study, they may differ across others with shorter versus longer times since diagnosis. Researchers may wish to consider splitting analyses by time groups (e.g., one, five, ten years) and employing longitudinal designs to better understand the evolution of CRCI. Likewise, variations that stem from other personal (e.g., age, life events) and sociocultural (e.g., ethnicity, sociodemographic status) experiences may influence how these themes present across other individuals and require future purposive sampling and cohort research. Fourth, most (62.5%) participants perceived their overall health as "good to very good" and the sample was generally classified as "active" based on their self-reported PA; future studies are needed to confirm if the themes reported herein are similar or differ from those with young adults who do *not* view themselves as healthy or active. Fifth, there are inherent limitations to using self-report measures (e.g., social desirability, recall bias) whereby participants may have under- or over-estimated their perceived cognitive impairments and thus influenced who was invited for an interview. Also, since inclusion criteria for this study included scoring below a certain threshold on the FACT-Cog PCI subscale, if only one cognitive dimension (e.g., memory) was affected, it could have been masked with the overall PCI score. Sixth, the sample may be biased towards those with greater computer literacy and/or ability to spend time online given the methods used, suggesting the need to enhance accessibility of future virtual studies for those with CRCI. Finally, there is inherent subjectivity in thematic analysis wherein the researchers' own biases and assumptions could have affected identification and interpretation of the themes/subthemes presented, although several steps were undertaken to mitigate this risk (see Study Rigour above).

5. Conclusions

The results show that young adults with clinically meaningful CRCI face deleterious consequences for their daily and overall QoL and suggest they experience CRCI differently than older cancer cohorts (i.e., those whom current definitions of CRCI are currently based on). Moreover, the findings reveal that young adults use several cognitive–behavioural strategies including organization, cognitive training and relaxation, and PA, highlighting that "one size may not fit all" when it comes to managing CRCI. This provides support for continuing to investigate how different forms of self-management (in isolation and in combination) may elicit cognitive benefits to appeal to the preferences of a wider range of survivors. Findings from this study also add to the growing body of research exploring links between cognitive function and PA and suggest more high-quality experimental research is needed to test the putative mechanisms underlying potential benefits of PA as well as optimal PA dosages/contexts. Last, this study lays important groundwork for creating CRCI-self-management supports for this underrepresented population and reinforces that young adults would benefit from more systematic awareness, assessment, and monitoring of CRCI in healthcare.

Supplementary Materials: The following supporting information can be downloaded at: https://www.mdpi.com/article/10.3390/curroncol30060422/s1, File S1: Consolidated Criteria for Reporting Qualitative Research (COREQ) Checklist.

Author Contributions: Conceptualization, S.S. and J.B.; Methodology, S.S. and J.B.; Formal Analysis, S.S.; Investigation, S.S.; Resources, J.B.; Data Curation, S.S.; Writing—Original Draft Preparation, S.S.; Writing—Review & Editing, S.S. and J.B.; Visualization, S.S. and J.B.; Supervision, J.B.; Project Administration, S.S. All authors have read and agreed to the published version of the manuscript.

Funding: This research received no external funding. This manuscript was prepared while SS was supported by a SSHRC Canada Graduate Scholarship and JB was supported by a Canada Researcher Chair Tier II in Physical Activity Promotion for Cancer Prevention and Survivorship.

Institutional Review Board Statement: This study was approved by the University of Ottawa Research Ethics Board (H-05-21-6889-REG-6889).

Informed Consent Statement: Informed consent was obtained from all participants involved in the study.

Data Availability Statement: The authors have access to the data in Microsoft Excel and SPSS files. Participants were assured that their data would be kept confidential to the extent permitted by law and that only the research team would have access; thus, the data cannot be shared.

Acknowledgments: We are grateful to the organizations that helped circulate recruitment materials for this study, and for each participant who volunteered their time and effort to share their experiences in an interview.

Conflicts of Interest: The authors have no conflict of interest to declare.

References

1. Gupta, S.; Harper, A.; Ruan, Y.; Barr, R.; Frazier, A.L.; Ferlay, J.; Steliarova-Foucher, E.; Fidler-Benaoudia, M.M. International trends in the incidence of cancer among adolescents and young adults. *J. Natl. Cancer Inst.* **2020**, *112*, 1105–1117. [CrossRef] [PubMed]
2. Bleyer, A.; Ferrari, A.; Whelan, J.; Barr, R.D. Global assessment of cancer incidence and survival in adolescents and young adults. *Pediatr. Blood Cancer* **2017**, *64*. [CrossRef] [PubMed]
3. Quinn, G.P.; Goncalves, V.; Sehovic, I.; Bowman, M.L.; Reed, D.R. Quality of life in adolescent and young adult cancer patients: A systematic review of the literature. *Patient Relat. Outcome Meas.* **2015**, *6*, 19–51. [CrossRef] [PubMed]
4. Lange, M.; Licaj, I.; Clarisse, B.; Humbert, X.; Grellard, J.M.; Tron, L.; Joly, F. Cognitive complaints in cancer survivors and expectations for support: Results from a web-based survey. *Cancer Med.* **2019**, *8*, 2654–2663. [CrossRef]
5. Lange, M.; Joly, F.; Vardy, J.; Ahles, T.; Dubois, M.; Tron, L.; Winocur, G.; De Ruiter, M.B.; Castel, H. Cancer-related cognitive impairment: An update on state of the art, detection, and management strategies in cancer survivors. *Ann. Oncol.* **2019**, *30*, 1925–1940. [CrossRef]
6. Janelsins, M.C.; Kohli, S.; Mohile, S.G.; Usuki, K.; Ahles, T.A.; Morrow, G.R. An update on cancer- and chemotherapy-related cognitive dysfunction: Current status. *Semin. Oncol.* **2011**, *38*, 431–438. [CrossRef]
7. Collins, B.; Mackenzie, J.; Tasca, G.A.; Scherling, C.; Smith, A. Persistent cognitive changes in breast cancer patients 1 year following completion of chemotherapy. *J. Int. Neuropsychol. Soc.* **2014**, *20*, 370–379. [CrossRef]

8. Janelsins, M.C.; Heckler, C.E.; Peppone, L.J.; Kamen, C.; Mustian, K.M.; Mohile, S.G.; Magnuson, A.; Kleckner, I.R.; Guido, J.J.; Young, K.L.; et al. Cognitive complaints in survivors of breast cancer after chemotherapy compared with age-matched controls: An analysis from a nationwide, multicenter, prospective longitudinal study. *J. Clin. Oncol.* **2017**, *35*, 506–514. [CrossRef]
9. Dewar, E.O.; Ahn, C.; Eraj, S.; Mahal, B.A.; Sanford, N.N. Psychological distress and cognition among long-term survivors of adolescent and young adult cancer in the USA. *J. Cancer Surv.* **2021**, *15*, 776–784. [CrossRef]
10. Epelman, C.L. The adolescent and young adult with cancer: State of the art—Psychosocial aspects. *Curr. Oncol. Rep.* **2013**, *15*, 325–331. [CrossRef]
11. Brower, K.; Schmitt-Boshnick, M.; Haener, M.; Wilks, S.; Soprovich, A. The use of patient-reported outcome measures in primary care: Applications, benefits and challenges. *J. Patient-Reported Outcomes* **2021**, *5*, 84. [CrossRef] [PubMed]
12. Aaronson, N.K.; Ahmedzai, S.; Bergman, B.; Bullinger, M.; Cull, A.; Duez, N.J.; Filiberti, A.; Flechtner, H.; Fleishman, S.B.; de Haes, J.C.J.M.; et al. The European Organisation for Research and Treatment of Cancer QLQ-C30: A quality-of-life instrument for use in international clinical trials in oncology. *J. Natl. Cancer Inst.* **1993**, *85*, 365–376. [CrossRef] [PubMed]
13. Wagner, L.S.J.; Butt, Z.; Lai, J.; Cella, D. Measuring patient self-reported cognitive function: Development of the Functional Assessment of Cancer Therapy–Cognitive Function instrument. *J. Support. Oncol.* **2009**, *7*, 32–39.
14. Broadbent, D.E.; Cooper, P.F.; FitzGerald, P.; Parkes, K.R. The Cognitive Failures Questionnaire (CFQ) and its correlates. *Br. J. Clin. Psychol.* **1982**, *21*, 1–16. [CrossRef] [PubMed]
15. Henneghan, A.M.; Van Dyk, K.; Kaufmann, T.; Harrison, R.; Gibbons, C.; Heijnen, C.; Kesler, S.R. Measuring self-reported cancer-related cognitive impairment: Recommendations from the Cancer Neuroscience Initiative Working Group. *J. Natl. Cancer Inst.* **2021**, *113*, 1625–1633. [CrossRef]
16. Bray, V.J.; Dhillon, H.M.; Vardy, J.L. Systematic review of self-reported cognitive function in cancer patients following chemotherapy treatment. *J. Cancer Surv.* **2018**, *12*, 537–559. [CrossRef]
17. Brunet, J.; Sharma, S. A scoping review of studies exploring physical activity and cognition among persons with cancer. *J. Cancer Surv.* **2023**, manuscript submitted.
18. Zeng, Y.; Cheng, A.S.; Liu, X.; Chan, C.C. Cervical cancer survivors' perceived cognitive complaints and supportive care needs in mainland China: A qualitative study. *BMJ Open* **2017**, *7*, e014078. [CrossRef]
19. Henderson, F.M.; Cross, A.J.; Baraniak, A.R. 'A new normal with chemobrain': Experiences of the impact of chemotherapy-related cognitive deficits in long-term breast cancer survivors. *Health Psychol. Open* **2019**, *6*, 1–10. [CrossRef]
20. Crotty, M. *The Foundations of Social Research: Meaning and Perspective in the Research Process*; SAGE Publications: Thousand Oaks, CA, USA, 1998.
21. Selamat, M.H.; Loh, S.Y.; Mackenzie, L.; Vardy, J. Chemobrain experienced by breast cancer survivors: A meta-ethnography study investigating research and care implications. *PLoS ONE* **2014**, *9*, e108002. [CrossRef]
22. Erickson, K.I.; Kramer, A.F. Aerobic exercise effects on cognitive and neural plasticity in older adults. *Br. J. Sports Med.* **2009**, *43*, 22–24. [CrossRef] [PubMed]
23. Groot, C.; Hooghiemstra, A.M.; Raijmakers, P.G.; van Berckel, B.N.; Scheltens, P.; Scherder, E.J.; van der Flier, W.M.; Ossenkoppele, R. The effect of physical activity on cognitive function in patients with dementia: A meta-analysis of randomized control trials. *Ageing Res. Rev.* **2016**, *25*, 13–23. [CrossRef] [PubMed]
24. Jia, R.X.; Liang, J.H.; Xu, Y.; Wang, Y.Q. Effects of physical activity and exercise on the cognitive function of patients with Alzheimer disease: A meta-analysis. *BMC Geriatr.* **2019**, *19*, 181. [CrossRef]
25. Zheng, G.; Xia, R.; Zhou, W.; Tao, J.; Chen, L. Aerobic exercise ameliorates cognitive function in older adults with mild cognitive impairment: A systematic review and meta-analysis of randomised controlled trials. *Br. J. Sports Med.* **2016**, *50*, 1443–1450. [CrossRef]
26. Den Heijer, A.E.; Groen, Y.; Tucha, L.; Fuermaier, A.B.; Koerts, J.; Lange, K.W.; Thome, J.; Tucha, O. Sweat it out? The effects of physical exercise on cognition and behavior in children and adults with ADHD: A systematic literature review. *J. Neural Transm.* **2017**, *124*, 3–26. [CrossRef] [PubMed]
27. Lambez, B.; Harwood-Gross, A.; Golumbic, E.Z.; Rassovsky, Y. Non-pharmacological interventions for cognitive difficulties in ADHD: A systematic review and meta-analysis. *J. Psychiatr. Res.* **2020**, *120*, 40–55. [CrossRef] [PubMed]
28. Suarez-Manzano, S.; Ruiz-Ariza, A.; De La Torre-Cruz, M.; Martinez-Lopez, E.J. Acute and chronic effect of physical activity on cognition and behaviour in young people with ADHD: A systematic review of intervention studies. *Res. Dev. Disabil.* **2018**, *77*, 12–23. [CrossRef]
29. Galiano-Castillo, N.; Arroyo-Morales, M.; Lozano-Lozano, M.; Fernandez-Lao, C.; Martin-Martin, L.; Del-Moral-Avila, R.; Cantarero-Villanueva, I. Effect of an Internet-based telehealth system on functional capacity and cognition in breast cancer survivors: A secondary analysis of a randomized controlled trial. *Support. Care Cancer* **2017**, *25*, 3551–3559. [CrossRef]
30. Gokal, K.; Munir, F.; Ahmed, S.; Kancherla, K.; Wallis, D. Does walking protect against decline in cognitive functioning among breast cancer patients undergoing chemotherapy? Results from a small randomised controlled trial. *PLoS ONE* **2018**, *13*, e0206874. [CrossRef]
31. Myers, J.S. Chemotherapy-related cognitive impairment: The breast cancer experience. *Oncol. Nurs. Forum* **2012**, *39*, E31–E40. [CrossRef]

32. Campbell, K.L.; Zadravec, K.; Bland, K.A.; Chesley, E.; Wolf, F.; Janelsins, M.C. The effect of exercise on cancer-related cognitive impairment and applications for physical therapy: Systematic review of randomized controlled trials. *Phys. Ther.* **2020**, *100*, 523–542. [CrossRef] [PubMed]
33. Tong, A.; Sainsbury, P.; Craig, J. Consolidated criteria for reporting qualitative research (COREQ): A 32-item checklist for interviews and focus groups. *Int. J. Qual. Health Care* **2007**, *19*, 349–357. [CrossRef] [PubMed]
34. Dyk, K.V.; Crespi, C.M.; Petersen, L.; Ganz, P.A. Identifying cancer-related cognitive impairment using the FACT-Cog perceived cognitive impairment. *JNCI Cancer Spectr.* **2020**, *4*, pkz099. [CrossRef] [PubMed]
35. Ware, J.E., Jr.; Sherbourne, C.D. The MOS 36-item short-form health survey (SF-36). I. Conceptual framework and item selection. *Med. Care* **1992**, *30*, 473–483. [CrossRef] [PubMed]
36. Godin, G.; Shephard, R.J. A simple method to assess exercise behavior in the community. *Can. J. Appl. Sport. Sci.* **1985**, *10*, 141–146.
37. Godin, G. The Godin-Shephard leisure-time physical activity questionnaire. *Health Fitness J. Can.* **2011**, *4*, 18–22.
38. Jacobs, D.R., Jr.; Ainsworth, B.E.; Hartman, T.J.; Leon, A.S. A simultaneous evaluation of 10 commonly used physical activity questionnaires. *Med. Science Sports Exerc.* **1993**, *25*, 81–91. [CrossRef]
39. Amireault, S.; Godin, G.; Lacombe, J.; Sabiston, C.M. The use of the Godin-Shephard Leisure-Time Physical Activity Questionnaire in oncology research: A systematic review. *BMC Med. Res. Methodol.* **2015**, *15*, 60. [CrossRef]
40. Fontana, A.; Frey, J.H. The interview: From neutral stance to political involvement. In *The SAGE Handbook of Qualitative Research*, 3rd ed.; Denzin, N.K., Lincoln, Y.S., Eds.; SAGE Publications: Thousand Oaks, CA, USA, 2005; pp. 695–727.
41. Glaser, B.G.; Strauss, A.L. *The Discovery of Grounded Theory: Strategies for Qualitative Research*; Aldine Publishing: Chicago, IL, USA, 1967.
42. Saunders, B.; Sim, J.; Kingstone, T.; Baker, S.; Waterfield, J.; Bartlam, B.; Burroughs, H.; Jinks, C. Saturation in qualitative research: Exploring its conceptualization and operationalization. *Qual. Quant.* **2018**, *52*, 1893–1907. [CrossRef]
43. Braun, V.; Clarke, V. Using thematic analysis in psychology. *Qual. Res. Psychol.* **2006**, *3*, 77–101. [CrossRef]
44. Smith, J.A.; Osborn, M. Interpretative phenomenological analysis. In *Qualitative Psychology: A Practical Guide to Research Methods*; Smith, J.A., Ed.; SAGE Publications: London, UK, 2003; pp. 51–80.
45. Smith, B.; McGannon, K.R. Developing rigor in qualitative research: Problems and opportunities within sport and exercise psychology. *Int. Rev. Sport. Exerc. Psychol.* **2018**, *11*, 101–121. [CrossRef]
46. Vizer, L.M.; Mikles, S.P.; Piepmeier, A.T. Cancer-related cognitive impairment in survivors of adolescent and young adult non-central nervous system cancer: A scoping review. *Psycho-Oncology* **2022**, *31*, 1275–1285. [CrossRef] [PubMed]
47. Dahl, A.A.; Fossa, S.D.; Lie, H.C.; Loge, J.H.; Reinertsen, K.V.; Ruud, E.; Kiserud, C.E. Employment status and work ability in long-term young adult cancer survivors. *J. Adolesc. Young Adult Oncol.* **2019**, *8*, 304–311. [CrossRef]
48. Brock, H.; Friedrich, M.; Sender, A.; Richter, D.; Geue, K.; Mehnert-Theuerkauf, A.; Leuteritz, K. Work ability and cognitive impairments in young adult cancer patients: Associated factors and changes over time-results from the AYA-Leipzig study. *J. Cancer Surviv.* **2022**, *16*, 771–780. [CrossRef] [PubMed]
49. Ketterl, T.G.; Syrjala, K.L.; Casillas, J.; Jacobs, L.A.; Palmer, S.C.; McCabe, M.S.; Ganz, P.A.; Overholser, L.; Partridge, A.; Rajotte, E.J.; et al. Lasting effects of cancer and its treatment on employment and finances in adolescent and young adult cancer survivors. *Cancer* **2019**, *125*, 1908–1917. [CrossRef]
50. Boykoff, N.; Moieni, M.; Subramanian, S.K. Confronting chemobrain: An in-depth look at survivors' reports of impact on work, social networks, and health care response. *J. Cancer Surviv.* **2009**, *3*, 223–232. [CrossRef]
51. Cheung, Y.T.; Shwe, M.; Tan, Y.P.; Fan, G.; Ng, R.; Chan, A. Cognitive changes in multiethnic Asian breast cancer patients: A focus group study. *Ann. Oncol.* **2012**, *23*, 2547–2552. [CrossRef]
52. Munir, F.; Burrows, J.; Yarker, J.; Kalawsky, K.; Bains, M. Women's perceptions of chemotherapy-induced cognitive side affects on work ability: A focus group study. *J. Clin. Nurs.* **2010**, *19*, 1362–1370. [CrossRef]
53. Von Ah, D.; Habermann, B.; Carpenter, J.S.; Schneider, B.L. Impact of perceived cognitive impairment in breast cancer survivors. *Eur. J. Oncol. Nurs.* **2013**, *17*, 236–241. [CrossRef]
54. Dhillon, H.M.; Tannock, I.F.; Pond, G.R.; Renton, C.; Rourke, S.B.; Vardy, J.L. Perceived cognitive impairment in people with colorectal cancer who do and do not receive chemotherapy. *J. Cancer Surviv.* **2018**, *12*, 178–185. [CrossRef]
55. Pullens, M.J.; De Vries, J.; Van Warmerdam, L.J.; Van De Wal, M.A.; Roukema, J.A. Chemotherapy and cognitive complaints in women with breast cancer. *Psycho-Oncology* **2013**, *22*, 1783–1789. [CrossRef] [PubMed]
56. Ganz, P.A.; Kwan, L.; Castellon, S.A.; Oppenheim, A.; Bower, J.E.; Silverman, D.H.; Cole, S.W.; Irwin, M.R.; Ancoli-Israel, S.; Belin, T.R. Cognitive complaints after breast cancer treatments: Examining the relationship with neuropsychological test performance. *J. Natl. Cancer Inst.* **2013**, *105*, 791–801. [CrossRef] [PubMed]
57. Schilder, C.M.; Seynaeve, C.; Linn, S.C.; Boogerd, W.; Beex, L.V.; Gundy, C.M.; Nortier, J.W.; van de Velde, C.J.; van Dam, F.S.; Schagen, S.B. Self-reported cognitive functioning in postmenopausal breast cancer patients before and during endocrine treatment: Findings from the neuropsychological TEAM side-study. *Psycho-Oncology* **2012**, *21*, 479–487. [CrossRef]
58. Yang, Y.; Hendrix, C.C. Cancer-related cognitive impairment in breast cancer patients: Influences of psychological variables. *Asia-Pac. J. Oncol. Nurs.* **2018**, *5*, 296–306. [CrossRef]
59. Pearce, S.; Whelan, J.; Kelly, D.; Gibson, F. Renegotiation of identity in young adults with cancer: A longitudinal narrative study. *Int. J. Nurs. Stud.* **2020**, *102*, 103465. [CrossRef]

60. Huysse-Gaytandjieva, A.; Groot, W.; Pavlova, M.; Joling, C. Low self-esteem predicts future unemployment. *J. Appl. Econ.* **2015**, *18*, 325–346. [CrossRef]
61. Statistics Canada. A Generational Portrait of Canada's Aging Population from the 2021 Census. Available online: https://www12.statcan.gc.ca/census-recensement/2021/as-sa/98-200-X/2021003/98-200-X2021003-eng.cfm (accessed on 2 April 2023).
62. Stone, D.S.; Ganz, P.A.; Pavlish, C.; Robbins, W.A. Young adult cancer survivors and work: A systematic review. *J. Cancer Surviv.* **2017**, *11*, 765–781. [CrossRef]
63. Hampstead, B.M.; Gillis, M.M.; Stringer, A.Y. Cognitive rehabilitation of memory for mild cognitive impairment: A methodological review and model for future research. *J. Int. Neuropsychol. Soc.* **2014**, *20*, 135–151. [CrossRef]
64. Mayo, S.J.; Rourke, S.B.; Atenafu, E.G.; Vitorino, R.; Chen, C.; Kuruvilla, J. Computerized cognitive training in post-treatment hematological cancer survivors: A feasibility study. *Pilot. Feasibility Stud.* **2021**, *7*, 36. [CrossRef]
65. Conklin, H.M.; Ogg, R.J.; Ashford, J.M.; Scoggins, M.A.; Zou, P.; Clark, K.N.; Martin-Elbahesh, K.; Hardy, K.K.; Merchant, T.E.; Jeha, S.; et al. Computerized cognitive training for amelioration of cognitive late effects among childhood cancer survivors: A randomized controlled trial. *J. Clin. Oncol.* **2015**, *33*, 3894–3902. [CrossRef]
66. Simons, D.J.; Boot, W.R.; Charness, N.; Gathercole, S.E.; Chabris, C.F.; Hambrick, D.Z.; Stine-Morrow, E.A. Do "brain-training" programs work? *Psychol. Sci. Public. Interest.* **2016**, *17*, 103–186. [CrossRef] [PubMed]
67. Mackenzie, L.; Marshall, K. Effective non-pharmacological interventions for cancer related cognitive impairment in adults (excluding central nervous system or head and neck cancer): Systematic review and meta-analysis. *Eur. J. Phys. Rehabil. Med.* **2022**, *58*, 258–270. [CrossRef] [PubMed]
68. Yan, X.; Wei, S.; Liu, Q. Effect of cognitive training on patients with breast cancer reporting cognitive changes: A systematic review and meta-analysis. *BMJ Open.* **2023**, *13*, e058088. [CrossRef] [PubMed]
69. Gooch, M.; Mehta, A.; John, T.; Lomeli, N.; Naeem, E.; Mucci, G.; Toh, Y.L.; Chan, A.; Bota, D.A.; Torno, L. Feasibility of cognitive training to promote recovery in cancer-related cognitive impairment in adolescent and young adult patients. *J. Adolesc. Young Adult Oncol.* **2022**, *11*, 290–296. [CrossRef]
70. Milbury, K.; Chaoul, A.; Biegler, K.; Wangyal, T.; Spelman, A.; Meyers, C.A.; Arun, B.; Palmer, J.L.; Taylor, J.; Cohen, L. Tibetan sound meditation for cognitive dysfunction: Results of a randomized controlled pilot trial. *Psycho-Oncology* **2013**, *22*, 2354–2363. [CrossRef]
71. Johns, S.A.; Von Ah, D.; Brown, L.F.; Beck-Coon, K.; Talib, T.L.; Alyea, J.M.; Monahan, P.O.; Tong, Y.; Wilhelm, L.; Giesler, R.B. Randomized controlled pilot trial of mindfulness-based stress reduction for breast and colorectal cancer survivors: Effects on cancer-related cognitive impairment. *J. Cancer Surviv.* **2016**, *10*, 437–448. [CrossRef]
72. Duval, A.; Davis, C.G.; Khoo, E.L.; Romanow, H.; Shergill, Y.; Rice, D.; Smith, A.M.; Poulin, P.A.; Collins, B. Mindfulness-based stress reduction and cognitive function among breast cancer survivors: A randomized controlled trial. *Cancer* **2022**, *128*, 2520–2528. [CrossRef]
73. Alvarez, J.; Meyer, F.L.; Granoff, D.L.; Lundy, A. The effect of EEG biofeedback on reducing postcancer cognitive impairment. *Integr. Cancer Ther.* **2013**, *12*, 475–487. [CrossRef]
74. Freeman, L.W.; White, R.; Ratcliff, C.G.; Sutton, S.; Stewart, M.; Palmer, J.L.; Link, J.; Cohen, L. A randomized trial comparing live and telemedicine deliveries of an imagery-based behavioral intervention for breast cancer survivors: Reducing symptoms and barriers to care. *Psycho-Oncology* **2015**, *24*, 910–918. [CrossRef]
75. Lambert, M.; Wurz, A.; Smith, A.M.; Fang, Z.; Brunet, J. Preliminary evidence of improvement in adolescent and young adult cancer survivors' brain health following physical activity: A proof-of-concept sub-study. *Brain Plast.* **2021**, *7*, 97–109. [CrossRef]
76. Wurz, A.; Ayson, G.; Smith, A.M.; Brunet, J. A proof-of-concept sub-study exploring feasibility and preliminary evidence for the role of physical activity on neural activity during executive functioning tasks among young adults after cancer treatment. *BMC Neurol.* **2021**, *21*, 300. [CrossRef] [PubMed]
77. Bryant, A.L.; Deal, A.M.; Battaglini, C.L.; Phillips, B.; Pergolotti, M.; Coffman, E.; Foster, M.C.; Wood, W.A.; Bailey, C.; Hackney, A.C.; et al. The effects of exercise on patient-reported outcomes and performance-based physical function in adults with acute leukemia undergoing induction therapy: Exercise and QUality of life in Acute Leukemia (EQUAL). *Integr. Cancer Ther.* **2018**, *17*, 263–270. [CrossRef] [PubMed]
78. Morielli, A.R.; Boule, N.G.; Usmani, N.; Tankel, K.; Joseph, K.; Severin, D.; Fairchild, A.; Nijjar, T.; Courneya, K.S. Effects of exercise during and after neoadjuvant chemoradiation on symptom burden and quality of life in rectal cancer patients: A phase II randomized controlled trial. *J. Cancer Surviv.* **2021**. [CrossRef]
79. Salerno, E.A.; Rowland, K.; Kramer, A.F.; McAuley, E. Acute aerobic exercise effects on cognitive function in breast cancer survivors: A randomized crossover trial. *BMC Cancer* **2019**, *19*, 371. [CrossRef] [PubMed]
80. Shiffman, S.; Stone, A.A.; Hufford, M.R. Ecological momentary assessment. *Ann. Rev. Clin. Psychol.* **2008**, *4*, 1–32. [CrossRef]
81. Diamond, A.; Ling, D.S. Conclusions about interventions, programs, and approaches for improving executive functions that appear justified and those that, despite much hype, do not. *Dev. Cogn. Neurosci.* **2016**, *18*, 34–48. [CrossRef] [PubMed]
82. Hillman, C.H.; McAuley, E.; Erickson, K.I.; Liu-Ambrose, T.; Kramer, A.F. On mindful and mindless physical activity and executive function: A response to Diamond and Ling (2016). *Dev. Cogn. Neurosci.* **2019**, *37*, 100529. [CrossRef] [PubMed]
83. Gheysen, F.; Poppe, L.; DeSmet, A.; Swinnen, S.; Cardon, G.; De Bourdeaudhuij, I.; Chastin, S.; Fias, W. Physical activity to improve cognition in older adults: Can physical activity programs enriched with cognitive challenges enhance the effects? A systematic review and meta-analysis. *Int. J. Behav. Nutr. Phys. Act.* **2018**, *15*, 63. [CrossRef]

84. Waddington, E.E.; Heisz, J.J. Orienteering experts report more proficient spatial processing and memory across adulthood. *PLoS ONE* **2023**, *18*, e0280435. [CrossRef]
85. Bo, W.; Lei, M.; Tao, S.; Jie, L.T.; Qian, L.; Lin, F.Q.; Ping, W.X. Effects of combined intervention of physical exercise and cognitive training on cognitive function in stroke survivors with vascular cognitive impairment: A randomized controlled trial. *Clin. Rehabil.* **2019**, *33*, 54–63. [CrossRef]
86. Melis, M.; Schroyen, G.; Leenaerts, N.; Smeets, A.; Sunaert, S.; Van der Gucht, K.; Deprez, S. The impact of mindfulness on cancer-related cognitive impairment in breast cancer survivors with cognitive complaints. *Cancer* **2023**, *129*, 1105–1116. [CrossRef] [PubMed]
87. Cantarero-Villanueva, I.; Fernandez-Lao, C.; Cuesta-Vargas, A.I.; Del Moral-Avila, R.; Fernandez-de-Las-Penas, C.; Arroyo-Morales, M. The effectiveness of a deep water aquatic exercise program in cancer-related fatigue in breast cancer survivors: A randomized controlled trial. *Arch. Phys. Med. Rehabil.* **2013**, *94*, 221–230. [CrossRef] [PubMed]
88. Cox, E.; Bells, S.; Timmons, B.W.; Laughlin, S.; Bouffet, E.; de Medeiros, C.; Beera, K.; Harasym, D.; Mabbott, D.J. A controlled clinical crossover trial of exercise training to improve cognition and neural communication in pediatric brain tumor survivors. *Clin. Neurophysiol.* **2020**, *131*, 1533–1547. [CrossRef] [PubMed]
89. Galiano-Castillo, N.; Cantarero-Villanueva, I.; Fernandez-Lao, C.; Ariza-Garcia, A.; Diaz-Rodriguez, L.; Del-Moral-Avila, R.; Arroyo-Morales, M. Telehealth system: A randomized controlled trial evaluating the impact of an internet-based exercise intervention on quality of life, pain, muscle strength, and fatigue in breast cancer survivors. *Cancer* **2016**, *122*, 3166–3174. [CrossRef]
90. Galvao, D.A.; Taaffe, D.R.; Spry, N.; Joseph, D.; Newton, R.U. Combined resistance and aerobic exercise program reverses muscle loss in men undergoing androgen suppression therapy for prostate cancer without bone metastases: A randomized controlled trial. *J. Clin. Oncol.* **2010**, *28*, 340–347. [CrossRef]
91. Henke, C.C.; Cabri, J.; Fricke, L.; Pankow, W.; Kandilakis, G.; Feyer, P.C.; de Wit, M. Strength and endurance training in the treatment of lung cancer patients in stages IIIA/IIIB/IV. *Support. Care Cancer* **2014**, *22*, 95–101. [CrossRef]
92. Howell, C.R.; Krull, K.R.; Partin, R.E.; Kadan-Lottick, N.S.; Robison, L.L.; Hudson, M.M.; Ness, K.K. Randomized web-based physical activity intervention in adolescent survivors of childhood cancer. *Pediatr. Blood Cancer* **2018**, *65*, e27216. [CrossRef]
93. Janelsins, M.C.; Peppone, L.J.; Heckler, C.E.; Kesler, S.R.; Sprod, L.K.; Atkins, J.; Melnik, M.; Kamen, C.; Giguere, J.; Messino, M.J.; et al. YOCAS(c)(R) yoga reduces self-reported memory difficulty in cancer survivors in a nationwide randomized clinical trial: Investigating relationships between memory and sleep. *Integr. Cancer Ther.* **2016**, *15*, 263–271. [CrossRef]
94. Larkey, L.K.; Roe, D.J.; Smith, L.; Millstine, D. Exploratory outcome assessment of Qigong/Tai Chi Easy on breast cancer survivors. *Complement. Ther. Med.* **2016**, *29*, 196–203. [CrossRef]
95. Miki, E.; Kataoka, T.; Okamura, H. Feasibility and efficacy of speed-feedback therapy with a bicycle ergometer on cognitive function in elderly cancer patients in Japan. *Psycho-Oncology* **2014**, *23*, 906–913. [CrossRef]
96. Oh, B.; Butow, P.N.; Mullan, B.A.; Clarke, S.J.; Beale, P.J.; Pavlakis, N.; Lee, M.S.; Rosenthal, D.S.; Larkey, L.; Vardy, J. Effect of medical Qigong on cognitive function, quality of life, and a biomarker of inflammation in cancer patients: A randomized controlled trial. *Support. Care Cancer* **2012**, *20*, 1235–1242. [CrossRef] [PubMed]
97. Park, J.H.; Park, K.D.; Kim, J.H.; Kim, Y.S.; Kim, E.Y.; Ahn, H.K.; Park, I.; Sym, S.J. Resistance and aerobic exercise intervention during chemotherapy in patients with metastatic cancer: A pilot study in South Korea. *Ann. Palliat. Med.* **2021**, *10*, 10236–10243. [CrossRef] [PubMed]
98. Poier, D.; Bussing, A.; Rodrigues Recchia, D.; Beerenbrock, Y.; Reif, M.; Nikolaou, A.; Zerm, R.; Gutenbrunner, C.; Kroz, M. Influence of a multimodal and multimodal-aerobic therapy concept on health-related quality of life in breast cancer survivors. *Integr. Cancer Ther.* **2019**, *18*, 1–10. [CrossRef] [PubMed]
99. Saarto, T.; Penttinen, H.M.; Sievanen, H.; Kellokumpu-Lehtinen, P.L.; Hakamies-Blomqvist, L.; Nikander, R.; Huovinen, R.; Luoto, R.; Kautiainen, H.; Jarvenpaa, S.; et al. Effectiveness of a 12-month exercise program on physical performance and quality of life of breast cancer survivors. *Anticancer. Res.* **2012**, *32*, 3875–3884. [PubMed]
100. Vadiraja, H.S.; Rao, M.R.; Nagarathna, R.; Nagendra, H.R.; Rekha, M.; Vanitha, N.; Gopinath, K.S.; Srinath, B.S.; Vishweshwara, M.S.; Madhavi, Y.S.; et al. Effects of yoga program on quality of life and affect in early breast cancer patients undergoing adjuvant radiotherapy: A randomized controlled trial. *Complement. Ther. Med.* **2009**, *17*, 274–280. [CrossRef]
101. Van Weert, E.; May, A.M.; Korstjens, I.; Post, W.J.; van der Schans, C.P.; van den Borne, B.; Mesters, I.; Ros, W.J.; Hoekstra-Weebers, J.E. Cancer-related fatigue and rehabilitation: A randomized controlled multicenter trial comparing physical training combined with cognitive-behavioral therapy with physical training only and with no intervention. *Phys. Ther.* **2010**, *90*, 1413–1425. [CrossRef]
102. Zimmer, P.; Baumann, F.T.; Oberste, M.; Schmitt, J.; Joisten, N.; Hartig, P.; Schenk, A.; Kuhn, R.; Bloch, W.; Reuss-Borst, M. Influence of personalized exercise recommendations during rehabilitation on the sustainability of objectively measured physical activity levels, fatigue, and fatigue-related biomarkers in patients with breast cancer. *Integr. Cancer Ther.* **2018**, *17*, 306–311. [CrossRef]
103. Rosenstock, I.M. Why people use health services. *Milbank Q.* **1966**, *44*, 94–127. [CrossRef]
104. Hanin, Y.L. Emotions and Athletic Performance: Individual Zones of Optimal Functioning Model. In *European Yearbook of Sport Psychology*; FEPSAC: Brussels, Belgium, 1997; pp. 29–72.

105. Hanin, Y.L. Individual zones of optimal functioning (IZOF) model: Emotions-performance relationships in sport. In *Emotions in Sport*; Hanin, Y.L., Ed.; Human Kinetics: Champaign, IL, USA, 2000.
106. Cutter, G.R.; Liu, Y. Personalized medicine: The return of the house call? *Neurol. Clin. Pract.* **2012**, *2*, 343–351. [CrossRef]

Disclaimer/Publisher's Note: The statements, opinions and data contained in all publications are solely those of the individual author(s) and contributor(s) and not of MDPI and/or the editor(s). MDPI and/or the editor(s) disclaim responsibility for any injury to people or property resulting from any ideas, methods, instructions or products referred to in the content.

Article

Reproductive Outcomes in Young Breast Cancer Survivors Treated (15–39) in Ontario, Canada

Moira Rushton [1,*], Jessica Pudwell [2], Xuejiao Wei [3], Madeleine Powell [2], Harriet Richardson [4,5] and Maria P. Velez [2,3,4,*]

1. Division of Medical Oncology, The Ottawa Hospital Cancer Centre, Ottawa, ON K1H 8L6, Canada
2. Department of Obstetrics and Gynecology, Queen's University, Kingston, ON K7L 3N6, Canada
3. ICES, Queen's University, Kingston, ON K7L 3N6, Canada
4. Department of Public Health Sciences, Queen's University, Kingston, ON K7L 3N6, Canada
5. Division of Canadian Cancer Trials Group, Queen's Cancer Research Institute, Kingston, ON K7L 3N6, Canada
* Correspondence: moirushton@toh.ca (M.R.); maria.velez@queensu.ca (M.P.V.)

Abstract: We conducted a population-based, retrospective, matched-cohort study to examine the impact of breast cancer diagnosis and treatment on fertility outcomes. Relative risks of infertility, childbirth, premature ovarian insufficiency (POI; age < 40) and early menopause (age < 45) were calculated using modified Poisson regression. Our primary cohort included young women (15–39) with early stage BC diagnosed 1995–2014. Five cancer-free patients were matched to each BC patient by birth year and census subdivision. The BC cohort was further divided by treatment with chemotherapy vs. no chemotherapy treatment. 3903 BC patients and 19,515 cancer-free women. BC patients treated with chemotherapy were at increased risk of infertility (RR 1.81; 95% CI 1.60–2.04), and POI (RR 6.25; 95% CI 5.15–7.58) and decreased childbirth (RR 0.85; 95% CI 0.75–0.96), compared to women without cancer. BC patients who did not receive chemotherapy were also at increased risk of infertility (RR 1.80 95% CI 1.48–2.18) and POI (RR 2.12 95% CI 1.37–3.28). All young BC survivors face an increased risk of diagnosed infertility and POI relative to women without cancer, independent of chemotherapy. These results emphasize the importance of pre-treatment fertility counselling for young women diagnosed with BC.

Keywords: breast cancer; infertility; early menopause; POI; AYA

1. Introduction

Breast cancer (BC) is the most common malignancy affecting women under age 40 accounting for ~5% of all breast cancer cases [1,2]. Adolescents and Young Adults (AYAs) aged 15–39 years at the time of cancer diagnosis are a unique population in terms of both the biology of their cancers and the way they experience their cancer journey [3]. Young women with breast cancer have unique concerns regarding fertility, pregnancy and contraception and report having difficulty obtaining information in this regard [3,4]. During the course of a curative-intent treatment plan, early stage (I–III) breast cancer patients will receive a combination of surgery, radiation and systemic therapy. Standard adjuvant treatment is multi-modal and can include hormonal therapy, chemotherapy, and targeted anti-HER2 therapy [5–7]. In addition to the systemic therapy options offered to all breast cancer patients, AYA patients are often offered ovarian suppression (surgical or pharmacological) for management of ER positive breast cancer due to increased long-term survival achieved with this strategy [7,8].

AYA breast cancer survivors have an increased risk of subsequent infertility diagnosis and/or premature ovarian insufficiency (POI). We have previously reported that compared with non-cancer AYAs, breast cancer survivors have increased risk of infertility diagnosis (RR 1.46; 95% CI 1.30–1.65) and POI (RR 4.37; 95% CI 3.88–4.93) [9,10]. Several mechanisms may play a role. Chemotherapy is one potential explanation, due to its toxic effect on ovarian follicles leading to POI [11–14] and has been shown to cause POI in 20–80% of AYA women depending on their age, the use of other treatment in addition to chemotherapy, and physician follow-up [15]. Additionally, women with estrogen sensitive cancers or carriers of BRCA1/2 gene mutations may be advised to have bilateral oophorectomy for ovarian suppression or ovarian cancer prevention, respectively, [4,8,16].

The issue of pregnancy after breast cancer is a growing concern. Women are delaying childbearing and family planning such that a greater proportion of AYA breast cancer survivors will be nulliparous. The median age at first pregnancy is steadily rising in Western nations and reached 27 in the United States in 2019 [17]. In clinical practise, patients want to clearly understand their risks of infertility, pregnancy and POI after breast cancer treatment. While we have already studied the risk of POI and diagnosed infertility in AYA cancer survivors, the impact of specific treatment modalities is less well characterized. We hypothesized that breast cancer treatment will increase risk of infertility and POI in young women. The objective of this study was to examine the impact of breast cancer diagnosis and treatment on reproductive outcomes in young breast cancer survivors compared with a matched non-cancer cohort in Ontario, Canada.

2. Materials and Methods

2.1. Study Design

We conducted a population-based, retrospective, matched-cohort study on breast cancer patients in Ontario, Canada diagnosed between 1 January 1995–31 December 2014. Ethics approval was obtained from Queen's University Health Sciences Research Ethics Board, Kingston, Ontario (OBGY-296-16 #6019934, Initial clearance on 12DEC2016).

2.2. Data Sources

The cohorts were identified using health administrative databases in Ontario, Canada that contain patient-level information on cancer diagnosis, cancer drug administration as well as inpatient and outpatient data, cancer registry data, and demographics. De-identified databases were accessed on June 11, 2020 through ICES (www.ices.on.ca) and all data sources were linked through a unique encrypted identifier and analyzed at ICES. ICES is an independent, non-profit research institute funded by an annual grant from the Ontario Ministry of Health and Long-Term Care. As a prescribed entity under Ontario's privacy legislation, ICES is authorized to collect and use health care data for the purposes of health system analysis, evaluation and decision support. Secure access to these data is governed by policies and procedures that are approved by the Information and Privacy Commissioner of Ontario.

Datasets used to construct the matched cohorts in this study included: Discharge Abstract Database (DAD); National Ambulatory Care Reporting System (NACRS); OHIP database; Same-Day Surgery; Registered Persons Database(RPD); Immigration Refugees and Citizenship Canada Permanent Resident (IRCC-PR) database; ICES derived cohort MOMBABY; ICES Physician Database; Postal Code Conversion File; Cancer Care Ontario Activity Level Reporting; Ontario Cancer Registry (OCR); and the New Drug Funding Program. Details on the databases utilized in this study are presented in the supplemental methods found in Supplementary Material.

2.3. Cohort Creation

Women aged 15–39 who were diagnosed with early stage (I–III) breast cancer between January 1, 1995 and December 31, 2014 were included. The index date for analysis was date of breast cancer surgery (e.g., lumpectomy, mastectomy). This index date was selected to ensure all captured cases were treated with curative intent. Exclusion criteria included: Any prior cancer diagnosis or a second primary cancer diagnosis within 12 months of the index date, women who died within 3 years of diagnosis/index date, stage IV breast cancer at time of diagnosis, prior diagnosis of infertility or menopause, history of prior tubal ligation, bilateral oophorectomy and/or hysterectomy or those same procedures up to 36 months after index date, and missing geographical census data. BC patients who did not have 5 matched controls were also excluded. We further categorized the BC cohort into those treated with or without intravenous chemotherapy. See Figure 1 for cohort inclusion/exclusion flow chart.

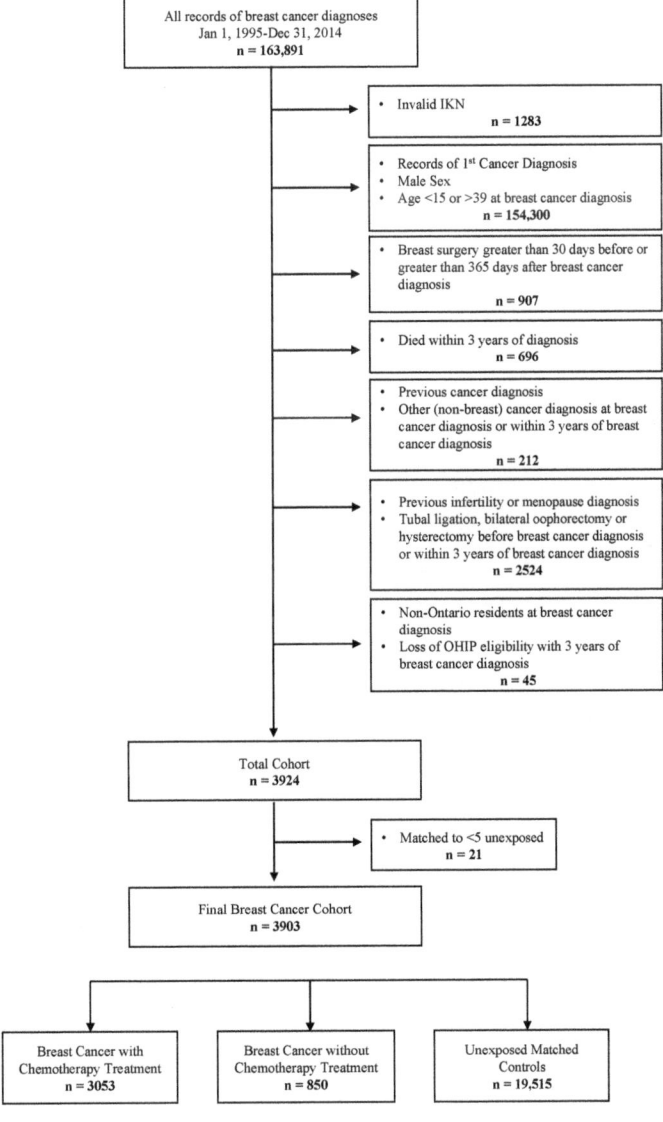

Figure 1. Flow chart demonstrating inclusion and exclusion ceiteria foe cohort design. IKN = ICES Key Number.

Five cancer-free women from the general population who had no cancer diagnosis prior to the index date were randomly selected without replacement, and were matched on year of birth and census subdivision. Individuals in the cancer-free cohort were assigned an index date based on the date of surgery for their matched case. The cancer-free cohort was subject to the same exclusion criteria as the BC cohort. Individuals who died within 3 years of index date were excluded to remove those with early cancer relapse and/or competing morbidity not otherwise captured in our cohort creation and avoid the bias this may bring to fertility/infertility diagnoses.

2.4. Covariates

Age at cancer diagnosis/index, income quintile, rurality index, immigration status, previous pregnancy, and history of endometriosis (ICD-9 617) or polycystic ovarian syndrome (ICD-9 256) were included in the analysis. Data on hormone receptors (estrogen, progesterone), HER2 amplification, and hormonal therapy treatments were not available.

2.5. Endpoints

Individuals in both cohorts were followed from the index date until the occurrence of the primary or secondary outcome or until censored. Censoring occurred at the time of a new primary cancer diagnosis, hysterectomy date, bilateral oophorectomy date, tubal ligation date, loss of Ontario Health Insurance Plan (OHIP) eligibility, death, or maximum follow-up date of 31 December 2019.

Outcomes of interest were: (1) diagnosed infertility defined as the presence of a physician billing code ICD-9 628 in the OHIP database after one year of cancer diagnosis; (2) childbirth defined as delivery of an infant, live or stillborn over 20 weeks gestational age (MOMBABY database); and (3) POI defined as the presence of a physician billing code for menopause (ICD-9 627) before age 40; and early menopause (menopause diagnosis-ICD-9 627–before age 45).

2.6. Statistical Analysis

Descriptive statistics were performed to report baseline characteristics of the cohort. Standardized differences between selected variables were reported for women with and without breast cancer and those differences > 0.10 were considered statistically meaningful in accordance with ICES reporting standards [18]. Modified Poisson regression was used to calculate the relative risk (RR) between exposures and outcomes of interest, adjusted for age at breast cancer surgery, immigrant status, neighbourhood income quintile and prior parity. All RRs are reported with the point estimate along with 95% confidence intervals (CI). The analyses were performed using SAS version 9.4 (Cary, NC, USA) at ICES Queen's University.

3. Results

3.1. Patient Characteristics

We identified 3903 women age 15–39 who were diagnosed with early stage breast cancer from 1995–2014 and met our study inclusion criteria for our BC cohort. These were matched to 19,515 cancer-free individuals. Median follow-up time was 12.8 years. Median age for the study population was 36.0 (IQR 33–38) and 78.2% of breast cancer patients received intravenous chemotherapy. Baseline characteristics are described in Table 1. Age was similar distributed as per study design. Women with breast cancer were more likely than women without breast cancer to have given birth before the index date, 50.2% vs. 39.7%. There were less immigrant women in the BC group than Canadian born women. History of PCOS or endometriosis was similar in BC and cancer-free individuals.

Table 1. Baseline Characteristics and standardized differences between 3903 women age 15–39 years with breast cancer and 19,515 cancer-free women in Ontario, Canada from 1995–2014.

Variable	Value	Chemo No N = 850	Chemo Yes N = 3053	All BC combined N = 3903	Non-Cancer Group N = 19,515	Std Difference *
Age at surgery	Mean (SD)	35.0 (4.1)	35.0 (3.7)	35.0 (3.8)	35.0 (3.9)	0
	Median (Q1–Q3)	36 (33–38)	36 (33–38)	36 (33–38)	36 (33–38)	0
	Min–Max	15–40	18–40	15–40	15–41	
Age group	15–24 - n (%)	18 (2.1%)	38 (1.2%)	56 (1.4%)	302 (1.5%)	0.01
	25–29 - n (%)	78 (9.2%)	265 (8.7%)	343 (8.8%)	1705 (8.7%)	0
	30–34 - n (%)	195 (22.9%)	829 (27.2%)	1024 (26.2%)	5151 (26.4%)	0
	35–41 - n (%)	559 (65.8%)	1921 (62.9%)	2480 (63.5%)	12,357 (63.3%)	0
Parity	Nulliparous - n (%)	500 (58.8%)	1444 (47.3%)	1944 (49.8%)	11,777 (60.3%)	0.21
	Parous - n (%)	350 (41.2%)	1609 (52.7%)	1959 (50.2%)	7738 (39.7%)	0.21
Neighbourhood income quintile	1 - Lowest quintile - n (%)	147 (17.3%)	520 (17.0%)	667 (17.1%)	3944 (20.2%)	0.08
	2 - n (%)	154 (18.1%)	593 (19.4%)	747 (19.1%)	3780 (19.4%)	0.01
	3 - n (%)	195 (22.9%)	657 (21.5%)	852 (21.8%)	3807 (19.5%)	0.06
	4 - n (%)	173 (20.4%)	652 (21.4%)	825 (21.1%)	4134 (21.2%)	0
	5 - Highest quintile - n (%)	181 (21.3%)	631 (20.7%)	812 (20.8%)	3850 (19.7%)	0.03
Immigrant	No - n (%)	663 (78.0%)	2391 (78.3%)	3054 (78.2%)	14,319 (73.4%)	0.11
	Yes - n (%)	187 (22.0%)	662 (21.7%)	849 (21.8%)	5196 (26.6%)	0.11
Rurality	Rural - n (%)	811 (95.4%)	2903 (95.1%)	3714 (95.2%)	18583 (95.2%)	0
	Urban - n (%)	39 (4.6%)	150 (4.9%)	189 (4.8%)	932 (4.8%)	0
Prior Endometriosis	No - n (%)	835 (98.2%)	2993 (98.0%)	3828 (98.1%)	19,261 (98.7%)	0.05
	Yes - n (%)	15 (1.8%)	60 (2.0%)	75 (1.9%)	254 (1.3%)	0.05
Prior PCOS	No - n (%)	829 (97.5%)	3010 (98.6%)	3839 (98.4%)	19,282 (98.8%)	0.04
	Yes - n (%)	21 (2.5%)	43 (1.4%)	64 (1.6%)	233 (1.2%)	0.04

* Differences are between all breast cancer combined and non-cancer patients. Values greater than 0.10 are considered statistically different.

3.2. Infertility

Infertility occurred in 9.1% of breast cancer patients who received chemotherapy, 11.8% of breast cancer patients who did not receive chemotherapy, and in 7.0% of the cancer-free (non-cancer) group. In the Poisson regression model (Figure 2), all cancer patients had an increased RR of infertility diagnosis compared to the non-cancer group with similar adjusted RRs for those treated with chemotherapy (1.81, 95% 1.60–2.04) and those who were not (1.80, 95% CI 1.48–2.18).

3.3. Childbirth

Fewer breast cancer survivors gave birth during follow up than the cancer-free group 9.1% vs. 12.8%. When survivors were categorized into those treated with chemotherapy vs. those were not, 8.4% and 11.6% gave birth during follow-up respectively. In the multivariable model (Figure 2), birth was less likely in the group of breast cancer patients that received chemotherapy, RR 0.85 (95% CI 0.75–0.96).

3.4. Premature Ovarian Insufficiency and Early Menopause

POI occurred in 5.4% of breast cancer survivors vs. 1.2% of the cancer-free group. Early menopause occurred in 10.5% of BC patients vs. 3.4% of cancer-free patients. Amongst BC patients treated with chemotherapy, 6.2% experienced POI and 11.0% experienced early menopause compared with 2.5% and 8.4% of those who did not receive chemotherapy. In the multivariable model, the risk of POI or early menopause was significantly increased for all breast cancer patients, regardless of treatment with chemotherapy, compared to the non-cancer group. For those who received chemotherapy the RR of POI and early menopause was 6.25 (95% CI 5.15–7.58) and 4.43 (95% CI 4.00–4.91), respectively. For those who did not receive chemotherapy the RR of POI and early menopause was 2.12 (95% CI 1.37–3.28) and 2.55 (95% CI 2.08–3.11), respectively.

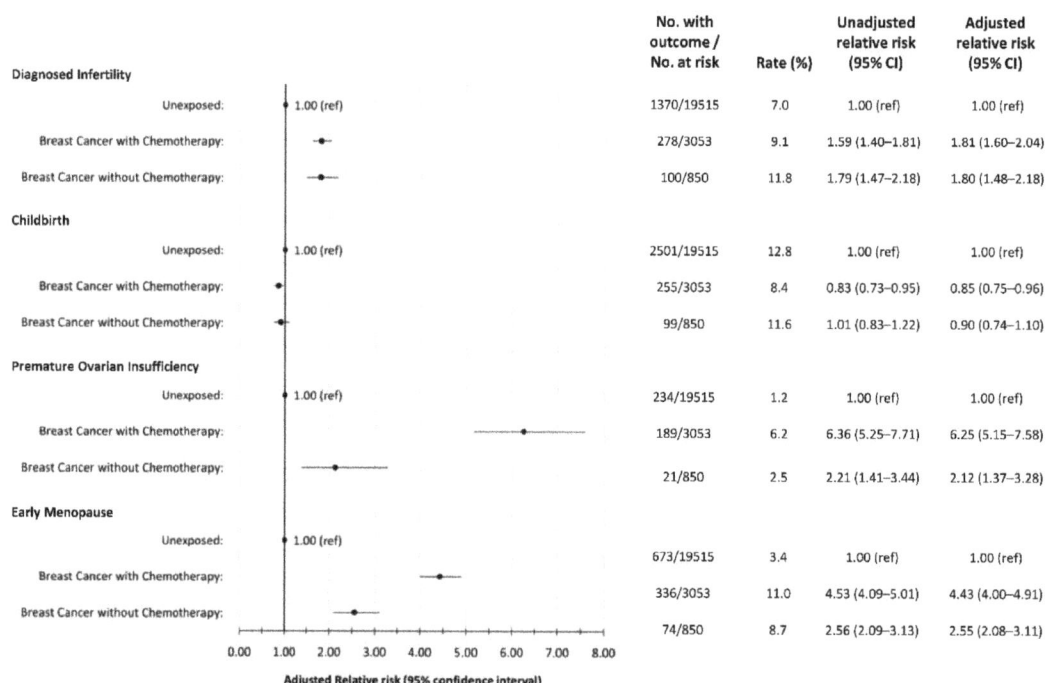

Figure 2. Forest plot depicting rates and relative risks (RR) with 95% confidence intervals for each outcome of interest by exposure and treatment group.

4. Discussion

In this study we found that all breast cancer patients are at increased risk of diagnosed infertility, not just those treated with chemotherapy. When compared with an age matched cohort, breast cancer patients treated with chemotherapy have a lower likelihood of giving birth during follow-up compared to women without cancer. BC patients who were not treated with chemotherapy did not have a statistically significant difference in childbirth. The risk of experiencing menopause after a breast cancer diagnosis increases with chemotherapy treatment. Notably, even without chemotherapy treatment there was an increased risk of POI and early menopause among breast cancer survivors.

Breast cancer is the most common malignancy affecting young women of childbearing age. Unfortunately, in young women, breast cancer is more likely to be high risk and require treatment with neoadjuvant or adjuvant chemotherapy [19] as evidenced in our study where 78% had chemotherapy included in their treatment plan. During the stress of a new cancer diagnosis, long-term health concerns, including fertility preservation, are often overlooked. A 2014 study from the United States estimated that nearly 50% of young women (age < 45) diagnosed with breast cancer, ~10,000 per year, are at risk of infertility due to breast cancer treatment [20]. Based on our findings this is likely an underestimate as we found an increased risk of infertility in all breast cancer survivors, not just those treated with chemotherapy. Current guidelines from the American Society of Clinical Oncology (ASCO) recommend embryo and/or oocyte cryopreservation or use of gonadotropin (GnRH) analogues during chemotherapy for fertility preservation [21]. Guidelines, however, do not always make it into clinical practice. A recent examination of the same Ontario population found that only 4% of AYA breast cancer patients diagnosed 2000–2017 were referred to a gynecologist for pre-chemotherapy fertility counselling [22]. While these rates improved over time, even the most contemporary results saw only 10.7% of patients referred for pre-chemotherapy counselling.

Counselling patients on the risk of infertility post breast cancer diagnosis is challenging. Our study provides a population-based estimate of infertility risk, childbirth and premature/early menopause in breast cancer patients compared to women without cancer. A similar population based age-matched cohort study from Norway in 2011 demonstrated much lower rates of pregnancy in breast cancer patients (diagnosed from 1967–2004) than was seen in our population with a HR of 0.35 (95% CI 0.27–0.44) compared to women without cancer [23]. A 2021 meta-analysis of pregnancy and pregnancy outcomes after cancer diagnosis of 39 studies including 112,840 BC patients found a 60 % lower rates of pregnancy in BC survivors compared to the general population (RR 0.40; 95% CI 0.32–0.49, $p < 0.001$) [24]. The differences from these large studies and ours may reflect changes in clinical practise or societal differences in family planning and child-rearing between populations. Fertility rates in general have been declining in Canada steadily since 2008, reaching a record low in 2020 of 1.4 live births per adult female age 15–39 [25]. It also demonstrates the importance of performing these analyses in different populations and time periods to understand the contemporary risks facing breast cancer survivors.

In terms of POI, to our knowledge this is the first study to assess the risk of POI at the population-based level in AYA with BC and the effect of chemotherapy. While it is accepted that chemotherapy possesses an increased rate of POI in 20–80% of AYA [26], our study supports an increased risk of POI even in patients without chemotherapy, likely related to the use of endocrine therapy. However, other contributing factors for this association need to be investigated such as defects in homologous recombination (e.g., BRCA1, BRCA2, PALB2, ATM, CHEK2) known to increase risk of breast cancer [27]. BRCA1 and 2 mutations are known to increase risk of POI due to impaired DNA repair mechanisms [28]. While accepted as a consequence of treatment, POI carries health risks for bone and cardiovascular health. Understanding these risks is important for both patients and providers for long-term health outcomes of these patients.

Our study has some important strengths including a large sample size, the inclusion of three reproductive outcomes (infertility diagnosis, childbirth, and POI) and the categorization of BC patients according to chemotherapy treatment (yes/no). This is the largest published study to date focusing on infertility diagnosis in relation to cancer treatment as the primary outcome considering cancer treatments; other large studies have focused on childbirth rates as the primary fertility outcome.

The main limitations of this study stem from the design and use of population-based data which is coded in administrative databases. There is the potential for information bias in this study, since the classification of infertility and menopause outcomes are likely under-reported, since many patients will not seek care for these concerns and therefore, they will not be captured in the health administrative database. We expect this under-reporting (misclassification) to be non-differential between exposure groups, and thus, the relative risks for these outcomes may be attenuated, such that the real effect estimates for breast cancer and infertility or menopause may be even larger than those reported in this article. Due to limitations of the data we were also unable to access information on several important variables which may have led to unmeasured confounding. Specifically, data on estrogen receptor status, endocrine therapy, and specifics of chemotherapy treatment was unavailable. It will be important to continue research in this field to understand whether or not fertility outcomes are impacted by breast cancer stage, subtype and contemporary treatment approaches.

5. Conclusions

This population-based cohort study found a significant association between chemotherapy treatment for AYA breast cancer and increased risk of Infertility and POI. There was also a novel finding that women with breast cancer who did not receive chemotherapy were also at a higher risk of Infertility and POI relative to women without cancer; an important detail to inform the care and counselling of AYA breast cancer patients. Further investigation into other mechanisms that can contribute to POI in women with breast cancer is needed. Oncofertility [29] is an important area which requires more attention to optimize care and education of young women with breast cancer.

Supplementary Materials: The following supporting information can be downloaded at: https://www.mdpi.com/article/10.3390/curroncol29110677/s1, supplemental methods

Author Contributions: Conceptualization, M.R., J.P., H.R., and M.P.V. methodology, M.R., J.P., H.R., X.W. and M.P.V.; software, X.W.; formal analysis, X.W.; data curation, X.W.; writing—original draft preparation, M.R.; writing—review and editing, J.P., X.W., M.P., H.R. and M.P.V.; visualization, J.P., X.W.; supervision, M.P.V.; project administration, J.P.; funding acquisition, M.P.V. All authors have read and agreed to the published version of the manuscript.

Funding: This research was funded by CIHR Institute of Gender and Health, Grant number WCH 169726.

Institutional Review Board Statement: The study was conducted in accordance with the Declaration of Helsinki, and approved by Queen's University Health Sciences Research Ethics Board, Kingston, Ontario (OBGY-296-16 #6019934, Initial clearance on 12 December 2016).

Data Availability Statement: The data set from this study is held securely in coded form at ICES. While data-sharing agreements prohibit ICES from making the data set publicly available, access may be granted to those who meet prespecified criteria for confidential access, available at www.ices.on.ca/DAS. The full data set creation plan and underlying analytic code are available from the authors upon request, understanding that the computer programmes may rely upon coding templates or macros.

Acknowledgments: This study was supported by ICES, which is funded by an annual grant from the Ontario Ministry of Health (MOH) and the Ministry of Long-Term Care (MLTC). This study also received funding from the Canadian Institute for Health Research (CIHR). Parts of this material are based on data and information compiled and provided by MOH, Ontario Health (Cancer Care Ontario), the Canadian Institute of Hospital Information (CIHI), and the Ontario Health Insurance Program (OHIP). Additionally, parts or whole of this material are based on data and/or information compiled and provided by Immigration, Refugees and Citizenship Canada (IRCC) current to 2019. The analyses, conclusions, opinions, and statements expressed herein are solely those of the authors and do not reflect those of the funding or data sources including the IRCC; no endorsement is intended nor should be inferred.

Conflicts of Interest: M.R.: Advisory Board: Gilead, Pfizer, Viatris, Exact Sciences. The rest authors declare no conflict of interest.

References

1. National Cancer Institute. Cancer Stat Facts: Cancer Among Adolescents and Young Adults (AYAs) (Ages 15–39). Available online: https://seer.cancer.gov/statfacts/html/aya.html (accessed on 2 March 2022).
2. National Cancer Institute. Cancer Stat Facts: Female Breast Cancer. Available online: http://seer.cancer.gov/statfacts/html/breast.html (accessed on 2 March 2022).
3. Canadian Partnership Against Cancer. Adolescents & Young Adults with Cancer: A System Performance Report. Toronto (ON): Canadian Partnership Against Cancer. 15 April 2017. Available online: https://s22457.pcdn.co/wp-content/uploads/2019/01/Adolescents-and-young-adults-with-cancer-EN.pdf (accessed on 14 April 2021).
4. Hickey, M.; Peate, M.; Saunders, C.M.; Friedlander, M. Breast cancer in young women and its im-pact on reproductive function. Human reproduction update. *Hum. Reprod. Update* **2009**, *15*, 323–339. [CrossRef] [PubMed]
5. Breast.PDF [Internet]. Available online: https://www.nccn.org/professionals/physician_gls/pdf/breast.pdf (accessed on 24 October 2021).
6. Henry, N.L.; Somerfield, M.R.; Abramson, V.G.; Allison, K.H.; Anders, C.K.; Chingos, D.T.; Hurria, A.; Openshaw, T.H.; Krop, I.E. Role of patient and disease factors in adjuvant systemic therapy decision making for early-stage, operable breast cancer: American Society of Clinical Oncology endorsement of Cancer Care Ontario guide-line recommendations. *Am. J. Clin. Oncol.* **2016**, *34*, 2303–2311. [CrossRef] [PubMed]
7. Burstein, H.J.; Lacchetti, C.; Anderson, H.; Buchholz, T.A.; Davidson, N.E.; Gelmon, K.A.; Giordano, S.H.; Hudis, C.A.; Solky, A.J.; Stearns, V.; et al. Adjuvant endocrine therapy for women with hormone receptor-positive breast cancer: ASCO clini-cal practice guideline focused update. *J. Clin. Oncol.* **2019**, *37*, 423–438. [CrossRef] [PubMed]
8. Francis, P.A.; Pagani, O.; Fleming, G.F.; Walley, B.A.; Colleoni, M.; Láng, I.; Gómez, H.L.; Tondini, C.; Ciruelos, E.; Burstein, H.J.; et al. Tai-loring adjuvant endocrine therapy for premenopausal breast cancer. *NEJM* **2018**, *379*, 122–137. [CrossRef]

9. Velez, M.P.; Richardson, H.; Baxter, N.N.; McClintock, C.; Greenblatt, E.; Barr, R.; Green, M. Risk of infertility in female adolescents and young adults with cancer: A population-based cohort study. *Hum. Reprod.* **2021**, *36*, 1981–1988. [CrossRef] [PubMed]
10. Baillargeon, A.; Pudwell, J.; McClintock, C.; Velez, M.P. Premature ovarian insufficiency in female adolescent and young adult survivors of cancer: A population-based cohort study. *J. Obstet. Gynaecol. Can.* **2021**, *43*, 658. [CrossRef]
11. Imai, A.; Furui, T. Chemotherapy-induced female infertility and protective action of gonadotro-pin-releasing hormone analogues. *JOG* **2007**, *27*, 20–24.
12. Levine, J.M.; Kelvin, J.F.; Quinn, G.; Gracia, C.R. Infertility in reproductive-age female cancer survivors. *Cancer* **2015**, *121*, 1532–1539. [CrossRef]
13. Partridge, A.H.; Ruddy, K.J. Fertility and adjuvant treatment in young women with breast cancer. *Breast* **2007**, *16*, 175–181. [CrossRef]
14. Morarji, K.; McArdle, O.; Hui, K.; Gingras-Hill, G.; Ahmed, S.; Greenblatt, E.M.; Warner, E.; Sridhar, S.; Ali, A.M.F.; Azad, A.; et al. Ovarian Function after Chemotherapy in Young Breast Cancer Survivors. *Curr. Oncol.* **2017**, *24*, 494–502. [CrossRef]
15. Del Mastro, L.; Catzeddu, T.; Venturini, M. Infertility and pregnancy after breast cancer: Current knowledge and future perspectives. *Cancer. Treat. Rev.* **2006**, *32*, 417–422. [CrossRef] [PubMed]
16. Burstein, H.J.; Lacchetti, C.; Anderson, H.; Buchholz, T.; Davidson, N.E.; Gelmon, K.E.; Giordano, S.H.; Hudis, C.A.; Solky, A.J.; Stearns, V.; et al. Adjuvant Endocrine Therapy for Women With Hormone Receptor–Positive Breast Cancer: American Society of Clinical Oncology Clinical Practice Guideline Update on Ovarian Suppression. *J. Clin. Oncol.* **2016**, *34*, 1689–1701. [CrossRef] [PubMed]
17. Marton, J.A.; Hamilton, B.E.; Osterman, M.J.K.; Driscoll, A.K. Births: Final report from 2019. *CDC Natl. Rep. Vital Stat.* **2021**, *70*, 4.
18. Austin, P.C. Using the Standardized Difference to Compare the Prevalence of a Binary Variable Be-tween Two Groups in Observational Research, *Commun. Stat.* **2009**, *38*, 1228–1234.
19. Murphy, B.L.; Day, C.N.; Hoskin, T.L.; Habermann, E.B.; Boughey, J.C. Adolescents and Young Adults with Breast Cancer have More Aggressive Disease and Treatment Than Patients in Their Forties. *Ann. Surg. Oncol.* **2019**, *26*, 3920–3930. [CrossRef]
20. Trivers, K.F.; Fink, A.K.; Partridge, A.H.; Oktay, K.; Ginsburg, E.S.; Li, C.; Pollack, L.A. Estimates of Young Breast Cancer Survivors at Risk for Infertility in the U.S. *Oncol.* **2014**, *19*, 814–822. [CrossRef]
21. Oktay, K.; Harvey, B.; Partridge, A.H.; Quinn, G.; Reinecke, J.; Taylor, H.S.; Wallace, W.H.; Wang, E.T.; Loren, A.W. Fertility Preservation in Patients With Cancer: ASCO Clinical Practice Guideline Update. *J. Clin. Oncol.* **2018**, *36*, 1994–2001. [CrossRef]
22. Korkidakis, A.; Lajkosz, K.; Green, M.; Strobino, D.; Velez, M.P. Patterns of Referral for Fertility Preservation Among Female Adolescents and Young Adults with Breast Cancer: A Population-Based Study. *J. Adolesc. Young- Adult. Oncol.* **2019**, *8*, 197–204. [CrossRef]
23. Stensheim, H.; Cvancarova, M.; Møller, B.; Fosså, S.D. Pregnancy after adolescent and adult cancer: A population-based matched cohort study. *Int. J. Cancer* **2011**, *129*, 1225–1236. [CrossRef]
24. Lambertini, M.; Blondeaux, E.; Bruzzone, M.; Perachino, M.; Anderson, R.A.; de Azambuja, E.; Poorvu, P.D.; Kim, H.J.; Villarreal-Garza, C.; Pistilli, B.; et al. Pregnancy After Breast Cancer: A Systematic Review and Meta-Analysis. *J. Clin. Oncol.* **2021**, *39*, 3293–3305. [CrossRef]
25. Statistics Canada: Crude Birth Rate, Age-Specific Fertility Rates and Total Fertility Rates (Live Births). Available online: https://www150.statcan.gc.ca/n1/en/catalogue/13100418 (accessed on 14 April 2021).
26. Gargus, E.; Deans, R.; Anazodo, A.; Woodruff, T.K. Management of Primary Ovarian Insufficiency Symptoms in Survivors of Childhood and Adolescent Cancer. *J. Natl. Compr. Cancer. Netw.* **2018**, *16*, 1137–1149. [CrossRef] [PubMed]
27. den Brok, W.D.; Schrader, K.A.; Sun, S.; Tinker, A.V.; Zhao, E.Y.; Aparicio, S.; Gelmon, K.A. Ho-mologous recombination deficiency in breast cancer: A clinical review. *JCO Precis. Oncol.* **2017**, *1*, 1–13. [PubMed]
28. Miao, Y.; Wang, P.; Xie, B.; Yang, M.; Li, S.; Cui, Z.; Fan, Y.; Li, M.; Xiong, B. BRCA2 deficiency is a potential driver for human primary ovarian insufficiency. *Cell. Death. Dis.* **2019**, *10*, 474. [CrossRef] [PubMed]
29. Woodruff, T.K. Oncofertility: A grand collaboration between reproductive medicine and oncolo-gy. *Reproduction* **2015**, *150*, S1–S10. [CrossRef]

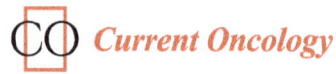

Commentary

Adolescents and Young Adults with Cancer and the Desire for Parenthood—A Legal View from a Swiss Perspective in Consideration of the Relevance of Cancer Support Organizations

Isabel Baur [1,2,*], Sina Staudinger [2,3] and Ariana Aebi [1,2]

1. Competence Center of Medicine-Ethics-Law Helvetiae, University of Zurich, 8032 Zurich, Switzerland; ariana.aebi@ius.uzh.ch
2. The Association "AYA Cancer Support CH", 8041 Zurich, Switzerland; sina.staudinger@ius.uzh.ch
3. Committee for Protection against Sexual Harassment, University of Zurich, 8032 Zurich, Switzerland
* Correspondence: isabel.baur@ius.uzh.ch

Abstract: This commentary focuses on the challenges and possibilities that adolescents and young adults with cancer (AYA) desiring parenthood face under Swiss law. The regulation of reproductive medicine procedures is stricter in Switzerland than in some other countries. Health insurance is compulsory, but the interventions that are covered are in constant flux. Recent changes pertain to the possibilities of future AYA parenthood and keeping up to date with practical and legal ramifications is taxing even for health professionals. AYA facing treatment decisions are uniquely vulnerable and dependent on comprehensive, clear, current, and country-specific information regarding risks and options pertaining to their fertility. This commentary provides a short overview of the Swiss legal framework related to reproductive medicine, highlighting its access restrictions and prohibitions, as well as recent changes. While the importance of patient, peer, caregiver, and interest groups supporting people affected by health conditions has long been recognized in many countries, an AYA organization was only recently established in Switzerland. Such organizations are vital for providing accurate, country-specific information and support, while individualized medical guidance, informed by the most current legal framework and its consequences, remains essential in addressing AYAs' specific needs in connection with the desire to have children.

Keywords: AYA oncology; treatment; models of care; long-term follow-up; survivorship; fertility; cancer association; peer group

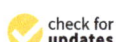

Citation: Baur, I.; Staudinger, S.; Aebi, A. Adolescents and Young Adults with Cancer and the Desire for Parenthood—A Legal View from a Swiss Perspective in Consideration of the Relevance of Cancer Support Organizations. *Curr. Oncol.* **2023**, *30*, 10124–10133. https://doi.org/10.3390/curroncol30120736

Received: 30 August 2023
Revised: 3 November 2023
Accepted: 22 November 2023
Published: 27 November 2023

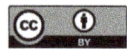

Copyright: © 2023 by the authors. Licensee MDPI, Basel, Switzerland. This article is an open access article distributed under the terms and conditions of the Creative Commons Attribution (CC BY) license (https://creativecommons.org/licenses/by/4.0/).

1. Introduction

Globally, approximately 1.2 million adolescents and young adults aged 15 to 39 years are diagnosed with cancer every year [1,2]. There is currently no consistent definition of the age range of AYA. According to common definitions, adulthood begins at around 20 years of age and young adulthood ends—depending on the point of view—at 24, 35 or 39 years. Since AYA have only recently been recognized as a distinct patient group in Switzerland, and since there is still no research in this area in Switzerland taking into account legal aspects, the authors have chosen this patient group. In the context of challenges regarding the fertility of AYA, an age range up to 39 years is justified [3]. In the past decade, AYA have become recognized as a vulnerable patient group [4]. In Switzerland—where AYA have long been unrecognized as a distinct patient group—calculations have shown that approximately 1770 AYA are newly diagnosed with cancer each year [5]. Due to progress in cancer treatment, over 80% of AYA diagnosed with cancer survive beyond 5 years, which leads to a continual increase in the number of AYA survivors who have the potential to continue living for decades [2,4]. This requires that the health system guarantees access to treatment and follow-up care in various medical and psychosocial areas beyond oncology [3].

The need to regard AYA as a distinct patient group affected by a broad spectrum of cancers stems from their life stage, their specific psychosocial needs, and the effects as well as long-term consequences of the cancers and their treatments, as well as the potential years of life lost [2]. AYA are at a stage in life where they may be very conscious of their body and appearance and would, under normal circumstances, develop a positive body image, start leaving home and establish independence, increase contact with peers, and start dating or making important career and family decisions [2,6]. It is essential to take into account that a cancer diagnosis—especially concerning younger AYA—affects not a mature but a maturing personality, in a developmentally vulnerable period, and still in the process of finding their identity [7,8]. The diagnosis comes at a time when under normal circumstances the fear of dying would have no place, with the diagnosis interfering with life overall and future planning [9]. Long-term and late effects among AYA survivors cover a range of physical issues (due to changes in appearance), secondary malignancies (for example, due to radiotherapy), cardiovascular diseases, endocrine dysfunctions (such as thyroid dysfunction or diabetes), neurocognitive deficits, impaired fertility, sexual dysfunction, body disfigurement, a lower level of physical functioning, and psychological and social issues (due to disruptions in social life, increased dependence or a premature confrontation with mortality), as well as challenges in finances and career [2,6]. In connection with the desire for parenthood, it should be mentioned that half of all male childhood cancer survivors suffer from infertility as a late consequence of treatment [10]. The lived experience of young survivors regarding decisions about fertility and parenthood has received insufficient attention in the literature to date. There is a clear unmet need to provide age-appropriate information regarding fertility and parenthood options [11]. Furthermore, an AYA's cancer diagnosis may also affect relatives, partners or caregivers, as well as potential future partners [2,12].

As legal volunteers for the non-profit organization "AYA Cancer Support CH", the authors have repeatedly been confronted with the legal challenges associated with survivors' desire to have children. This commentary provides a broad overview of the current practice in Switzerland from a legal perspective. In Switzerland, medical insurance is compulsory and covers interventions that meet certain criteria, such as cost-effectiveness, the definition of which is a matter of ongoing debate. Medically assisted reproduction is more strictly regulated in Switzerland than in other countries, which has implications for AYA, requiring measures for human reproduction and fertility preservation due to the impact of chemotherapy. This paper answers questions such as the following: To what extent are human reproduction measures for AYA possible, be it legally or practically, in Switzerland? How are costs covered, e.g., in connection with egg storage? Due to cancer support organizations becoming increasingly relevant in Switzerland, where peer, family, and caregiver support groups have been less common in the past than they have been in other countries, this commentary aims to bridge the gap between legal practice and constraints and the role of non-profit organizations to support AYA with lived experiences of cancer and their partners considering a current or future wish to become a parent.

2. Materials and Methods

This commentary is based on a systematic literature search and the personal experiences of the three authors and co-founders of the AYA organization "AYA Cancer Support CH". International AYA-related studies, topic-specific literature, and Swiss legal opinion publications as well as Swiss case law and court rulings were used, taking into account current developments and innovations in legislation. The choice of literature was at the discretion of the authors. Most of the literature analyzed is relevant to the field and scientifically based. In isolated cases, e.g., with regard to supportive measures, sources relevant to practice were also used.

3. AYA, Fertility and Childbearing

3.1. Introduction

Involuntary childlessness—for a variety of reasons—may place a considerable burden on people of all genders [13]. Although cancer therapy can severely limit fertility, many AYA do not consider dealing with a possible future desire to have children when confronted with a cancer diagnosis. Rather, the disease and its treatment take center stage and disrupt the planned life course. In the general public in Switzerland, the mean age for giving birth for the first time is 31 for the person carrying the child [14]. This points to the fact that the discussion about having children usually follows at a later stage in life.

For people affected by cancer at a later stage in life, the desire to have children may already be present at the time of diagnosis or efforts may already have been made to become pregnant. At this stage of life, the topics of the desire to have children and fertility already lead to considerations of whether cryopreservation should be considered at the time of diagnosis. Fertility can be limited by impending cancer therapy, which can lead to full infertility. However, this is not always the case, as different therapies entail different consequences in terms of fertility. Nevertheless, with a view to the future, the retrieval and cryopreservation of oocytes or sperm early on may greatly improve the chance of preserving fertility [15].

In addition to medical questions and decisions in the context of a cancer diagnosis, for a physician, it would be particularly important to also discuss the topics of "sexuality", "fertility" and "desire for children" with young patients. Sexuality and fertility are often dismissed in society and problems in this area tend to receive little attention. Nevertheless, it is of utmost importance that physicians address the issues, outline the various consequences, and provide information so that a conscious decision can be made for or against fertility-preserving measures [16]. The inclusion of various options is of great importance in this decision-making process. This is because even if a therapy is to be used and the treatment is expected to have little or no effect on fertility, scenarios with less favorable or different outcomes need to be considered up front. For example, it may be necessary to switch therapies due to treatment resistance, cancer progression, or the intolerability of side-effects. It is the duty of the physician to inform young patients of the choices and potential consequences. These decisions and burdens should not be underestimated in the overall process of treatment. The issue of fertility in AYA requires collaboration and cooperation among specialists in oncology, reproductive medicine, and pediatrics, as appropriate. Certain considerations may be obvious and self-evident to specialists; however, they must be communicated and discussed with the patient in concrete terms in order to enable the patient to grant truly comprehensive informed consent [15].

3.2. Legal Framework in Switzerland

3.2.1. Current Situation in Switzerland

In Switzerland, approximately 6200 women made use of reproductive medicine options (in vitro methods) in 2020 [17]. The common reasons why couples remain involuntarily childless and make use of medically assisted reproduction vary. For example, the first pregnancy resulting in childbirth increasingly occurs in those over 35 years old because the reconciliation of work and family life is difficult. Another reason can be found in genetic diseases that could be transmitted to the newborn [13]. These reasons may also apply to AYA. However, AYA face additional challenges. In the following sections, the legal situation in Switzerland with regard to the possible use of medical reproductive procedures is outlined.

The following figure (Figure 1) provides an initial overview of the relevant laws in Switzerland:

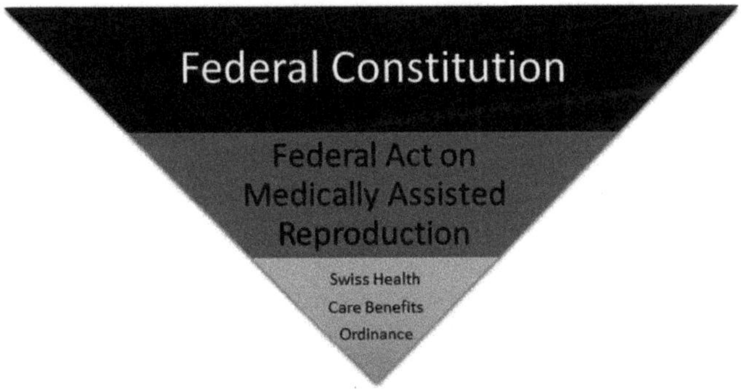

Figure 1. Visualization of the hierarchy levels of the different laws.

3.2.2. Federal Constitution and Legislative Level

The Federal Constitution (FC) [18] is the constitution of the Swiss Confederation and is hierarchically at the highest level of the Swiss legal system. Laws or ordinances of the Confederation as well as the cantons and the communes are subordinate to the Federal Constitution [19]. The desire to have children is recognized as an elementary element of personality development and is protected by the fundamental right of personal freedom, which is protected by the Confederation in Art. 10 para. 2. In concrete terms, this protection means that, on the one hand, access to methods of reproductive medicine is guaranteed, and on the other hand, human beings are to be protected from abuses of reproductive medicine. Human dignity in dealing with human germinal and genetic material takes precedence at all times. The Confederation has the competence to regulate the handling of human germinal and genetic material (Art. 119 para. 2 FC). It is prohibited to use medically assisted reproduction in order to conduct research or to induce certain characteristics in a child (Art. 119 para. 2 lit. c FC).

Furthermore, the Constitution forms the basis of specific substantive requirements for the use of reproductive medicine, which are specified by the Federal Act on Medically Assisted Reproduction (RMA) [20].

3.2.3. Access Restrictions and Prohibitions

Both the FC and the RMA contain restrictions and limitations on access. The declared aim of the restrictions is to ensure the best interests of the child. This is because medically assisted reproduction may only be used if the best interests of the child, as the overriding good, are safeguarded (Art. 3 para. 1 RMA). The scope, meaning and understanding of what the best interests of the child entail are not legally defined [13] and are subject to social views and developments.

In order to do justice to the best interests of the child, various prohibitions are contained in both the FC and the RMA, which are handled less restrictively in other countries. Of particular relevance for AYA is that both embryo donation and all forms of surrogacy are prohibited in Switzerland (Art. 119 para. 2 lit. d FC). Furthermore, according to Art. 4 RMA, egg donation is prohibited. However, artificial insemination, in vitro fertilization with embryo transfer, and gamete transfer are generally permitted (Art. 2 lit. a RMA, Art. 5 and Art. 5b RMA). In particular, surrogacy and egg donation are the subject of a lively social and professional debate [13,21]. Especially for young female AYA, the prohibition of surrogacy has implications if there is a desire to have children and the woman's fertility has become limited or fully impaired. In this case, it is not permitted for another person to carry a child by means of egg donation or with the egg of the AYA concerned.

In addition to the prohibitions described above, Swiss law also imposes various restrictions on access to reproductive medical procedures. The procedures are reserved for couples with whom a future child is deemed to be able to establish a parent–child relationship in accordance with the Swiss Civil Code, and who, based on their age and personal circumstances, are capable of caring for such a future child until it reaches the age of majority (Art. 3 para. 2 lit. a and b RMA). If this is considered to be established, the reproductive procedure must serve to overcome the infertility of the couple, if other methods of treatment do not lead to the desired outcome or if there is a risk of transmission of a serious disease (Art. 5 lit a and b RMA). Only married heterosexual and—only since 1 July 2022—homosexual couples can make use of sperm donation (Art. 3 para. 3 RMA).

3.3. AYA and the Desire to Have Children

After the preceding explanations, the question arises as to what extent AYA can make use of reproductive medicine in Switzerland. According to the current law, germ cells may be preserved (Art. 15 RMA). Progress in reproductive medicine has led to a continued improvement in the possibilities of preserving germ cells. From a legal point of view, germ cells can in principle be preserved for five years and, at the request of the person concerned, the preservation may be extended by a maximum of five years (Art. 15 para. 1 RMA). A longer preservation period is also possible if a medical treatment is carried out which the person concerned must undergo, or if he/she must perform an activity that may lead to infertility or damage to his/her genetic material (Art. 15 para. 2 RMA). So-called cryopreservation refers to the method by which vital cells (male or female) or fertilized oocytes or embryos can be frozen [22]. There are different methods, especially "slow freezing" and "vitrification"; while the choice of the method is considered less decisive, the factors of the time of collection and the time of possible use of the frozen cells are considered crucial. Even the duration of storage is considered less relevant. From a technical point of view, the freezing and thawing process plays a more important part [22].

The storage of germ cells is agreed upon with a contract: a so-called cryo-contract (deposit contract according to Art. 472 Code of Obligations [23]). In this contract, the custodian is charged with the safekeeping of a movable object (unfertilized extracorporeal germ cells) entrusted to him or her by the depositor. Use without the depositor's consent is prohibited. The contract is usually renewed annually [22]. An annual storage fee is payable for the service. In addition, there are costs for ovarian stimulation and egg retrieval. Compulsory health insurance does not usually cover these costs and so storage must be self-financed by the person concerned. However, since July 2019, there has been an exception for fertility-preserving measures for men and women up to 40 years of age suffering from cancer (Art. 1 Swiss Health Care Benefits Ordinance (KLV) [24] in connection with Annex 1 No. 3 KLV). This provision may be considered an important step in the perception and concrete support of AYA in Switzerland. The exception indicates that the legislator and the public are developing an awareness of the AYA patient group as well as their specific needs.

For AYA with the desire to father offspring through reproductive medicine, the provision of Art. 15 RMA is of particular importance. On the one hand, a reproductive procedure can be used to circumvent infertility caused by cancer therapy. Medical treatments leading to infertility, surgical interventions, radiological treatments, chemotherapies or potentially fertility-toxic medication are to be thought of [22]. On the other hand, there are also cancers that can be transmitted to offspring. In these cases, reproductive medicine can avert this risk to the extent that the germ cells are specifically selected in an in vitro procedure to avoid this risk (Art. 5a RMA). Regarding future medical treatment leading to damage to the genetic material or to a permanent loss of fertility, it is possible to preserve germ cells beyond the ten-year storage period.

In addition to the medical support options described above, it should be mentioned that the possibility of adoption must also be considered. The legal requirements for adoption are also regulated nationally and are considered strict in Switzerland in comparison to other countries (Art. 264 ff. Swiss Civil Code [25]). A detailed explanation of the legal basis with regard to adoption would go beyond the scope of this commentary.

3.4. AYA Organisations

The above-mentioned legal and medical challenges regarding parenthood after a cancer diagnosis can be quite complex, and a lack of knowledge about possible measures and possibilities could even lead to an unfulfilled desire for parenthood. In order to counteract this lack of information as well as other possible long-term consequences of cancer, support by organizations tailored to the needs of AYA during and after treatment as well as for their relatives, partners, friends and caregivers is essential. Psychosocial and behavioral interventions may assist AYA in returning to their social roles as a parent, spouse, student, worker or friend, and provide support with finding specific and relevant cancer-related information, as well as measures for specific problems, such as coping with the future, possible impaired fertility, fatigue, fear of relapses, or challenges concerning the resumption of work or education [6,26]. Peer support among AYA in dealing with long-term consequences, sharing their lived experience in an age-appropriate way, and talking to someone in the same situation about specific problems is vital [6,27]. AYA have to face different questions due to their stage in life, such as the following: How much should they tell new acquaintances, including an employer or someone they are newly dating, about their illness or long-term impacts [6]? Where can they find medical and psychological support once their treatment ends [26]? How should they deal with friends lost due to cancer [26]? Does cancer during pregnancy effect the unborn child? What happens during breastfeeding while having breast cancer? These are all questions where AYA could benefit from the experiences of other AYA who have already experienced these situations.

There are many different organizations worldwide for AYA. Table 1 is an attempt to categorize some of these organizations, although the list is in no way exhaustive and certain organizations may include services that would also make them fall in more than one category:

Table 1. List of AYA organizations.

AYA Organization Categories	Examples
Local advocacy and support organizations	Cancer Fight Club [28] (Canada), Ulman Cancer Fund for Young Adults [29] (USA), Shine [30] (UK), Canteen [31] (Australia), etc.
Organizations for specific AYA	Pink Pearl [32] (young women), Sharsheret [33] (Jewish AYA), Hope for Two [34] (pregnant AYA), etc.
Organizations for specific AYA cancer types	YSC [35] (breast cancer), Tigerlily Foundation [36] (breast cancer), Testicular Cancer Society [37], National Ovarian Cancer Coalition [38], etc.
Research and education organizations	SAYAO [39], Smart Patients [40], Ovarian Cancer Research Alliance [41], etc.
Web-based social-media platforms or apps	Stupid Cancer [42], Stop Cancer [43], Cancerversity [44] (for young women of color), GRYT Health Cancer Community [45] (Application), Young Adult Cancer Connection [46]

As shown by the incredible number of users on the two largest web-based social media platforms [47], Stop Cancer (with over 30,000 followers on Facebook) [48] and Stupid Cancer (with almost 315,000 followers on Facebook) [49], organizations that utilize digital measures have gained massive relevance when it comes to supporting AYA. Through using technologies that AYA as digital natives are familiar with (Facebook, Youtube, etc.). Web-based social networking websites help AYA to connect with each other and therefore give an opportunity for peer involvement as well as social support through peer interaction, where AYA can exchange the above-mentioned fears or social issues [6,26]. Social digital media platforms allow a multi-perspective exchange that can cover topics ranging from social security to clinical information, for example, on side effects and personal experiences,

16. Glazer, T.S.; Schulte, F. Barriers to Oncofertility Care among Female Adolescent Cancer Patients in Canada. *Curr. Oncol.* **2022**, *29*, 1583–1593. [CrossRef] [PubMed]
17. Federal Statistical Office. Medically Assisted Reproduction. 22 March 2022. Available online: http://www.bfs.admin.ch/bfs/de/home/statistiken/gesundheit/gesundheitszustand/reproduktive/medizinisch-unterstuetzte-fortpflanzung.html (accessed on 18 July 2023).
18. Federal Constitution of the Swiss Confederation of 18 April 1999, SR 101. Available online: https://www.fedlex.admin.ch/eli/cc/1999/404/en (accessed on 18 July 2023).
19. Relationship Cantonal Law and Constitutional Law. Available online: https://www.parlament.ch/de/über-das-parlament/wie-funktioniert-das-parlament/parlamentsrecht/bundesverfassung (accessed on 18 July 2023).
20. Federal Act on Medically Assisted Reproduction (RMA) of 8 December 11998, SR 810.11. Available online: https://www.fedlex.admin.ch/eli/cc/2000/554/en (accessed on 18 July 2023).
21. Federal Office of Public Health. Available online: http://www.bag.admin.ch/bag/en/home/medizin-und-forschung/fortpflanzungsmedizin.html (accessed on 18 July 2023).
22. Dörr, B. Art. 15 Konservierung von Keimzellen. In *Handkommentar Fortpflanzungsmedizin*; Büchler, A., Rütsche, B., Eds.; Stämpfli Verlag: Bern, Switzerland, 2020; p. 522.
23. Federal Act on the Amendment of the Swiss Civil Code, Part Five: The Code of Obligations of 30 March 1911, SR 220. Available online. https://www.fedlex.admin.ch/eli/cc/27/317_321_377/en (accessed on 18 July 2023).
24. Regulation of the Federal Department of Home Affairs on Benefits in Compulsory Health Care Insurance (Swiss Health Care Benefits Ordinance, KLV) of 29 September 1995, SR 832.112.31. Available online: https://www.fedlex.admin.ch/eli/cc/1995/4964_4964_4964/de?print=true (accessed on 18 July 2023).
25. Swiss Civil Code of 10 December 1907, SR 210. Available online: https://www.fedlex.admin.ch/eli/cc/24/233_245_233/en (accessed on 18 July 2023).
26. Moody, L.; Turner, A.; Osmond, J.; Hooker, L.; Kosmala-Anders, J.; Batehup, L. Web-based self-management for young cancer survivors: Consideration of user requirements and barriers to implementation. *J. Cancer Surviv.* **2015**, *9*, 188–200. [CrossRef]
27. Matsui, M.; Taku, K.; Tsutsumi, R.; Ueno, M.; Seto, M.; Makimoto, A.; Yuza, Y. Role of Peer Support in Posttraumatic Growth Among Adolescent and Young Adult Cancer Patients and Survivors. *J. Adolesc. Young Adult Oncol.* **2023**, *12*, 503–511. [CrossRef] [PubMed]
28. CancerFightClub, an Initiative from across Montreal and Quebec. Available online: http://www.cancerfightclub.com (accessed on 18 July 2023).
29. Ulman Cancer Fund for Young Adults. Available online: http://www.ulmanfoundation.org (accessed on 18 July 2023).
30. Shine Cancer Support. Available online: http://www.shinecancersupport.org (accessed on 18 July 2023).
31. Canteen. Available online: http://www.canteen.org.au (accessed on 18 July 2023).
32. Pink Pearl Canada. Available online: http://www.pinkpearlcanada.org (accessed on 18 July 2023).
33. Sharasheret. Available online: http://www.sharsheret.org (accessed on 18 July 2023).
34. Hope for Two, the Pregnant with Cancer Network. Available online: http://www.hopefortwo.org (accessed on 18 July 2023).
35. YSC, Young Survival Coalition. Available online: http://www.youngsurvival.org (accessed on 18 July 2023).
36. Tigerlily Foundation. Available online: http://www.tigerlilyfoundation.org (accessed on 18 July 2023).
37. Testicular Cancer Society. Available online: https://testicularcancersociety.org/ (accessed on 18 July 2023).
38. National Ovarian Cancer Coalition. Available online: https://www.ovarian.org (accessed on 20 October 2023).
39. SAYAO. Society for Adolescent and Young Adult Oncology. Available online: http://www.sayao.org (accessed on 18 July 2023).
40. Smart Patients Young Adults Community. Available online: http://www.smartpatients.com (accessed on 18 July 2023).
41. Ovarian Cancer Research Alliance. Available online: https://ocrahope.org/ (accessed on 18 July 2023).
42. Stupid Cancer, Get Busy Living, Established 2007. Available online: http://www.stupidcancer.org (accessed on 18 July 2023).
43. Stop Cancer "A Spark of Life for the Young". Available online: http://www.stop-cancer.co.il/a-spark-of-life-for-the-young (accessed on 18 July 2023).
44. Cancerversity. Available online: http://www.cancerversity.com (accessed on 18 July 2023).
45. GRYT Health Cancer Community. Available online: http://www.apps.apple.com/us/app/gryt-health-cancer-community/id1219349562 (accessed on 18 July 2023).
46. Young Adult Cancer Connection, Meet Your Cell Mates. Available online: http://www.yacancerconnection.org (accessed on 18 July 2023).
47. Ben-Aharon, I.; Goshen-Lago, T.; Fontana, E.; Smyth, E.; Guren, M.; Caballero, C.; Lordick, F. Social networks for young patients with cancer: The time for system agility. *Lancet Oncol.* **2019**, *20*, 765, Erratum in *Lancet Oncol.* **2019**, *20*, e346. [CrossRef] [PubMed]
48. Facebook-Page of Stop Cancer. Available online: http://www.facebook.com/halasartan (accessed on 18 July 2023).
49. Facebook-Page of Stupid Cancer. Available online: http://www.facebook.com/stupidcancer (accessed on 18 July 2023).
50. Competence Center for Medicine-Ethics-Law Helvetiae. Available online: http://www.merh.uzh.ch (accessed on 18 July 2023).
51. PhD Program Biomedical Ethics and Law. Available online: http://www.bmel.uzh.ch (accessed on 18 July 2023).
52. All.Can Switzerland. Available online: http://www.allcan-schweiz.ch (accessed on 18 July 2023).
53. Supervised by, Dr. Martin Inderbitzin, Founder of mysurvivalstory.org. Available online: https://www.mysurvivalstory.org/ (accessed on 18 July 2023).

54. For Example of the Krebsliga Beider Basel, Who Also Provide an AYA Program. Available online: http://www.basel.krebsliga.ch/beratung-unterstuetzung/jung-und-krebs (accessed on 18 July 2023).
55. AYA Cancer Support Instagram Account. Available online: http://www.www.instagram.com/ayacancersupport.ch (accessed on 18 July 2023).
56. AYA Cancer Support Facebook Account. Available online: http://www.www.facebook.com/groups/ayacancersupport.ch (accessed on 18 July 2023).
57. Darabos, K.; Berger, A.J.; Barakat, L.P.; Schwartz, L.A. Cancer-Related Decision-Making Among Adolescents, Young Adults, Caregivers, and Oncology Providers. *Qual. Health Res.* **2021**, *31*, 2355–2363. [CrossRef] [PubMed]
58. Norton, W.; Wright, E. Barriers and Facilitators to Fertility-Related Discussions with Teenagers and Young Adults with Cancer: Nurses' Experiences. *J. Adolesc. Young Adult Oncol.* **2020**, *9*, 481–489. [CrossRef] [PubMed]
59. Ruiz, S.; Mintz, R.; Sijecic, A.; Eggers, M.; Hoffman, A.; Woodard, T.; Bjonard, K.L.; Hoefgen, H.; Sandheinrich, T.; Omurtag, K.; et al. Websites about, not for, adolescents? A systematic analysis of online fertility preservation information for adolescent and young adult cancer patients. *J. Cancer Surviv.* **2023**. [CrossRef] [PubMed]
60. Nahata, L.; Anazodo, A.; Cherven, B.; Logan, S.; Meacham, L.R.; Meade, C.D.; Zarnegar-Lumley, S.; Quinn, G.P. Optimizing health literacy to facilitate reproductive health decision-making in adolescent and young adults with cancer. *Pediatr. Blood Cancer* **2023**, *70* (Suppl. S5), e28476. [CrossRef] [PubMed]
61. Marino, J.L.; Peate, M.; McNeil, R.; Orme, L.M.; McCarthy, M.C.; Glackin, A.; Sawyer, S.M. Experiences of Family and Partner Support in Fertility Decision-Making Among Adolescents and Young Adults with Cancer: A National Australian Study. *J. Adolesc. Young Adult Oncol.* 2023; *ahead of print*. [CrossRef] [PubMed]

Disclaimer/Publisher's Note: The statements, opinions and data contained in all publications are solely those of the individual author(s) and contributor(s) and not of MDPI and/or the editor(s). MDPI and/or the editor(s) disclaim responsibility for any injury to people or property resulting from any ideas, methods, instructions or products referred to in the content.

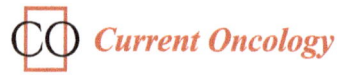

Article

Exercise Preferences in Young Adults with Cancer—The YOUEX Study

Annelie Voland [1,†], Verena Krell [2,3,†], Miriam Götte [4], Timo Niels [5], Maximilian Köppel [1] and Joachim Wiskemann [1,*]

1. Department of Medical Oncology, National Center for Tumor Diseases, Heidelberg University Hospital, 69120 Heidelberg, Germany
2. Department of Sports Medicine, Charité—Universitätsmedizin Berlin, 10115 Berlin, Germany
3. Department of Sports Medicine, Humboldt—Universität zu Berlin, 10115 Berlin, Germany
4. West German Cancer Center, University Hospital Essen, 45122 Essen, Germany
5. Department I of Internal Medicine, Center of Integrated Oncology Aachen Bonn Cologne Düsseldorf, University Hospital of Cologne, 50937 Cologne, Germany
* Correspondence: joachim.wiskemann@nct-heidelberg.de
† These authors contributed equally to this work.

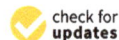

Abstract: (1) Background: Strong evidence supports the persuasive positive effects of exercise for cancer patients and survivors. Different approaches of exercise programs have been established; however, the special interests of young adults (YAs) with cancer have rarely been considered in exercise interventions. Therefore, the study YOUng EXercisers (YOUEX) aimed to investigate exercise preferences in YAs. (2) Methods: YOUEX was a three-arm, patient preference-based non-randomized, longitudinal, pre–post exercise intervention, offering three different exercise modules to YAs during or after acute therapy (Module 1: online supervised group-based (M1); Module 2: online unsupervised (M2); Module 3: in-person supervised (M3)). The intervention period was 12 weeks with another 12-week follow-up period, the modules could be changed or amended after 6 and 12 weeks. (3) Results: 92 YAs were allocated to the study. At baseline, 50 YAs (54%) chose M2, 32 YAs (35%) M1 and 10 YAs (11%) M3. The analysis revealed high acceptability and feasibility of the online exercise programs (M1, M2). There was a high impact of the COVID-19 pandemic on the execution of M3. YAs showed diverse preferences in module selection due to differences in, e.g., cancer therapy status or favored level of supervision. (4) Conclusions: YAs need personalized exercise programs that consider their individual interests and needs. Online exercise programs can be a promising addition to existing exercise opportunities. They are an effective way to increase physical activity levels in YAs.

Keywords: exercise; oncology; adolescents and young adults (AYA); breast cancer; physical activity; online exercise programs; COVID-19

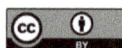

1. Introduction

A strong body of evidence demonstrates the beneficial psychological and physiological effects of physical activity (PA) and exercise in cancer patients and survivors before, during and after treatment. Hundreds of exercise interventions have revealed the reduction in highly prevalent cancer- and treatment-related side effects, such as fatigue [1,2], physical disabilities [3,4], polyneuropathy [5–7], or lymphedema [8,9]. Several systematic reviews and meta-analyses have shown the positive effects on overall quality of life [10–12]. Moreover, regular PA during and after cancer treatment is associated with improved treatment efficacy [13] and increased cancer-specific survival rates [14]. Based on the high amount of evidence, the American College of Sports Medicine (ACSM) defined specific exercise guidelines for individual side effects in oncology. They recommend to reduce sedentary time [15] and to reach at least 150 min of moderate-intensity exercise (or 75 min of vigorous-intensity exercise) and two strength-training sessions per week [16]. These recommendations correspond to the World Health Organization guidelines on physical activity and sedentary behavior [17]. However, to date, the vast majority of studies have been conducted with cancer patients over the age of 50 years, underrepresenting young adults and their special needs and preferences [18,19]. A review by Munsie et al. [20] highlights the lack of high-quality studies that examine the effects of physical activity in this cohort.

Commonly, the term 'adolescents and young adults' (AYA) includes individuals between the ages of 15–39 years. Today, cancer occurs about 66,000 times in AYA per year in Europe [21]. Due to improvements in treatment and care, the five-year relative survival of AYA diagnosed with cancer is 80–85%. However, long treatment regimens and periods of isolation away from their peer groups compromise their physical and psychological well-being. Further, long-term sequelae of cancer treatments can range from mild to severe. Late effects involve, for example, cardiovascular diseases, lung problems, high risk for osteoporosis or increased risks to develop other types of cancer later in life [18,22]. In light of the special life situation of AYA, the adoption and implementation of exercise programs need to involve adjustments according to the various factors, such as physical and mental health, financial position, time, and family role [23]. At present, there are very few specialized exercise programs that focus on the interests and needs of AYA. Most of them are tailored for children undergoing cancer treatment or childhood cancer survivors [24–29]. According to reports of the German Foundation for Young Adults with Cancer, there is a lack of attractive exercise programs for young adults with cancer aged 18–39 (YAs) as well as a lack of research about their feasibility and efficacy [30]. Although most YAs are highly interested in PA support and increasing PA levels [31], only a few studies have examined the feasibility and acceptance of exercise programs in YA [19].

With a focus on YAs, we developed a health care research study, called YOUEX (YOUng EXercisers) that addresses and investigates the needs and preferences of YAs aged 18–39 years to participate in a structured exercise program. Therefore, we implemented three different exercise modules that included different online tools or in-person training sessions. The YOUEX study is based on a comprehensive evaluation design and is supported by the German Foundation for Young Adults with Cancer.

The goal of the YOUEX study was to investigate the feasibility, acceptance and individual module selection of the three exercise modules by YAs with cancer to gain knowledge about how exercise programs should be structured for this young target group.

2. Materials and Methods

2.1. Study Design

We conducted a three-arm, patient preference-based non-randomized longitudinal pre-post exercise intervention for YAs with cancer with three eligible exercise modules. The main intervention period was 12 weeks with another 12-week follow-up period. We defined four time points for the intervention evaluation (T0: baseline; T1: after 6 weeks of intervention; T2: 12 weeks of intervention; T3: follow-up 24 weeks). The study protocol was approved by the ethics committee of the medical faculty at Heidelberg University (S-932/2020). The study was registered at clinicaltrials.gov (NCT05613699).

2.2. Participants and Recruitment

Participants were eligible if they were aged between 18–39 years, had a cancer diagnosis within the past five years and confirmed the study letter of consent. Exclusion criteria were the lack of physical exercise clearance from the attending oncologist (e.g., in case of fragile bone metastases), subjectively perceived cancer-related cognitive impairment, current participation in another exercise intervention or insufficient German language skills. We recruited patients via social media, clinical websites, flyers and from survivor groups of the German Foundation for Young Adults with Cancer from September 2020 to April 2021. Interested patients were contacted via e-mail or telephone for further information and to check inclusion criteria.

2.3. YOUEX Exercise Intervention Modules

Patients who fulfilled the inclusion criteria and provided informed consent received a comprehensive exercise consultation via phone or in person at the exercise department of the National Center of Tumor Disease (NCT), Heidelberg, or the department of sports medicine at Charité—Universitätsmedizin, Berlin. In the first consultation, study coordinators collected information about the cancer diagnosis and therapy, cancer- and cancer-treatment-related side effects, medical history, past and current physical activity levels and patient's preferences to exercise. Further, they explained to the participants that they were free to choose one of three different exercise programs. The different modules were developed in exchange with the German Foundation for Young Adults with Cancer. Based on a survey that was carried out by the foundation and asked young adults for their wishes regarding different exercise options, the following three modules were developed:

1. Module 1 (M1): supervised, group-based, online exercise program once a week
2. Module 2 (M2): unsupervised, individual home-based training with an online-training app at least once per week
3. Module 3 (M3): participation in a supervised, in-person exercise program close to place of residence at least once per week

At baseline (T0), patients choose one of the three exercise modules. The selected module had to be followed obligatory for the first six weeks. After 6 weeks (T1), the initial module could be replaced or amended by another study module. This or these selected module(s) had to be followed for another six weeks. The same procedure was repeated after 12 weeks (T2) of the exercise intervention. The main intervention ended after 12 weeks (T2). Thereafter, participants could voluntarily maintain one or up to three modules for another unsupervised 12-week time period. The follow-up ended at the 24-week time point (T3).

The supervised M1 took place once per week at a fixed, pre-scheduled time, via an online video conference platform. The training sessions lasted 60 min. They always started with a general 10 min warm-up, followed by a 40 to 45 min workout with specific exercises and finished with a 5 to 10 min stretching or relaxation part. The main workout focused on a different aspect of exercise each week (e.g., resistance training for lower extremities, sensorimotor training, home-based endurance training). The aim was for the YAs to learn exercises that they could do independently at home. For participants starting with M1, the study coordinator further recommended independent physical activity, such as walking or cycling, 1–2 times per week or to maintain the current volume of PA. Exercise recommendations for M2 were personalized and included primarily a combination of endurance and resistance training, 2–3 times a week, depending on the patient's needs. Endurance training should be performed with moderate intensity for at least 30 min duration (or less, if the patient needed to adopt the exercise recommendations due to their current health status). The type of endurance exercise (e.g., walking, cycling, swimming) was chosen according to the individual interest of the patient. Resistance training consisted of various strength exercises for the large muscle groups (at least two each for lower and upper extremities and two for trunk muscles) and was aimed to improve muscular strength. Additional types of exercise (e.g., sensorimotor training) were added if therapy-related side effects were present. If necessary, exercise trainers conducted one introductory training session as a video conference to check for exercise techniques and answer any individual questions. Thereafter, M2 was executed as application-guided home-based intervention. M3 was executed in a certified exercise facility of the network OnkoAktiv and supervised by special qualified exercise trainers. The weekly recommendation was to participate in a personalized in-person exercise program 1–2 per week plus independent physical activity (or to maintain the current level of PA). Evolution of the training load was recommended in each of the three modules if this was possible for the patients.

Due to the differences in the three modules regarding frequency and content, the overall exercise recommendations in all study modules were guided by the present exercise guidelines of the ACSM, aiming to reach at least 150 min of moderate PA per week plus two strength-training sessions per week [16]. The subjects are asked to independently carry out that part of the overall recommendations that cannot be achieved via the module.

2.4. Outcomes and Study Instruments

2.4.1. Physical Activity

Physical activity levels were determined by the standardized Godin–Shephard Leisure-Time Questionnaire [32]. The questionnaire was used to ask for pre-diagnosis-, post-diagnosis- and pre–post-intervention physical activity levels within three categories: light, moderate and vigorous physical activity in minutes per week. Participants were categorized in a sufficiently active and insufficiently active subgroup with a threshold of 150 min of moderate or 75 min of vigorous physical activity per week (or a combination of both) based on the ACSM guidelines.

2.4.2. Module Selection and Exercise Preferences

The YOUEX study is based on a comprehensive evaluation questionnaire that focused on the main outcomes: module selection and exercise preferences. The individual module selections were queried and documented at the first three time points (T0, T1, T2). Reasons for any module selection and why other modules were not selected was collected through open answer questions while multiple answers were possible. The subgroups of the initial module selection were analyzed according treatment and employment status. Further, we asked for module preferences under COVID-19-free conditions.

2.4.3. Impact of the COVID-19 Pandemic

The questionnaire about the impact of COVID-19 was self-developed and used internally in other studies at the National Center of Tumor Diseases (NCT), Heidelberg, but has not been published. The COVID-19 questionnaire consisted of six items and surveyed the impact of COVID-19 on a patient's current job situation, leisure-time activities, physical activity levels, self-efficacy, anxiety and mental health. Further, we asked whether COVID-19 had any effect on the participant's module selection. The COVID-19 questionnaire was submitted later during the ongoing study due to the COVID-19 lockdown in November 2020. Therefore, not all participants completed the COVID-19 questionnaire.

2.5. Statistical Analysis

The statistical analysis followed an exploratory approach applying descriptive and inferential statistics using the programs IBM SPSS Statistics 28 and Microsoft Excel 2016. The inference statistical pre-analysis for the normal distribution hypothesis was conducted using Shapiro–Wilk test and optical representation by histograms and Q-Q-diagrams. For inference statistics, non-parametric Wilcoxon, Friedman and Pearson chi-square tests were applied. We also conducted the Dunn–Bonferroni test as an equivalent post hoc procedure to the Friedman test. Correlations between the categorical variables were estimated applying Cramer's V. A 95% confidence interval was defined for all significance tests and all tests were two-sided. Due to the exploratory approach, procedures for multiple test adjustments were dispensed [33]. Effect sizes for median differences were calculated using the Pearson correlation coefficient r. To measure the effect size of the Friedman test, we used Kandell's W. Cramer's V, Pearson's r and Kandell's W were reported according to the interpretation by Cohen (small ≥ 0.1; medium ≥ 0.3; large ≥ 0.5) [34].

2.6. Qualitative Analysis

The qualitative data were analyzed by structured content analysis in Microsoft Excel 2016. We coded all open answers and sorted them into categories based on Kuckartz et al. [35]. Then, we counted the number of codes (quantitative) and sorted them according to their number of occurrences.

3. Results

From September 2020 to April 2021, 106 young adults contacted us regarding participation in YOUEX across all social media platforms which were deployed for recruitment. One-hundred and four of those met the inclusion criteria and 92 patients confirmed the letter of consent and started at baseline (T0). Figure 1 shows the flow diagram from enrollment to analysis including the number of and reasons for dropouts.

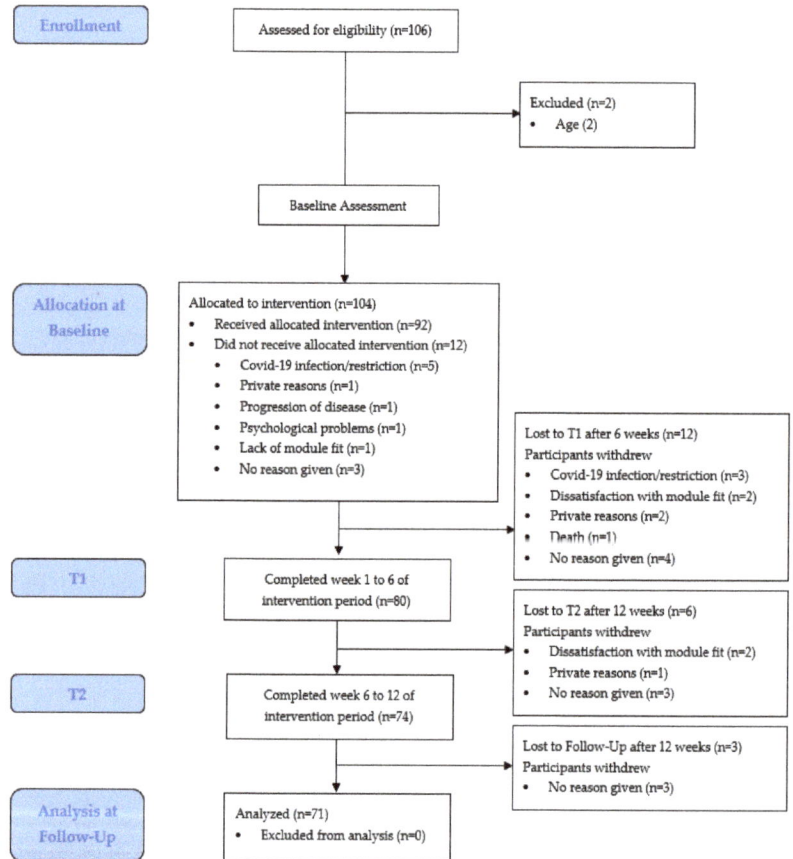

Figure 1. Flow diagram from enrollment to analysis, including dropouts.

3.1. Patient Characteristics

Ninety-four percent of participants ($n = 86$) were women and the average age among all participants was 32 years (min: 19; max: 39). The distribution of cancer types was 55% breast, 19% (non-)Hodgkin lymphoma and 15% other cancer types (e.g., ovarian, skin, colon, cervix, testicles, lung). Overall, 18 YAs (20%) underwent acute tumor therapy (chemotherapy or radiation) at baseline. There were no smokers among the participants (see Table 1).

Table 1. Patient characteristics at baseline.

Characteristics	n (%)	Mean ± SD	Median	Range
Age (years)	92	31.9 ± 4.9	32.5	19–39
Gender				
Female	86 (93.5)			
Male	6 (6.5)			
Body composition				
Height (cm)	92	169.9 ± 7.1	170.0	146–190
Weight (kg)	92	68.2 ± 11.5	66.5	48–102
BMI (kg/m^2)	92	23.6 ± 3.8	23.3	17.5–35.7
Disease				
Breast cancer	51 (55.4)			
(Non-)Hodgkin lymphoma	17 (18.5)			
Sarcoma	4 (4.3)			
Leukemia	3 (3.3)			
Brain tumor	3 (3.3)			
Other	14 (15.2)			
Disease progression				
Metastasis	17 (18.5)			
Relapse	13 (14.1)			
Treatment				
Surgery	68 (73.9)			
Chemotherapy				
Total	84 (91.3)			
Ongoing	18 (19.6)			
Radiotherapy				
Total	49 (53.3)			
Ongoing	1 (1.1)			
Immunotherapy				
Total	10 (10.9)			
Ongoing	5 (5.4)			
Hormone therapy				
Total	35 (38.0)			
Ongoing	26 (28.3)			
Other therapy				
Total	22 (23.9)			
Antibody	15 (16.3)			
Stem cell transplantation	5 (5.4)			
Other	2 (2.2)			
Education				
Middle school	2 (2.2)			
Vocational training	9 (9.8)			
University entrance qualification	24 (26.1)			
University degree	54 (58.7)			
Other degree	3 (3.3)			
Employment				
Employed, currently working	36 (39.1)			
Employed but on medical leave	35 (38.0)			
Still in education	17 (18.5)			
Housewife/houseman	1 (1.1)			
Retired	2 (2.2)			
Unemployed	1 (1.1)			
Family situation				
Married/permanent relationship	57 (62.0)			
Single	32 (34.8)			
Divorced	2 (2.2)			

Table 1. Cont.

Characteristics	n (%)	Mean ± SD	Median	Range
Smoking behavior				
Smoker	0 (0)			
Non-smoker	92 (100)			
Social media usage behavior				
Smartphone/tablet (h/week)	90	12.5 ± 8.5	10.7	1–42
PC (h/week)	91	11.8 ± 15.1	4	0–60
Frequency of social media use (h/week)				
Instagram	91	3.4 ± 1.0	4	1–4
Facebook	91	2.6 ± 1.2	3	1–4
YouTube	91	2.3 ± 0.8	2	1–4
Twitter	91	1.2 ± 0.5	1	1–4
Tik Tok	91	1.1 ± 0.4	1	1–4
Twitch	91	1.1 ± 0.3	1	1–4
NCCN Distress [1]	91	6.18 ± 2.1	6	1–10

[1] National Comprehensive Cancer Network (NCCN) Distress thermometer: scale 0 (not stressed at all) to 10 (extremely stressed) [36].

3.2. Physical Activity

During the primary intervention period the mean amount of light physical activity did not differ significantly between the time points (see Table 2). Significant improvements were found in both, moderate PA level (chi-square (3) = 23.556, $p < 0.001$, $n = 70$, W = 0.11) and vigorous PA level (chi-square (3) = 18.995, $p < 0.001$, $n = 69$, W = 0.09) across the time points. There was also a significant improvement in the total duration of PA (chi-square (3) = 18.199, $p < 0.001$, $n = 66$, W = 0.09). Using the Dunn–Bonferroni test, a significant differences in the duration of PA between post-diagnosis and T1 (moderate PA: $z = 0.821$, $p = 0.001$, $r = 0.10$; total PA; $z = 0.758$, $p < 0.005$, $r = 0.09$) and between post-diagnosis and T2 (moderate PA: $z = 0.750$, $p < 0.005$, $r = 0.09$; vigorous PA: $z = 0.696$, $p < 0.01$, $r = 0.08$; total PA: $z = 0.795$, $p < 0.005$, $r = 0.10$) were computed. The proportion of patients belonging to the sufficiently active subgroup increased from post-diagnosis (40%) to T1 (53%) to T2 (59%).

Table 2. Physical activity before and during YOUEX intervention.

	Pre-Diagnosis		Post-Diagnosis		T1		T2		p Value
	n	M ± SD	n	M ± SD	n	M ± SD	n	M ± SD	
Light PA (min/week)	69	154.8 ± 142.7	69	194.1 ± 176.2	69	205.9 ± 203.1	69	206.2 ± 236.4	0.270
Moderate PA (min/week)	70	83.4 ± 81.4	70	76.1 ± 95.4	70	119.4 ± 116.2 *,#	70	116.8 ± 94.8 *	<0.001
Vigorous PA (min/week)	69	86.1 ± 94.5	69	46.9 ± 71.7 #	69	68.3 ± 77.5	69	69.4 ± 65.6 *	<0.001
Total PA (min/week)	66	325.8 ± 210.9	66	322.0 ± 245.7	66	397.1 ± 256.3 *	66	399.9 ± 315.7 *	<0.001

significantly different to pre-diagnosis; * significantly different to post-diagnosis.

Compared to pre-diagnosis, the following significant differences were determined: The PA with vigorous intensity decreased significantly from pre-diagnosis to post-diagnosis ($z = 0.819$, $p = 0.001$, $r = 0.10$) and the PA with moderate intensity increased significantly from pre-diagnosis to T1 ($z = 0.621$, $p < 0.05$, $r = 0.10$). There was no significant change from pre-diagnosis to T2. Before diagnosis, 63% fulfilled the international physical activity recommendations of ACSM. This proportion dropped to 40% after diagnosis.

3.3. Module Selection and Exercise Preferences

3.3.1. Initial Module Selection at T0

With regard to module preferences at baseline (T0), 50 participants (54%) chose the online-training app (M2), 32 participants (35%) chose the supervised, group-based online exercise program (M1) and 10 participants (11%) chose the in-person exercise program (M3). However, due to the COVID-19 national lockdown and several restrictions on exercise facilities, M3 could not be served from November 2020 to March 2021. Participants who performed M3 at that time could switch to either M1 or M2. The most frequently mentioned reason for choosing M2 (56% of a total of 82 qualitative answers) was the flexibility in terms of time. The second most given reasons were both, personal reasons (e.g., "I want to lose weight") and the personalized training schedule (respectively 15% of 82 qualitative answers). The reasons for choosing M1 (a total of 56 qualitative answers were given) were the fixed training date (30%) and doing sports with other cancer patients (27%). Sixteen percent of the YAs indicated that M1 was easy to integrate into everyday life. The most common reason for choosing M3 (a total of 19 qualitative answers were given) was the individual supervision by an exercise therapist (47%). Additionally, fixed dates (26%), closeness to residence (16%) and social contact (11%) were mentioned in regard to M3.

3.3.2. Module Change at T1

Eighty from ninety-two participants completed the first 6 weeks of intervention and reached the first time point of intervention (T1). At T1, 43% ($n = 34$) of participants replaced or amended their initial module (see Figure 2). Eleven participants (14%) replaced their initial module, of which 55% ($n = 6$) chose M2, 27% ($n = 3$) chose M3 and 18% ($n = 2$) chose M1. Twenty-three participants (29%) amended the initial module of which thirteen patients added M2 to M1 (57%), six patients added M1 to M2 (26%), three patients added M2 to M3 (13%) and one patient added M3 to M1 (4%). Reasons for replacing or amending the group-based online exercise program (M1) were the wish to increase activity through adding another module (33% of 39 given answers) and the wish to receive more individual advice by an exercise therapist (26% of 39 given answers). YAs who chose the online-training-app (M2) (a total of 44 qualitative answers were given) named the wish for more interaction with trainers (27%), problems with COVID-19 restrictions (23%) and that they wanted to try another module (14%) as reasons for replacing or amending the initial module. The most common reason for replacing M3 (a total of 7 qualitative answers given) was COVID-19 restrictions (43%). Seventy-four from eighty participants reached the T2 (12 week) time point and the end of the main exercise intervention. Between T1 and T2, 71% took part in one module and 29% took part in two different modules.

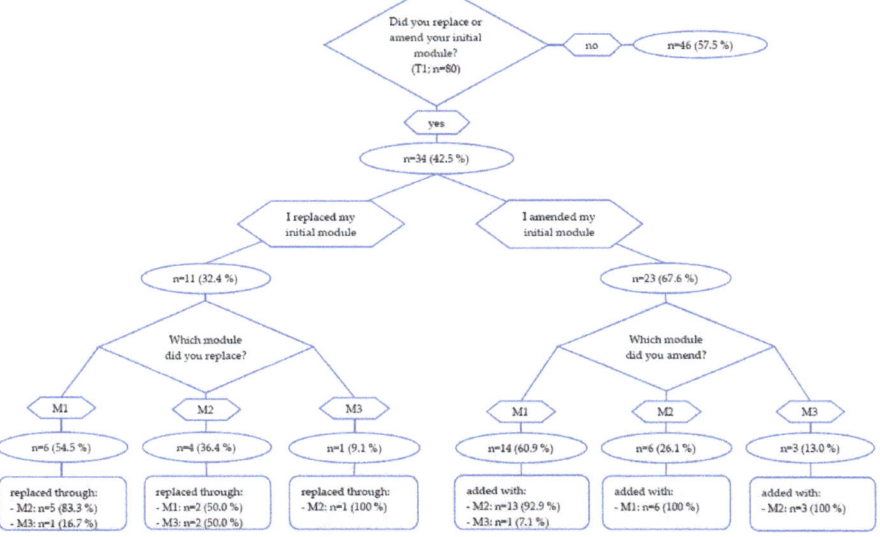

Figure 2. Module change at T1.

3.3.3. Subgroup Analysis of Patient Characteristics According to Module Selection at T0

Table 3 shows the patients' characteristics regarding treatment status and employment within the three exercise modules at T0. A total of 18 patients were undergoing acute therapy during their participation. These patients were distributed relatively evenly across the three modules (M1: 39%, M2: 33%, M3: 28%). Looking at distribution within the module selection, 50% of those who chose M3 were undergoing acute therapy during their participation, while only 22% from M1 and 12% from M2 were under ongoing therapy. The correlation analysis indicated a significant correlation between module selection and treatment status (chi-square (2) = 7.81, p = 0.02, V = 0.29). Of the 36 patients who were employed at the time of the intervention, the majority chose M2 (53%), 39% chose M1 and 8% chose M3. There was no significant correlation between module selection and employment status. Additionally, physical activity level, distress and social media behavior were analyzed but showed no significant correlations.

Table 3. Patient characteristics according to module selection at T0.

	M1 (n = 32)		M2 (n = 50)		M3 (n = 10)	
	n	%	n	%	n	%
Treatment status *						
During acute therapy	7	21.9	6	12.0	5	50.0
Before or after acute therapy	25	78.1	44	88.0	5	50.0
Employment						
Employed	14	43.8	19	38.0	3	30.0
On medical leave	14	43.8	17	34.0	4	40.0
Still in education	4	12.5	12	24.0	1	10.0
Not employed	0	0.0	2	4.0	2	20.0

* significant correlation with module selection.

3.4. Impact of COVID-19 Pandemic

Eighty-five percent of the participants reported that the COVID-19 pandemic influenced their module selection. Thirty-three percent expressed that they felt unsafe to exercise in local facilities and were afraid of infection. More than half of all surveyed (52%) mentioned that their module selection was influenced by severe COVID-19 restrictions within the exercise institutions. The results coincide with the interest in different modules under COVID-19-free circumstances (see Table 4 and Figure 3).

Table 4. Interest in different modules under COVID-19-free circumstances on a scale of 1 (very low interest) to 10 (very high interest).

	n (%)	Mean ± SD	Median	Range	Percentile	
					25	75
M1	68 (73.9)	5.1 ± 2.6	5.0	1 to 10	3.0	7.0
M2	68 (73.9)	7.2 ± 2.8	7.5	1 to 10	5.0	9.5
M3	68 (73.9)	8.4 ± 2.1	9.5	1 to 10	7.0	10.0

The analysis of the general impact of COVID-19 illustrates that the status and circumstances of employment changed in 60% of the participants due to the COVID-19 pandemic (e.g., changing to home office (26 YAs), changing to short-time work (4 YAs) or other changes (16 YAs) such as constant new regulations as a teacher or extension of parental leave). The impact of the COVID-19 pandemic on the physical activity level was diverse across the YA population. While 39 YAs (53%) stated that their PA level had been reduced a little to a lot due to the COVID-19 pandemic, 27 YAs (29%) reported that they became more active during the pandemic. Seventy-five percent of all the participants felt, that their quality of life was impaired, 70% of the YAs felt stressed, 40% felt anxious and 37% felt helpless because of the COVID-19 restrictions during the pandemic.

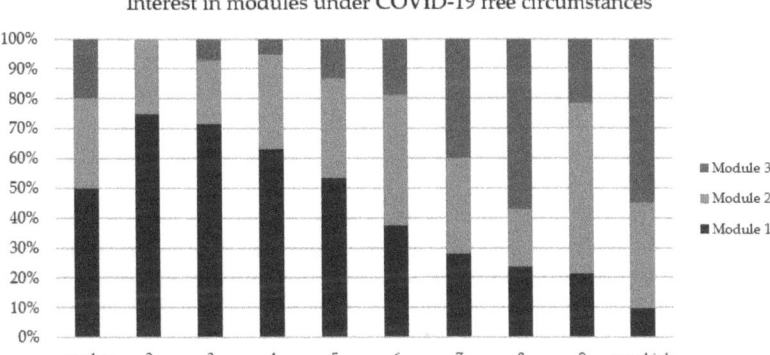

Figure 3. Interest in different modules under COVID-19-free circumstances on a scale of 1 (very low interest) to 10 (very high interest).

4. Discussion

The YOUEX study investigated the exercise preferences and module selections of young adults with cancer. Our analysis revealed high acceptability and feasibility of online training programs. The YOUEX participants showed diverse preferences in exercise selection due to differences in cancer therapy status, interests in exercise options and favored level of supervision.

4.1. Physical Activity

Only 40% of all YOUEX participants met the physical activity recommendations after cancer diagnosis and therefore 60% can be classified as insufficiently active. This highlights the importance of exercise programming for YAs, especially right after their cancer diagnosis and during treatment. Interestingly, the participations in one or more of the three study modules had a significant effect on YAs moderate and vigorous PA levels after 12 weeks of the study intervention. Both activity levels increased by about 35%. The number of patients who met the ACSM guidelines after 12 weeks increased from 40% to 59%. A comparison of the self-reported physical activity level before and after cancer diagnosis revealed a significant difference in exercise intensity. YAs decreased their vigorous exercise by about 40% after diagnosis. This phenomenon has also been described by different authors in older cancer patients [37–39].

The effectiveness of exercise programs has been investigated by many researchers in the field of exercise oncology [4,11,12,40]. Friedenreich et al. [14] underlined the importance of post-diagnosis PA levels in their current review and meta-analysis. The authors revealed a significant difference in the mortality rates in cancer patients for those with low vs. high post-diagnosis PA levels. The benefits of physical activity for YAs have also been stated in the review by Munsi et al. [20]. Further, several European studies investigated the positive effects of exercise interventions in children and adolescents [28,41,42], pointing out that monitoring PA levels is important to accomplish positive PA effects [37].

4.2. Module Selection and Exercise Preferences

The evaluation of module selection at baseline showed the highest interest in module 2 followed by module 1. However, the strong influence of the COVID-19 pandemic and the comprehensive restrictions have had a high impact on module selections. Since module 3 could not be offered during the majority of the study period, no clear statement can be made about the actual interest in the in-person exercise program. Nevertheless, the hypothetical question about module interest under COVID-19-free circumstances showed very high interest in M3. At the same time, study participants showed high interest in both online modules (M1 and M2). After 12 weeks, more YAs participated in the individual home-based program M2 than the fixed group-based program M1. The most named reasons for choosing M2 was the flexibility in terms of time and individual training programming, whereas M1 was chosen because of the fixed training date and being motivated by others.

Further, the module changes at T1 highlighted interesting findings. Less than half of the participants changed their initial module. The amendment or replacement of modules were related to different reasons such as increasing the physical activity, interest in other modules or the wish to receive more individual advice by exercise trainers. Interestingly, despite the possibility to amend the initial module, no increase in PA could be determined between T1 and T2. Overall, comparing the two online modules, M1 (supervised, group-based online exercise program) was less popular than M2 (home-based individual training via app). Around 60% of those who chose M1 at baseline decided to amend or replace that module after 6 weeks. Compared to M2, only around 30% wanted to replace or amend that module. All in all, only around 20% of the YAs took part in two different modules during the 12-week intervention. Adams and colleagues outlined in their study with 533 AYA that the majority of patients preferred home-based (79%) and online (47%), but less hospital-based (25%) programs. Further, a significant higher proportion of AYA preferred individually supervised programs (82%) rather than group-based programs (63%). Interestingly, most AYA preferred to exercise ≥ 30 min on ≥ 3 days per week [31]. Another digital health intervention showed that a group-based intervention with a mobile app was accepted by YAs and revealed significantly greater improvements in muscle strength but had limited reach due to the competing needs experienced [43]. A systematic review on social media interventions targeting exercise in people with non-communicable diseases (including cancer) investigated five RCTs that improved the exercise behaviors and concluded overall feasibility of social media intervention among specific populations [44].

Our analysis highlights that exercise preferences of YAs are highly individual and diverse. First of all, the demography of patient characteristics showed the high variety of different diagnosis, treatment status, employment status, family situations and physical activity levels among YAs. At the same time, the given reasons for choosing a module or for not choosing a module were very diverse, some were even contradictory (e.g., flexibility in terms of time vs. fixed training dates). The subgroup analysis in which patient characteristics of the three different module groups were examined, brought only little insights. A significant correlation between treatment status and module selection was found. YAs undergoing acute therapy seem to prefer supervised training; however, due to the little sample size, non-randomization and limitations in the context of COVID-19 pandemic, we cannot conclude any clear statement about which exercise program fits the individual treatment status. Further, neither employment status nor physical activity level, distress or social media usage behavior seemed to have a definite influence on module selection. We therefore conclude that in order to be able to respond to different needs of YAs, a wide range of exercise programs must be created.

4.3. Implementation of the YOUEX Exercise Programs and the Impact of COVID-19

The comparatively small number of young cancer cases in Germany [45] leads to the challenge that region-specific group trainings might not be accessible to all patients. However, the need for high-quality exercise programs during and after cancer therapy still applies for YAs. Exercise programs offered digitally could be a suitable solution to consolidate YAs nationwide. Different studies analyzing digital health interventions showed the feasibility and acceptance in YAs with cancer [43,46,47]. Similarly, this study indicated that the digitally offered modules 1 and 2 were well-accepted. Especially during the COVID-19 pandemic, online-programs have had many advantages. Compared to the only in-person program (M3), major benefits of M1 and M2 were the independency against pandemic restrictions and the low risk of infections. However, M2 was intended as an unsupervised home-based program. Different studies show significant positive effects of the supervised training interventions on treatment-related side effects compared to unsupervised training [11]. Additionally, the qualitative evaluation of M1 and M2 revealed some critical aspects of online programs from the patient's perspective. M1 was supervised in a group context but still a quarter of participants claimed that the training had not been individual enough. Still, online supervised training has its boundaries due to technical limitations (e.g., restricted field of vision). Further, one out of four patients in M2 (online, individual training plan) wished more personal interaction with the exercise therapist.

4.4. Limitations

Our study needs to be interpreted in light of several limitations. First, our data showed a great selection bias which resulted in a non-representable group of YAs. Our participants were mostly already active, with a high educational level, mostly women and non-smokers. We conclude that our reach was limited to the already interested, active group of potential YAs and people that were active on social media and engaged in self-help groups. In regard to the methodological approach, our study was a non-randomized intervention only, with no control group. A randomized, inactive control group could have shown causal differences in the patient-related outcomes and would have allowed a reasonable interpretation of our results. Further, when interpreting changes in the PA level it is imperative to consider that the study participants only subjectively estimated their PA level, there was no objectively measured method. Götte et al. highlighted that PA should be assessed by objective methods in pediatric cancer patients [48]. By using the Godin–Shepard Leisure-Time Questionnaire no distinction can be made between endurance or resistance training. Additionally, the study questionnaire did not cover the concrete PA levels at baseline and only asked for the pre- and post-diagnosis PA levels. In addition, there is a lack of data on the adherence of the participants to each module, which must be taken into account when interpreting the results. The different modules vary in terms of frequency, content and volume. A comparison of the modules with regard to the effects of each module on physical activity is therefore not possible. We also included a self-developed questionnaire about the impact of COVID-19, three months after we had started the patient recruitment. Overall, the YOUEX study was intensely impacted by the COVID-19 pandemic. The COVID-19 restrictions biased our measured outcomes (e.g., PA level), module selections and the entire execution of M3. The impact of COVID-19 on our study outcomes needs to be respected with important meaning.

4.5. Further Research

YOUEX has shown that social media tools are effective for participant recruitment in our young target group. However, it is not clear how to reach the broad range of YAs regarding their interest in PA participation, cancer diagnosis or treatment status. Further, the question of how to ensure adequate training stimuli for the right dose-effect in the context of online and/or home-based exercise programs remains unanswered and should be the subject of further research. Therefore, more data on the adherence of YAs participating in (online) exercise programs is needed. Additionally, the long-term effects of online exercise programs in YAs are yet to be evaluated and should be taken into account in future studies. Additionally, the question of how special exercise offers for YAs can be implemented into existing healthcare structures remains problematic. Further interventions should focus on the adaption, long-term implementation strategies and maintenance of exercise programs (including the long-term adherence of YAs) to provide a sustainable impact on PA levels and health-related improvements for this target group.

5. Conclusions

We found that young adults with cancer recruited via social media and different online websites have a wide range of interests and needs regarding exercise programs during and after cancer therapy. According to our findings, YAs need specific exercise programs that include their individual interests and needs. In this context, online exercise programs in different forms (e.g., group-based, individual program) can be an addition and/or an alternative to existing exercise options. It must be underlined, that such online programs were highly accepted in our study (which partly took place during lockdown periods in the COVID-19 pandemic) and can be effective in increasing YA's physical activity levels.

Author Contributions: Conceptualization, A.V. and J.W.; methodology, A.V. and J.W.; software, A.V.; validation, A.V., V.K., M.G., T.N. and M.K.; formal analysis, A.V. and V.K.; investigation, A.V., V.K., M.G., T.N. and M.K.; resources, J.W.; data curation, A.V. and V.K.; writing—original draft preparation, A.V. and V.K; writing—review and editing, M.G., T.N., M.K. and J.W.; visualization, A.V. and V.K.; supervision, J.W.; project administration, A.V.; funding acquisition, J.W. All authors have read and agreed to the published version of the manuscript.

Funding: This research was funded by the German Foundation of Young Adults with Cancer, grant number 17/10/2022.

Institutional Review Board Statement: The study was conducted in accordance with the Declaration of Helsinki, and approved by the Ethics Committee of the medical faculty at Heidelberg University (S-932/2020).

Informed Consent Statement: Written informed consent has been obtained from the patients to publish this paper.

Data Availability Statement: The datasets used and analyzed during the current study are available from the corresponding author upon reasonable request.

Conflicts of Interest: J.W. invented and founded the network OnkoAktiv and is currently a member of the association board. The other authors declare no conflict of interests. The funders had no role in the design of the study; in the collection, analyses, or interpretation of data; in the writing of the manuscript; or in the decision to publish the results.

References

1. Brandenbarg, D.; Korsten, J.H.W.M.; Berger, M.Y.; Berendsen, A.J. The effect of physical activity on fatigue among survivors of colorectal cancer: A systematic review and meta-analysis. *Support. Care Cancer* **2018**, *26*, 393–403. [CrossRef] [PubMed]
2. Wagoner, C.W.; Lee, J.T.; Battaglini, C.L. Community-based exercise programs and cancer-related fatigue: A systematic review and meta-analysis. *Support. Care Cancer* **2021**, *29*, 4921–4929. [CrossRef]
3. Gebruers, n.; Camberlin, M.; Theunissen, F.; Tjalma, W.; Verbelen, H.; Van Soom, T.; van Breda, E. The effect of training interventions on physical performance, quality of life, and fatigue in patients receiving breast cancer treatment: A systematic review. *Support. Care Cancer* **2019**, *27*, 109–122. [CrossRef] [PubMed]
4. Buffart, L.M.; Sweegers, M.G.; May, A.M.; Chinapaw, M.J.; van Vulpen, J.K.; Newton, R.U.; Galvão, D.A.; Aaronson, N.K.; Stuiver, M.M.; Jacobsen, P.B.; et al. Targeting exercise interventions to patients with cancer in need: An individual patient data meta-analysis. *J. Natl. Cancer Inst.* **2018**, *110*, 1190–1200. [CrossRef]
5. Müller, J.; Weiler, M.; Schneeweiss, A.; Haag, G.M.; Steindorf, K.; Wick, W.; Wiskemann, J. Preventive effect of sensorimotor exercise and resistance training on chemotherapy-induced peripheral neuropathy: A randomised-controlled trial. *Br. J. Cancer* **2021**, *125*, 955–965. [CrossRef]
6. Kleckner, I.R.; Kamen, C.; Gewandter, J.S.; Mohile, n.A.; Heckler, C.E.; Culakova, E.; Fung, C.; Janelsins, M.C.; Asare, M.; Lin, P.J.; et al. Effects of exercise during chemotherapy on chemotherapy-induced peripheral neuropathy: A multicenter, randomized controlled trial. *Support. Care Cancer* **2018**, *26*, 1019–1028. [CrossRef]
7. Zimmer, P.; Trebing, S.; Timmers-Trebing, U.; Schenk, A.; Paust, R.; Bloch, W.; Rudolph, R.; Streckmann, F.; Baumann, F.T. Eight-week, multimodal exercise counteracts a progress of chemotherapy-induced peripheral neuropathy and improves balance and strength in metastasized colorectal cancer patients: A randomized controlled trial. *Support. Care Cancer* **2018**, *26*, 615–624. [CrossRef]
8. Zhang, X.; Brown, J.C.; Paskett, E.D.; Zemel, B.S.; Cheville, A.L.; Schmitz, K.H. Changes in arm tissue composition with slowly progressive weight-lifting among women with breast cancer-related lymphedema. *Breast Cancer Res. Treat.* **2017**, *164*, 79–88. [CrossRef] [PubMed]
9. Rogan, S.; Taeymans, J.; Luginbuehl, H.; Aebi, M.; Mahnig, S.; Gebruers, N. Therapy modalities to reduce lymphoedema in female breast cancer patients: A systematic review and meta-analysis. *Breast Cancer Res. Treat.* **2016**, *159*, 1–14. [CrossRef]
10. Zhang, X.; Li, Y.; Liu, D. Effects of exercise on the quality of life in breast cancer patients: A systematic review of randomized controlled trials. *Support. Care Cancer* **2019**, *27*, 9–21. [CrossRef]
11. Sweegers, M.G.; Altenburg, T.M.; Chinapaw, M.J.; Kalter, J.; Verdonck-de Leeuw, I.M.; Courneya, K.S.; Newton, R.U.; Aaronson, N.K.; Jacobsen, P.B.; Brug, J.; et al. Which exercise prescriptions improve quality of life and physical function in patients with cancer during and following treatment? A systematic review and meta-analysis of randomised controlled trials. *Br. J. Sports Med.* **2018**, *52*, 505–513. [CrossRef]

12. Buffart, L.M.; Kalter, J.; Sweegers, M.G.; Courneya, K.S.; Newton, R.U.; Aaronson, n.K.; Jacobsen, P.B.; May, A.M.; Galvao, D.A.; Chinapaw, M.J.; et al. Effects and moderators of exercise on quality of life and physical function in patients with cancer: An individual patient data meta-analysis of 34 RCTs. *Cancer Treat. Rev.* **2017**, *52*, 91–104. [CrossRef] [PubMed]
13. Yang, L.; Morielli, A.R.; Heer, E.; Kirkham, A.A.; Cheung, W.Y.; Usmani, N.; Friedenreich, C.M.; Courneya, K.S. Effects of exercise on cancer treatment efficacy: A systematic review of preclinical and clinical studies. *Cancer Res.* **2021**, *81*, 4889–4895. [CrossRef] [PubMed]
14. Friedenreich, C.M.; Stone, C.R.; Cheung, W.Y.; Hayes, S.C. Physical activity and mortality in cancer survivors: A systematic review and meta-analysis. *JNCI Cancer Spectr.* **2019**, *4*, pkz080. [CrossRef]
15. Patel, A.V.; Friedenreich, C.M.; Moore, S.C.; Hayes, S.C.; Silver, J.K.; Campbell, K.L.; Winters-Stone, K.; Gerber, L.H.; George, S.M.; Fulton, J.E.; et al. American College of Sports Medicine Roundtable Report on Physical Activity, Sedentary Behavior, and Cancer Prevention and Control. *Med. Sci. Sports Exerc.* **2019**, *51*, 2391–2402. [CrossRef] [PubMed]
16. Campbell, K.L.; Winters-Stone, K.M.; Wiskemann, J.; May, A.M.; Schwartz, A.L.; Courneya, K.S.; Zucker, D.S.; Matthews, C.E.; Ligibel, J.A.; Gerber, L.H.; et al. Exercise Guidelines for Cancer Survivors: Consensus Statement from International Multidisciplinary Roundtable. *Med. Sci. Sports Exerc.* **2019**, *51*, 2375–2390. [CrossRef]
17. Bull, F.C.; Al-Ansari, S.S.; Biddle, S.; Borodulin, K.; Buman, M.P.; Cardon, G.; Carty, C.; Chaput, J.P.; Chastin, S.; Chou, R.; et al. World Health Organization 2020 guidelines on physical activity and sedentary behaviour. *Br. J. Sports Med.* **2020**, *54*, 1451–1462. [CrossRef]
18. Lewis, D.R.; Siembida, E.J.; Seibel, n.L.; Smith, A.W.; Mariotto, A.B. Survival outcomes for cancer types with the highest death rates for adolescents and young adults, 1975–2016. *Cancer* **2021**, *127*, 4277–4286. [CrossRef]
19. Pugh, G.; Below, N.; Fisher, A.; Reynolds, J.; Epstone, S. Trekstock RENEW: Evaluation of a 12-week exercise referral programme for young adult cancer survivors delivered by a cancer charity. *Support. Care Cancer* **2020**, *28*, 5803–5812. [CrossRef]
20. Munsie, C.; Ebert, J.; Joske, D.; Ackland, T. The benefit of physical activity in adolescent and young adult cancer patients during and after treatment: A systematic review. *J. Adolesc. Young Adult. Oncol.* **2019**, *8*, 512–524. [CrossRef]
21. Desandes, E.; Stark, D.P. Epidemiology of adolescents and young adults with cancer in Europe. *Tumors Adolesc. Young Adults* **2016**, *43*, 1–15. [CrossRef]
22. Barr, R.D.; Ferrari, A.; Ries, L.; Whelan, J.; Bleyer, W.A. Cancer in adolescents and young adults: A narrative review of the current status and a view of the future. *JAMA Pediatr.* **2016**, *170*, 495–501. [CrossRef] [PubMed]
23. Coccia, P.F.; Pappo, A.S.; Beaupin, L.; Borges, V.F.; Borinstein, S.C.; Chugh, R.; Dinner, S.; Folbrecht, J.; Frazier, A.L.; Goldsby, R.; et al. Adolescent and young adult oncology, version 2. *2018, NCCN clinical practice guidelines in oncology. J. Natl. Compr. Cancer Netw.* **2018**, *16*, 66–97. [CrossRef]
24. Beulertz, J.; Prokop, A.; Rustler, V.; Bloch, W.; Felsch, M.; Baumann, F.T. Effects of a 6-month, group-based, therapeutic exercise program for childhood cancer outpatients on motor performance, level of activity, and quality of life. *Pediatr. Blood Cancer* **2016**, *63*, 127–132. [CrossRef]
25. Braam, K.I.; van der Torre, P.; Takken, T.; Veening, M.A.; van Dulmen-den Broeder, E.; Kaspers, G.J. Physical exercise training interventions for children and young adults during and after treatment for childhood cancer. *Cochrane Database Syst. Rev.* **2013**, *4*, Cd008796. [CrossRef]
26. Le, A.; Mitchell, H.R.; Zheng, D.J.; Rotatori, J.; Fahey, J.T.; Ness, K.K.; Kadan-Lottick, N.S. A home-based physical activity intervention using activity trackers in survivors of childhood cancer: A pilot study. *Pediatr. Blood Cancer* **2017**, *64*, 387–394. [CrossRef]
27. Morales, J.S.; Valenzuela, P.L.; Herrera-Olivares, A.M.; Baño-Rodrigo, A.; Castillo-García, A.; Rincón-Castanedo, C.; Martín-Ruiz, A.; San-Juan, A.F.; Fiuza-Luces, C.; Lucia, A. Exercise interventions and cardiovascular health in childhood cancer: A meta-analysis. *Int. J. Sports Med.* **2020**, *41*, 141–153. [CrossRef]
28. Morales, J.S.; Valenzuela, P.L.; Rincón-Castanedo, C.; Takken, T.; Fiuza-Luces, C.; Santos-Lozano, A.; Lucia, A. Exercise training in childhood cancer: A systematic review and meta-analysis of randomized controlled trials. *Cancer Treat. Rev.* **2018**, *70*, 154–167. [CrossRef]
29. Shi, Q.; Zheng, J.; Liu, K. Supervised exercise interventions in childhood cancer survivors: A systematic review and meta-analysis of randomized controlled trials. *Children* **2022**, *9*, 824. [CrossRef]
30. Neuer Themenbereich "Bewegung & Sport bei Krebs" im JUNGEN KREBSPORTAL Online. Available online: https://junge-erwachsene-mit-krebs.de/neuer-themenbereich-bewegung-sport-bei-krebs-im-jungen-krebsportal-online/ (accessed on 8 August 2022).
31. Adams, S.C.; Petrella, A.; Sabiston, C.M.; Vani, M.F.; Gupta, A.; Trinh, L.; Matthew, A.G.; Hamilton, R.J.; Mina, D.S. Preferences for exercise and physical activity support in adolescent and young adult cancer survivors: A cross-sectional survey. *Support. Care Cancer* **2021**, *29*, 4113–4127. [CrossRef]
32. Godin, G.; Shephard, R.J. A simple method to assess exercise behavior in the community. *Can. J. Appl. Sport Sci.* **1985**, *10*, 141–146. [PubMed]
33. Bender, R.; Lange, S. Adjusting for multiple testing—When and how? *J. Clin. Epidemiol.* **2001**, *54*, 343–349. [CrossRef]
34. Cohen, J. *Statistical Power Analysis for the Behavioral Sciences*, 2nd ed.; Lawrence Erlbaum Associates: Hillsdale, NJ, USA, 1988.
35. Kuckartz, U. *Einführung in Die Computergestützte Analyse Qualitativer Daten*, 3rd ed.; Verlag für Sozialwissenschaften: Wiesbaden, Germany, 2010.

36. Mehnert, A.; Müller, D.; Lehmann, C.; Koch, U. Die deutsche Version des NCCN Distress-Thermometers. *Z. Psychiatr. Psychol. Und Psychother.* **2006**, *54*, 213–223. [CrossRef]
37. Stössel, S.; Neu, M.A.; Oschwald, V.; Söntgerath, R.; Däggelmann, J.; Eckert, K.; Hamacher, V.; Baumann, F.T.; Bloch, W.; Faber, J. Physical activity behaviour in children and adolescents before, during and after cancer treatment. *Sport Sci. Health* **2020**, *16*, 347–353. [CrossRef]
38. Christensen, J.F.; Simonsen, C.; Hojman, P. Exercise training in cancer control and treatment. *Compr. Physiol.* **2018**, *9*, 165–205. [CrossRef] [PubMed]
39. Voland, A.; Köppel, M.; Wiskemann, J. Evaluation des Netzwerk OnkoAktiv aus Patientenperspektive. *B&G Beweg. Gesundh.* **2022**, *38*, 103–109.
40. Sweegers, M.G.; Buffart, L.M.; van Veldhuizen, W.M.; Geleijn, E.; Verheul, H.M.W.; Brug, J.; Chinapaw, M.J.M.; Altenburg, T.M. How does a supervised exercise program improve quality of life in patients with cancer? A concept mapping study examining patients' perspectives. *Oncologist* **2019**, *24*, e374–e383. [CrossRef] [PubMed]
41. Saultier, P.; Vallet, C.; Sotteau, F.; Hamidou, Z.; Gentet, J.C.; Barlogis, V.; Curtillet, C.; Verschuur, A.; Revon-Riviere, G.; Galambrun, C.; et al. A randomized trial of physical activity in children and adolescents with cancer. *Cancers* **2021**, *13*, 121. [CrossRef]
42. Beller, R.; Bennstein, S.B.; Götte, M. Effects of exercise interventions on immune function in children and adolescents with cancer and HSCT recipients—A systematic review. *Front. Immunol.* **2021**, *12*, 746171. [CrossRef]
43. Devine, K.A.; Viola, A.; Levonyan-Radloff, K.; Mackowski, n.; Bozzini, B.; Chandler, A.; Xu, B.; Ohman-Strickland, P.; Mayans, S.; Farrar-Anton, A.; et al. Feasibility of FitSurvivor: A technology-enhanced group-based fitness intervention for adolescent and young adult survivors of childhood cancer. *Pediatr. Blood Cancer* **2020**, *67*, e28530. [CrossRef]
44. McKeon, G.; Papadopoulos, E.; Firth, J.; Joshi, R.; Teasdale, S.; Newby, J.; Rosenbaum, S. Social media interventions targeting exercise and diet behaviours in people with noncommunicable diseases (NCDs): A systematic review. *Internet Interv.* **2022**, *27*, 100497. [CrossRef]
45. Gondos, A.; Hiripi, E.; Holleczek, B.; Luttmann, S.; Eberle, A.; Brenner, H. Survival among adolescents and young adults with cancer in Germany and the United States: An international comparison. *Int. J. Cancer* **2013**, *133*, 2207–2215. [CrossRef] [PubMed]
46. Devine, K.A.; Viola, A.S.; Coups, E.J.; Wu, Y.P. Digital health interventions for adolescent and young adult cancer survivors. *JCO Clin. Cancer Inform.* **2018**, *2*, 1–15. [CrossRef] [PubMed]
47. Mendoza, J.A.; Baker, K.S.; Moreno, M.A.; Whitlock, K.; Abbey-Lambertz, M.; Waite, A.; Colburn, T.; Chow, E.J. A Fitbit and Facebook mHealth intervention for promoting physical activity among adolescent and young adult childhood cancer survivors: A pilot study. *Pediatr. Blood Cancer* **2017**, *64*, e26660. [CrossRef] [PubMed]
48. Götte, M.; Seidel, C.C.; Kesting, S.V.; Rosenbaum, D.; Boos, J. Objectively measured versus self-reported physical activity in children and adolescents with cancer. *PLoS ONE* **2017**, *12*, e0172216. [CrossRef] [PubMed]

Disclaimer/Publisher's Note: The statements, opinions and data contained in all publications are solely those of the individual author(s) and contributor(s) and not of MDPI and/or the editor(s). MDPI and/or the editor(s) disclaim responsibility for any injury to people or property resulting from any ideas, methods, instructions or products referred to in the content.

Article

Effects of an Exercise Intervention on Gait Function in Young Survivors of Osteosarcoma with Megaendoprosthesis of the Lower Extremity—Results from the Pilot Randomized Controlled Trial proGAIT

Simon Basteck [1,2], Wiebke K. Guder [3], Uta Dirksen [1,2], Arno Krombholz [4], Arne Streitbürger [3], Dirk Reinhardt [1,2] and Miriam Götte [1,2,*]

1. Department of Pediatric Hematology/Oncology, Clinic for Pediatrics III, West German Cancer Centre, University Hospital Essen, 45147 Essen, Germany
2. German Cancer Consortium (DKTK), Partner Site Essen, 45147 Essen, Germany
3. Department of Orthopedic Oncology, West German Cancer Center, University Hospital Essen, 45147 Essen, Germany
4. Faculty of Sport Science, Ruhr University Bochum, 44801 Bochum, Germany
* Correspondence: miriam.goette@uk-essen.de; Tel.: +49-201-723-8083

Abstract: Limb preservation with megaendoprosthesis in adolescents and young adults (AYA) with bone tumors is associated with functional limitations and gait abnormalities. The proGAIT trial evaluated the effectiveness of an exercise program on gait function and quality of life, functional scales (MSTS, TESS), functional mobility, and fatigue as secondary outcomes. Eleven AYA survivors of malignant osteosarcoma with a tumor endoprosthesis around the knee (mean age: 26.6 ($\pm$8.4) years) were randomized into an intervention group receiving an 8-week exercise program or into a control group. Gait function was assessed via 3D motion capture and analyzed using the Gait Profile Score (GPS) and the Gait Deviation Index (GDI). GDI and GPS scores of participants suggest deviations from a healthy reference group. The exercise intervention had small-to-medium positive effects on gait score GDI $|d| = 0.50$ (unaffected leg), $|d| = 0.24$ (affected leg), subjective functional scores TESS $|d| = 0.74$ and MSTS $|d| = 0.49$, and functional tests TUG and TUDS $|d| = 0.61$ and $|d| = 0.52$. None of these changes showed statistical significance. Promising intervention effects suggest that regular exercise could improve lower limb function and follow-up care for survivors; however, a powered RCT as a follow-up project needs to confirm the pilot findings.

Keywords: bone tumor; AYA; endoprosthesis; exercise; gait analysis; lower limb function

1. Introduction

The incidence of bone tumors is particularly high in adolescents and young adults (AYA) between 15 and 39 years of age [1]. Due to the development of new treatment methods, improved imaging techniques determining the disease extent, and improved surgical techniques, the overall survival of patients is above 60% [2–4]. These improved survival rates are bringing the focus on addressing psychological and physical long-term consequences and late effects, and underline the need of supportive concepts to ameliorate these negative effects. These approaches include behavior change interventions in the areas of adequate physical activity, healthy diet, smoking cessation, and alcohol consumption [5,6]. Previous research has shown that the quality of life is reduced in survivors of bone tumors, and the prevalence of somatic disease and psychological problems is high in comparison to matched comparison groups [7,8]. Modular megaendoprostheses have become a gold standard in the reconstruction of osteoarticular defects following tumor resections, while amputation can be avoided in the majority of patients [9]. Limb salvage has both functional and psychological benefits compared to amputation of the affected limb. However, studies suggest that former bone tumor patients have specific gait and functional limitations [10]. These also affect the quality of life of this patient cohort and their participation in daily, social, and professional life, and sports [11–13]. The most frequently reported limitations are regular pain, difficulties in participation in sports and other everyday life activities [14]. Initial interventions indicate positive effects of rehabilitative and exercise programs on the postural control and walk ratio of patients with bone or soft tissue sarcomas [15]. In addition, high evidence levels indicate that exercise is beneficial for cancer patients and survivors in general to reduce fatigue, anxiety and depression, and increase physical performance, quality of life, and bone health [16,17]. The group of adolescent and young adult bone tumor survivors and the effects of exercise in this cohort have only been studied in very few trials. Winter et al. [18] evaluated an individualized exercise program and found that it was feasible, safe, and tended to be beneficial to increase physical activity levels. The lack of data on bone tumor patients contrasts with the high need and burden of this group. It is well known that young adults in the process of structuring their private and educational life have a very special need for supportive services [19]. Limited mobility in everyday life, and the presence of late effects, can severely limit sports participation and participation in social life [11]. However, standardized methods to monitor patients during follow-up, to analyze their gait pattern, and to evaluate the effectiveness of appropriate exercise programs have not yet been established. The main objective of this randomized controlled pilot trial was to investigate the effects of an individualized 8-week exercise program on gait function in adolescents and young adults (AYA) with megaendoprosthesis of the lower extremities in their follow-up care.

2. Materials and Methods

2.1. Design

The inclusion criteria were: (1) a confirmed lower extremity bone tumor (osteosarcoma, Ewing sarcoma, chondrosarcoma), (2) had follow-up care at the University Hospital Essen, (3) aged between 15 and 45 years, and (4) had implantation surgery at least 12 months prior to the baseline assessment. Exclusion criteria were medical conditions that preclude participation in the testing and/or the intervention. The inclusion age range was extended over typical AYA definition to allow for an expanded pool of potential participants. The study population characteristics are summarized in Table 1. Written informed consent was required to participate in the study and the local Ethics Committee of the Faculty of Sport Science at Ruhr University Bochum approved this study (reference number EKS V 04/2021). Recruitment was performed in the period 1 August–16 October 2021 by contacting former patients with megaendoprosthesis of the lower extremity.

Table 1. Demographic characteristics of the study population at baseline.

Characteristic	IG			CG		
	Mean	SD	Range	Mean	SD	Range
Number of patients	6	-	-	5	-	-
Male/female	3/3	-	-	3/2	-	-
Tumor location (Proximal tibia/distal femur)	3/3	-	-	1/4	-	-
Age at gait analysis (years)	26.3	8.0	15–34	27.0	9.8	17–41
Age at surgery (years)	19.8	7.5	12–31	24.0	11.2	10–39
Follow-up (years)	6.5	6.1	1–16	3.0	2.3	1–7
Weight (kg)	69	12.4	52.0–82.0	76.1	25.9	60.0–122.0
Height (cm)	172.2	7.7	163–182	179.0	4.7	172.0–185.0
BMI (kg/m^2)	23.4	4.7	18.0–29.1	23.4	6.8	20.0–35.6
Leg Length Discrepancy (mm)	23.7	30.5	1.6–83.2	13.6	13.3	3.9–36.9

IG, intervention group; CG, control group; SD, standard deviation.

The proGAIT study (NCT04963517) was a randomized controlled trial (RCT). Randomization was carried out via minimization using the software minimPy version 2.0 by Dr. M. Saghaei [20]. Factors in the randomized allocation process were participants' resection length of the affected limb and participants' age. Both factors had two levels. The shortest reconstruction lengths were 100 mm or 120 mm for the distal femur and 115 mm or 135 mm for the proximal tibia. All longer resections were reconstructed using extension sleeves in a modular implant design. Sleeves were available in 30 mm, 40 mm, 60 mm, 80 mm, and 100 mm. Combinations were also used. Based on this, a classification between the shortest possible (<140mm) and longer ($\geq$140mm) resections/reconstructions for both localizations (distal femur, proximal tibia) was chosen. Different levels of age were classified with <30 years and $\geq$30 years. Participants were allocated to the study groups directly after their baseline visit.

2.2. Study Population and Surgery

All patients included in this study were reconstructed using a linked knee megaendoprosthesis (implantcast GmbH, Buxtehude, Germany, MUTARS system) following bone tumor resections of the distal femur or proximal tibia. Oncological tumor resections, disregarding the tumor site, aimed at the complete removal of the tumor that was surrounded by a healthy soft tissue margin, thus, in distal femur tumors that entailed the detachment and partial loss of the vastus medialis, vastus lateralis, vastus intermedius and adductor muscles. Both venters of the gastrocnemius muscle were severed close to their insertion in the distal femur. The patella and insertion of the patella tendon at the tuberosity of the tibia were retained. While the femoral insertion of both venters of the gastrocnemius muscle remained intact in proximal tibia resections, the patella ligament was detached from its insertion at the tibial tuberosity. The following muscles inserted at the proximal tibia were severed, leaving a margin of healthy muscle around the tumor: tibialis anterior, extensor digitorum and hallucis longus, soleus, tibialis posterior, flexor digitorum, and hallucis longus. An attachment tube covering the implant body of the proximal tibia megaendoprosthesis was used for the refixation of the patella ligament. Additionally, to improve the soft tissue coverage of the implant, patients were reconstructed using a local gastrocnemius flap.

However, since both the distal femur and proximal tibia resections were osteoarticular resections around the knee, they shared common characteristics as well: both cruciate and collateral ligaments needed to be severed, necessitating a reconstruction using a linked megaendoprosthesis. As a result, the long-term flexion of the knee joint was limited to 90° due to the metal-on-metal rotating-hinge coupling piece used in this patient collective.

Early rehabilitation included a period of six weeks with the partial weight bearing of 20 kg after the cementless implantation of megaendoprostheses of either site. However, while the knee joint flexion was increased by 30° each week immediately after distal femur resection, the refixation of the patella tendon and gastrocnemius flap on the attachment tube led to a four-week immobilization period of the knee joint using an extension brace. Thus, flexion was only increased by 30°, starting in week five after the surgery. Patients after proximal tibia replacement also commonly suffer from a weakness of dorsiflexion of the foot, which is supported by an ankle foot orthosis for several months after the operation until active dorsiflexion recovers. After the completion of adjuvant chemotherapy, all patients are eligible for a three-to-four-week inpatient rehabilitation program to recover socially, psychologically, and physically.

To control for different functional abilities and requirements during early rehabilitation after distal femur and proximal tibia resection, this study recruited patients only if their surgery was performed at least 12 months prior to the baseline evaluation. By that time, rehabilitation no longer needs to be site-specific, and varying site-specific early functional impairments had usually recovered. In addition, no spontaneous improvement without training was expected after 12 months [21].

2.3. Intervention

The intervention group (IG) received a personalized 8-week training consisting of exercises focusing on strength, coordination, balance, and mobility of the lower extremities to improve gait function according to the intervention schedule. In detail, the training sessions mainly involved strength exercises for leg extensor and flexor muscles as well as muscle groups responsible for leg add- and abduction. Another training aspect focused on proprioceptive training of the lower extremities and trunk stabilizers through balance training in different variations. All exercises were designed to be carried out with the participants' own individual bodyweight and minimal equipment expenses. Training sessions were supervised via the Zoom conference tool (Zoom Video Communications Inc., San Jose, CA, USA). The long-term aim was to encourage participants to engage in independent exercise, so the supervised session frequency for the IG decreased during the course of the study. Participants exercised twice a week for eight weeks overall. They received two supervised sessions per week in week 1 and 2. In week 3, 4, and 5, they received one supervised session per week and trained unsupervised a second time. This was followed by a period of unsupervised exercise in week 6 and 7. In the last week of the intervention, participants received 2 supervised sessions (intensification phase). Additionally, participants in the IG received a brochure with sport and exercise recommendations for their independent exercise. The control group only received a booklet with general information about physical activity and cancer, but no specific intervention recommendations for patients with endoprosthesis. They were also not encouraged to change their current physical activity behavior during the eight-week study period.

2.4. Assessments

To measure the effect of the intervention, all endpoints were assessed at baseline (before the randomization, T0) and after the 8-week intervention/control period (T1 at both appointments (baseline and post-intervention); the assessments were conducted in a standardized order. At first, participants filled in the questionnaires for the subjective rating of physical function, quality of life, and fatigue. For subjective physical function, we used the Musculoskeletal Tumor Society Score (MSTS) and the Toronto Extremity Salvage Score (TESS), which have widely been used for patients with lower extremity musculoskeletal sarcomas [22]. The MSTS scoring system was developed by Enneking et al. [23] and the lower extremity version assesses pain, function, emotional, support, walking, and gait problems on a 0–5 point scale (maximum overall score 30 points). The TESS [24] version for lower extremity sarcomas contains 30 questions to assess physical function in daily activities such as working, dressing, and mobility. Questions are rated on a 1–5 point scale and the total score is calculated as the percentage of the maximum score (leading to a total maximum score of 100 points). Quality of life was assessed with the EORTC QLQ-C30 questionnaire, developed by the European Organization for Research and Treatment of Cancer. It contains 30 questions in subscales (functional score and symptom score) and single items. All subscales and the individual items have a score range from 0 to 100 points. A higher score represents better function and a higher quality of life. However, in the symptom's subscale, a higher score represents a higher level of symptoms or problems. The EORTC QLQ-FA12 questionnaire was used to evaluate fatigue in the cohort. The EORTC questionnaires are commonly used in cancer patients, including sarcoma patients with lower extremity tumors [25,26]. Participants under the age of 18 years used the Pediatric Quality of Life Inventory (PedsQL) cancer and fatigue modules instead of the EORTC, which have been shown to be valid and reliable in this population [27]. Gait analysis is the most frequently used single physical performance test for bone tumor patients [28]. This was then conducted with a Vicon camera system including 8 cameras recording at 120 Hz at different projections along a runway to record marker positions in a three-dimensional space (Vicon Vantage V5, Oxford, UK). The Conventional Gait Model 2.3 (CGM 2.3) for the lower body, which is also integrated in the Vicon Nexus software, was used to calculate the kinematics of the segments and joints of the lower body of the participants. Each patient walked along a runway (15 m) 5 times in a self-selected walking speed. Five complete gait cycles for the left and right side were selected for further data processing. Gait cycles for each side were defined as the period between the touchdowns of the same foot. The touchdown was defined as the instant when the heel marker reaches the lowest value on the vertical z-coordinate. To assure the greatest possible comparability and minimum variation of intraindividual gait data due to different marker placements at baseline and follow-up measurements, participants' lower body marker locations were marked after gait analysis with a permanent skin marker. Every participant received a skin marker and was asked to redraw marker locations in case of fading.

After gait analysis, the patients proceeded to the physiological function assessment, which consisted of two functional tests and a knee joint range-of-motion assessment via manual goniometry to assess maximal active and passive knee flexions and extensions. Under consideration of the systematic review by Söntgerath et al. [28] the "timed up and go" test and the "timed up and downstairs" test were conducted. During the "timed up and go", the participants needed to stand up from a chair, walk a distance of 3 m, return, and sit down again. During the "timed up and downstairs", participants walked up and down 14 flights of stairs as fast as possible. The endpoint of both tests was the time the participants required to fulfill the task.

2.5. Data Analysis and Statistics

To evaluate and analyze the data from the 3D gait analysis in a clinical context, recent studies proposed different indices of overall gait pathology to merge the complex information contained in these highly interdependent 3D data into a single measure [29]. Belonging to the most commonly used gait indices, the Gait Profile Score (GPS) by Baker et al. [29] and the Gait Deviation Index (GDI) by Schwartz and Rozumalski [30] were the two indices used to analyze 3D data in this study. For the calculation of the GPS and GDI scores, the GDI-GPS-Calculator Version3.2 by Richard Baker was used. The different segment angles from the collected gait cycles were normalized over the gait cycle and extracted in 2% increments. For further calculation, gait cycles for each side were averaged. In the study, reference group gait data from healthy subjects (n = 13) in the same age range as the AYA participants were gathered and implemented into the GDI-GPS-Calculator Version 3.2; this was used as the reference dataset to provide valid values using the exact same method, researcher, and biomechanical lab. Four of the 13 healthy subjects were male, nine were female, and the age of the healthy reference group ranged from 22 to 39 years. Further data analysis was carried out using Python data analysis tools (Biomechanical ToolKit, Pandas, NumPy, SciPy, Matplotlib, Seaborn). The differences in the scores of the GPS and GDI between measurements (delta changes) were investigated for differences between CG and IG via an independent *t*-test followed by a calculation of the effect size expressed in Cohen's d. All changes in patient-reported outcomes as well as the physiological function outcomes between measurements (delta changes) were also compared via an independent t-test, and Cohen's d was calculated. The significance level for all statistical tests was determined as $\alpha = 0.05$.

3. Results

3.1. Patient Characteristics

Eleven participants with lower extremity osteosarcoma around the knee and endoprosthesis, aged between 15 and 41 years, and had implantation surgery at least 12 months before inclusion participated in this RCT. Six participants were allocated to the IG, whereas 5 participants were allocated to the CG (Table 1). No adverse events occurred during gait analysis and the physical performance assessment or during the intervention.

3.2. Gait Function at Baseline and Change during the Intervention

Gait analysis at baseline revealed that the gait of every participant deviated from a healthy reference group. Deviations were particularly larger in the affected leg than the unaffected leg. This can be seen in individual GDI, GPS, and GVS, as well as the averaged gait curves of all assessed gait variables from all participants throughout the entire gait cycle (see Figure 1). Larger deviations were noticed in the pelvis up/down, hip adduction/abduction, as well as the hip internal/external rotation variables. Furthermore, there were obvious deviations in the knee flexion/extension variable of the affected leg during the first half of the gait cycle in all participants. Summarizing the results of the intervention, Table 2 shows an overview of the relevant descriptive statistical parameters of all assessed outcome measures (gait scores, patient-reported outcomes, and physiological function assessment).

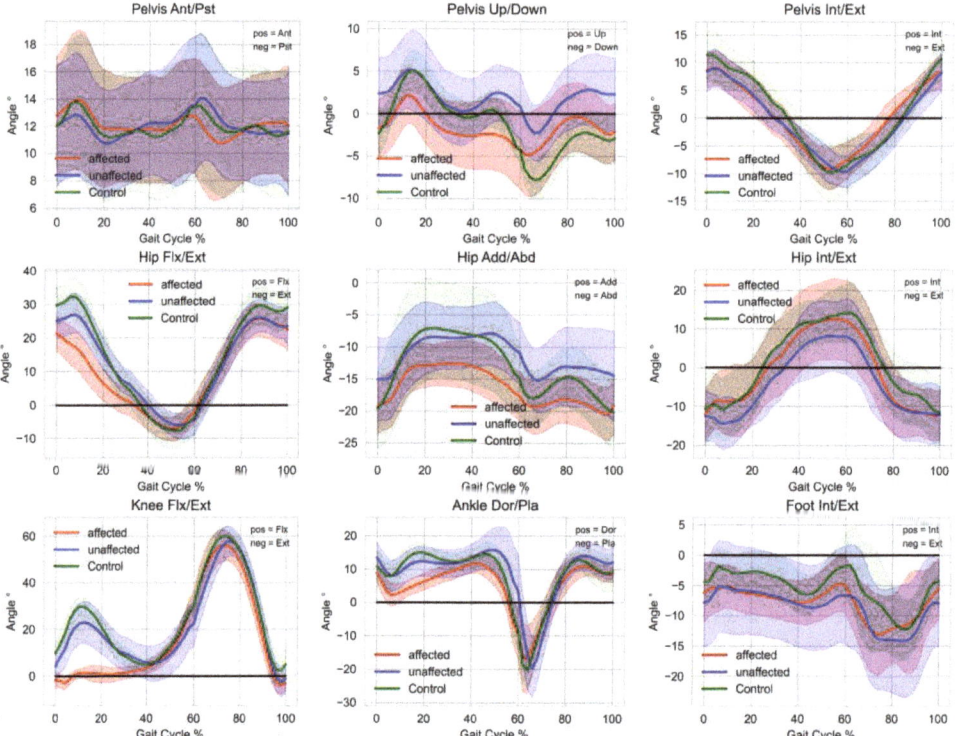

Figure 1. Averaged segment and joint angles throughout the entire gait cycle of all participants at baseline. Unaffected (red) and affected (blue) side of participants with endoprosthesis and a healthy reference group (green) showing the mean and SD (light color area). Healthy reference goup: n = 13, 4 male, 9 female, 22–39 years without tumor megaendoprosthesis.

Delta changes between CG and IG were not significant in all assessed gait scores (see Figure 2). Absolute d-values range between $|d| = 0.11$ (GPS (overall), small effect) and $|d| = 0.50$ (GDI (unaffected leg), medium effect). Additionally, a larger effect could be identified in the GPS (unaffected leg) variable ($|d| = 0.29$) compared to the GPS (affected leg) variable ($|d| = 0.19$).

Table 2. Overview of the relevant descriptive statistical parameters of all assessed outcome measures at baseline (T0) and after the intervention (T1).

			GDI (aff)	GDI (unaff.)	GPS (aff.)	GPS (unaff.)	GPS (Overall)	TESS	MSTS	QoL	Function	Symptom	Fatigue	TUG (sec)	TUDS (sec)	Knee Flexion Active (°)	Knee Flexion Passive (°)	Knee Extension Active (°)	Knee Extension Passive (°)
CG (n = 5)	T0	Mean	86.5	95.8	6.7	5.4	6.4	86.0	24.6	81.0	73.0	8.75	20.0	6.4	18.2	90.7	92.4	13.3	0.0
		Min	72.3	79.5	4.5	4.2	4.4	77.0	22.0	67.0	63.0	0.0	10.0	5.1	9.5	80.0	85.0	5.0	0.0
		Max	103.3	104.6	9.4	7.7	9.2	96.0	27.0	97.2	85.0	21.0	30.0	8.4	32.9	105.0	110.0	30.0	0.0
		95%-CI	72.9–100.2	82.7–108.9	4.6–8.9	3.6–7.1	4.3–8.6	75.4–96.6	22.2–27.0	67.1–95.0	57.2–88.8	0.0–22.8	8.3–31.7	4.7–8.2	6.3–30.0	58.6–122.7	79.9–104.9	0.0–49.2	-
	T1	Mean	84.8	95.0	6.9	5.5	6.6	85.2	25.0	84.3	78.5	9.0	12.6	5.9	17.1	86.0	95.2	14.0	2.0
		Min	71.9	78.0	5.5	3.9	4.9	73.0	21.0	67.0	59.0	3.0	0.0	4.0	7.9	70.0	85.0	0.0	0.0
		Max	93.2	108.8	9.1	8.1	9.3	94.	27.0	96.3	91.0	24.0	33.0	8.2	31.2	108.0	115.0	45.0	10.0
		95%-CI	74.8–94.9	78.6–111.5	5.1–8.7	3.3–7.7	4.5–8.6	74.5–95.9	22.1–28.0	70.3–98.2	54.9–100.0	0.0–25.0	0.0–31.1	3.7–8.1	6.2–28.1	68.9–103.1	79.7–110.7	0.0–36.1	0.0–7.6
IG (n = 6)	T0	Mean	78.5	88.4	8.1	6.2	7.7	87.0	24.5	79.1	84.8	11.4	7.2	6.5	16.5	87.5	97.5	26.3	1.7
		Min	67.6	76.2	5.9	5.0	5.9	75.0	19.0	50.0	68.0	5.0	0.0	4.1	9.9	66.0	70.0	10.0	0.0
		Max	90.0	95.4	10.5	8.1	10.2	99.0	28.0	92.6	94.0	19.0	27.0	8.8	33.6	110.0	120.0	50.0	10.0
		95%-CI	70.4–86.7	80.5–96.4	6.4–9.8	5.0–7.4	6.1–9.2	78.1–95.9	21.2–27.8	63.6–94.6	72.5–97.1	3.2–19.6	0.0–18.1	4.8–8.1	7.4–25.6	72.3–102.7	78.2–116.8	7.6–45.1	0.0–6.0
	T1	Mean	77.9	91.8	8.4	6.0	7.8	90.0	25.8	83.3	86.8	13.4	12.2	5.6	14.7	82.5	98.3	16.0	0.8
		Min	61.8	73.8	5.0	3.7	4.5	84.0	23.0	42.0	66.0	4.0	0.0	3.8	8.3	55.0	70.0	0.0	0.0
		Max	96.0	111.2	12.3	8.8	11.3	98.0	28.0	100.0	99.0	32.0	40.0	8.6	31.8	120.0	125.0	45.0	5.0
		95%-CI	64.8–91.0	75.8–107.9	5.6–11.2	3.8–8.3	5.1–10.4	83.1–96.9	23.3–28.4	60.6–100.0	69.1–100.0	0.0–29.4	0.0–27.2	4.0–7.3	5.5–23.9	59.8–105.2	75.2–121.4	0.0–37.2	0.0–3.0

Gait Deviation Index (GDI), Gait Profile Score (GPS), Toronto Extremity Salvage Score (TESS); Musculoskeletal Tumor Society Score (MSTS); Quality of Life assessment (QoL), Function, Symptom and Fatigue Scale; Timed up and go (TUG); Timed up and downstairs (TUDS). Mean values (mean), min. values (min), max. values (max), and 95% confidence intervals (95%-CI); aff = affected; unaff = unaffected (without prosthesis); sec = seconds; ° = angle degree.

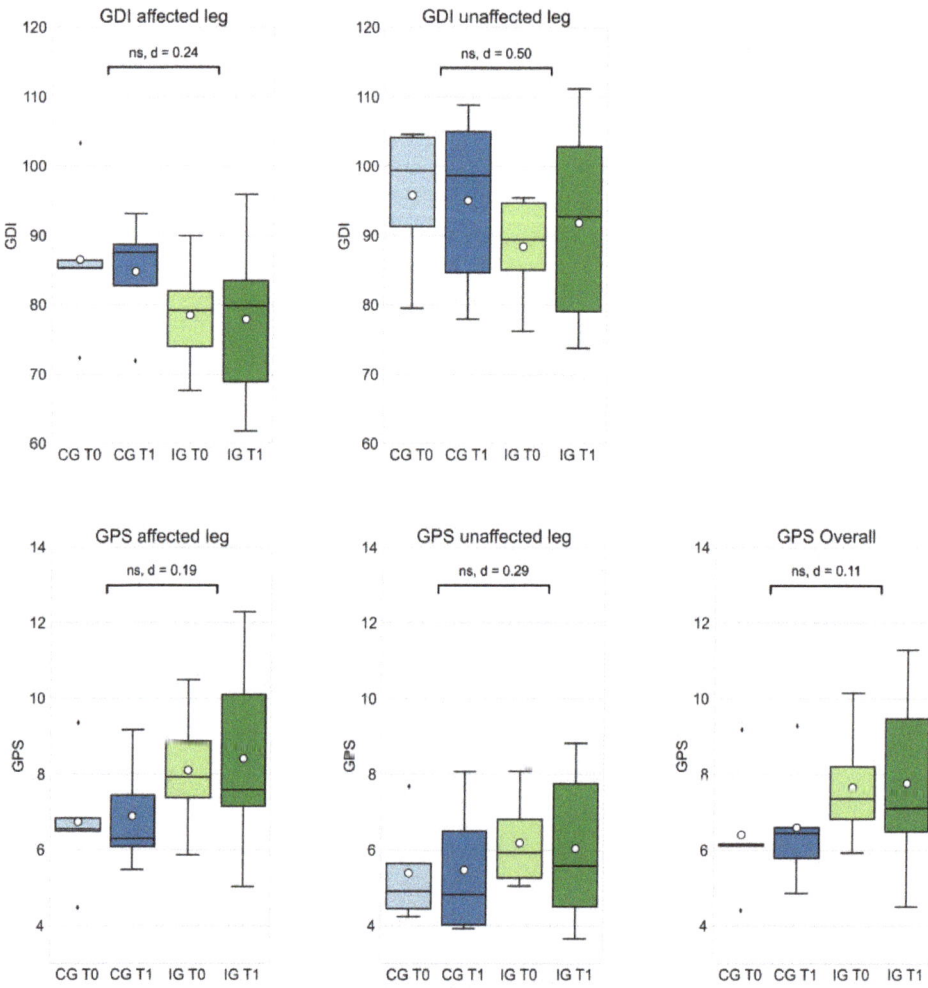

Figure 2. The Gait Deviation Index (GDI) and Gait Profile Score (GPS) of the control group at T0 (CG T0, light blue) and T1 (CG T1, dark blue) as well the intervention group at T0 (IG T0, light green) and T1 (IG T1, dark green). Box-whisker plot shows quartiles, mean (°), and outliers (♦); statistical annotations show significance (ns = not significant) and effect size (absolute Cohen's d); comparison of delta changes via independent t-test, $\alpha = 0.05$.

3.3. TESS and MSTS

Effect sizes ranged from small to large in patient-reported functional outcomes (TESS: $|d| = 0.74$; MSTS: $|d| = 0.49$). Delta changes in the patient-reported outcomes did not differ significantly in the comparison between IG and CG (see Figure 3).

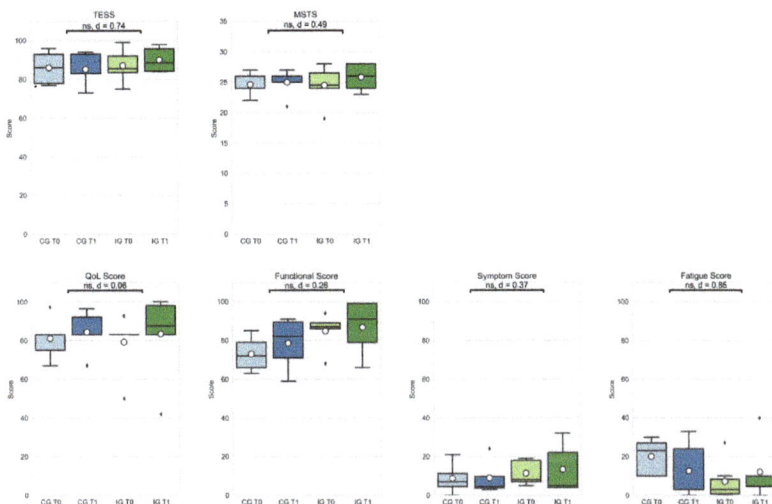

Figure 3. Patient-reported outcomes (Toronto Extremity Salvage Score (TESS); Musculoskeletal Society Score (MSTS); Quality of Life assessment—Function, Symptom, and Fatigue scores) of the control group at T0 (CG T0, light blue) and T1 (CG T1, dark blue) as well as the intervention group at T0 (IG T0, light green) and T1 (IG T1, dark green). Box-whisker plot showing quartiles, mean (°), and outliers (♦); statistical annotations showing significance (ns = not significant) and effect size (absolute Cohen's d); comparison delta changes via independent t-test, $\alpha = 0.05$.

3.4. Physical Function

Effect size for physiological function assessment measures (TUG, TUDS) were medium (TUG: $|d| = 0.61$; TUDS: $|d| = 0.52$). Delta changes did not differ significantly (see Figure 4).

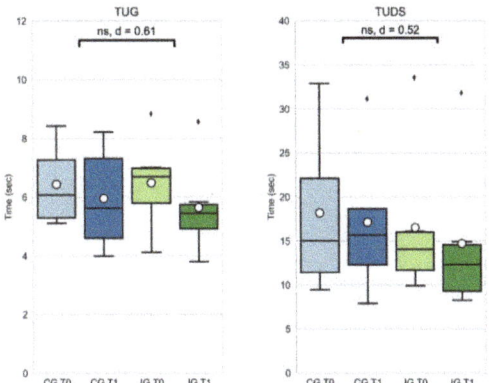

Figure 4. Timed up and go (TUG) and timed up and downstairs (TUDS) outcomes of the control group at T0 (CG T0, light blue) and T1 (CG T1, dark blue) as well as the intervention group at T0 (IG T0, light green) and T1 (IG T1, dark blue). Box-whisker plot showing quartiles, mean (°), and outliers (♦); statistical annotations showing significance (ns = not significant) and effect size (absolute Cohen's d); comparison of delta changes via independent t-test, $\alpha = 0.05$.

3.5. Quality of Life and Fatigue

Delta changes in outcomes regarding quality of life showed no significant differences, but small to large effect sizes (Quality of Life (QoL): $|d| = 0.06$; functional score: $|d| = 0.26$; symptom score: $|d| = 0.37$; fatigue score: $|d| = 0.85$).

4. Discussion

The objective kinematic parameters show deviations in the participants' gait data from healthy control group kinematics and appear on both the affected and unaffected side. This phenomenon seems reasonable because of the necessary interactions between both legs in the gait cycle. Those deviations are comparable to findings of Kim et al. [31], who investigated lower limb joint kinematics of former patients with distal femur and proximal tibia reconstructions. Larger deviations in the pelvic up-and-down motion most likely derive from leg length discrepancies between the affected and unaffected legs. Participants in the proGAIT study had leg length discrepancies ranging from 1.6 to 83.2 mm. These differences are normally compensated through orthopedic devices in the everyday life of participants. Especially in cases with increased LLD (>30 mm), participants usually wear a shoe raise on the affected side. Gait analysis was carried out without compensating footwear to minimize external influences and ensure comparability with the control group data, which were also gathered in barefoot trials. A future option would be a gait analysis involving compensating footwear for participants with increased LLD to allow a detailed look into other potential causes for gait abnormalities.

In addition, larger deviations from healthy gait seem to appear, especially in the knee flexion/extension of the participants' affected legs during the first half (stance phase to toe-off) of the gait cycle. After the phase of touchdown, the affected knee is nearly fully extended or even overextended in most participants. Compared to knee data from a healthy reference group, which show an initial flexion to about 20–30° after touchdown, this seems to be the most remarkable deviation in participants with endoprosthesis around the knee, which is also mentioned in a paper by Kim et al. [31]. A previous study by Rompen et al. [32] also describes this type of deviation. Some participants of the proGAIT study reported a feeling of instability in the knee when it is slightly bent, so full extension or overextension seems to be a way to compensate for this problem for most of the participants. A possible origin of hyperextension may be the lack of stabilization by the two gastrocnemius muscles, which are always disconnected in distal femoral replacements and at least unilaterally in proximal tibial replacements. The results of a study by Pesenti et al. [10] also suggest that overextension is typical in this cohort. After the touchdown of the affected leg, the quadriceps muscle-tendon units work eccentrically to absorb energy and to decelerate knee flexion. In case of quadriceps weakness or dysfunction after tumor surgery, this is compensated by the hip extensors which then help to bring the lower limb into a more extended position to passively stabilize the knee joint. Thus, hip flexion and extension also deviate in survivors of osteosarcoma with knee tumor endoprosthesis reconstruction compared to a healthy control group. The affected leg especially seems to be more extended at the hip joint throughout the entire gait cycle compared to healthy participants (see Figure 1). Furthermore, proGAIT data show reduced dorsiflexion in the ankle joint compared to the healthy reference group. These deviations seem to appear primarily in the stance phase of the affected leg. Kim et al. [31] hypothesized that this might be due to calf muscle activity stabilizing the tibia to compensate for the above-mentioned quadriceps weakness, and therefore, reduced knee stability. Furthermore, larger deviations can be seen in hip adduction and abduction, and hip internal and external rotation. It remains unclear from where these deviations derive. A meaningful interpretation of outcomes can only be made under the consideration of the gait assessment method, and especially the gait model which was used. The CGM 2.3 still lacks the ability to measure hip rotation and foot progression during dynamic trials with the help of medial markers at the knee and the malleoli, which are used only for the calibration trial. Thus, these results still need to be interpreted with caution.

The results presented in this study indicate positive effects of the intervention in all assessed gait scores, even though the delta differences between groups were statistically not significant (see Figure 2). Larger effects seem to occur in GDI and GPS of patients' unaffected legs. Due to long periods of physical inactivity [33] and the load restrictions of the affected leg before and after tumor surgery, it can be hypothesized that muscles, and potentially tendon and ligament structures in the unaffected limb, obtain a better trainability, and thus, respond better to an exercise intervention. Medium-to-large positive effects of the intervention can also be seen in patient-reported outcomes, TESS and MSTS (see Figure 3). The review of Kask et al. [22] summarized studies that examined functional outcomes in patients with lower-extremity soft tissue sarcomas and bone sarcomas, and calculated a mean overall TESS score of 86.7, which corresponds to the baseline TESS scores of the proGAIT cohort (CG: 86.0; IG: 87.0). The post-intervention TESS score in the IG group increased to 90.0, which is higher than in previous studies with lower extremity tumor patients [34,35], and indicates a comparably good function.

The objective functional results of the TUG and TUDS also improved in favor of the intervention group (see Figure 4), though these were also not statistically significant. However, an improved functional mobility in daily live facilitates everyday tasks, positively correlates with quality of life [13], and probably also influences physical activity behavior. For most outcomes, both groups showed improvements after the study period of 8 weeks. The IG, however, showed a decline in outcomes in the symptom and fatigue scale. Although in contrast with the general evidence regarding the effectiveness of exercise to reduce fatigue in cancer patients [16], for some patients, the transition to strenuous exercise may have resulted in an increased workload that was unfamiliar and also fatiguing for them. It can also be hypothesized that the duration of the intervention was too short, and that the results would be different if the supervision was in person and not via an online platform. It should be clear that an exercise intervention for this patient group should be well balanced and individually adjusted to avoid excessive physical load, especially on structures affected by former tumor resection surgery. Furthermore, previous chemotherapy treatment and corresponding late effects should be considered in the exercise planning. Improvements in the above-mentioned outcomes in both study groups are probably a result of the contamination of the CG. This is a well-known problem in exercise oncology studies, as described by Steins Bisschop et al. [36]. The CG received a booklet with general information about physical activity and cancer prior to the intervention period. Participation in gait analysis seemed to create awareness of the issue and potentially motivated participants to increase their physical activity and lower limb function.

The systematic review by Wilson et al. [37] did not identify any studies involving an exercise intervention in combination with an objective gait assessment in this context, although improvement in lower limb function, and thus, quality of life, is becoming an increasing issue for this patient group. A long-term prospective study by Egmond-van Dam et al. [38] with former bone tumor patients investigated long-term functional outcomes, focusing on the knee joint. They found no significant changes in functional outcome measures between 2 and 7 years after surgery. It, therefore, seems appropriate to test the effectiveness of an intervention that starts earlier.

The proGAIT study has several limitations. The overall sample size is small, so that even in the case of medium-to-large effect sizes, no statistical significance could be detected. Furthermore, the gait assessment time from surgery was different between participants and might be a reason for the varying effects of the exercise intervention in different participants. It could not be guaranteed that the markers were placed in exactly the same place before and after the intervention. However, intensive palpation seemed to have led to the correct placement. Some differences between IG and CG characteristics were noted that seem be present as a result of the small sample size. In the IG, half of participants had a history of proximal tibia tumor versus 20% in the CG. IG participants were younger at surgery, had a longer follow-up period since surgery, and had larger leg lengths discrepancies. However, since all intervention effects were calculated as the change to baseline, these clinical differences seem to be negligible in terms of outcomes. Another limitation regarding gait analysis and comparability with the above-mentioned studies is the lack of kinetic outcomes in gait analysis. This would have been an option to gain a more detailed look into typical gait deviations in the investigated group of former cancer patients.

5. Conclusions

The exploratory proGAIT randomized controlled trial shows promising positive effects—however, without statistical significance—of an 8-week exercise intervention on lower limb gait function in former patients with tumor endoprostheses around the knee. Additional powered clinical trials with larger samples sizes are needed to confirm these preliminary results. In a subsequent study, further questions need to be addressed, such as the ideal time after surgery to start the supervised gait exercise program, the most effective exercises in the program, and the preferred intensity and duration. Nonetheless, it should be noticed that exercise has already been shown to be beneficial for several groups of cancer patients and survivors, and existing guidelines in pediatric and adult oncology provide feasible and safe concepts to improve the mobility and physical performance and reduce symptoms [16,39,40]. Therefore, in addition to the required confirmatory studies, there is a particular need for the development of implementation approaches, such as the partially supervised online training from proGAIT. The long-term goal is to implement effective exercise concepts as the standard care for AYA survivors with a tumor endoprosthesis and survivors with other consequences of cancer treatment.

Author Contributions: Conceptualization, S.B., W.K.G., U.D., A.K., A.S., D.R. and M.G.; Formal analysis, S.B. and M.G.; Funding acquisition, D.R.; Investigation, S.B. and M.G.; Methodology, S.B., W.K.G., U.D., A.K., A.S., D.R. and M.G.; Project administration, U.D., A.K., A.S., D.R. and M.G.; Software, A.K.; Supervision, W.K.G., A.S., D.R. and M.G.; Validation, M.G.; Visualization, S.B. and M.G.; Writing—original draft, S.B. and M.G.; Writing—review and editing, W.K.G., U.D., A.K., A.S., D.R. and M.G. All authors have read and agreed to the published version of the manuscript.

Funding: This research received no external funding.

Institutional Review Board Statement: The study was conducted in accordance with the Declaration of Helsinki, and approved by the Ethics Committee of the Faculty of Sport Science at Ruhr University Bochum (reference number EKS V 04/2021).

Informed Consent Statement: Informed consent was obtained from all subjects involved in the study.

Data Availability Statement: The data are available from the corresponding author on reasonable request.

Acknowledgments: The authors would like to thank Tobias Weingarten and Daniel Hahn for their motion science expertise and support during the study, and Hahn for valuable suggestions in the manuscript. We would also like to thank all study participants for their time and interest in this study. We acknowledge support by the Open Access Publication Fund of the University of Duisburg-Essen.

Conflicts of Interest: The authors declare no conflict of interest.

References

1. Miller, K.D.; Fidler-Benaoudia, M.; Keegan, T.H.; Hipp, H.S.; Jemal, A.; Siegel, R.L. Cancer statistics for adolescents and young adults, 2020. *CA A Cancer J. Clin.* **2020**, *70*, 443–459. [CrossRef]
2. Meltzer, P.S.; Helman, L.J. New Horizons in the Treatment of Osteosarcoma. *N. Engl. J. Med.* **2021**, *385*, 2066–2076. [CrossRef] [PubMed]
3. Bölling, T.; Hardes, J.; Dirksen, U. Management of bone tumours in paediatric oncology. *Clin. Oncol. (R. Coll. Radiol.)* **2013**, *25*, 19–26. [CrossRef] [PubMed]
4. Grünewald, T.G.P.; Cidre-Aranaz, F.; Surdez, D.; Tomazou, E.M.; de Álava, E.; Kovar, H.; Sorensen, P.H.; Delattre, O.; Dirksen, U. Ewing sarcoma. *Nat. Rev. Dis. Primers* **2018**, *4*, 5. [CrossRef]
5. Pugh, G.; Gravestock, H.L.; Hough, R.E.; King, W.M.; Wardle, J.; Fisher, A. Health Behavior Change Interventions for Teenage and Young Adult Cancer Survivors: A Systematic Review. *J. Adolesc. Young Adult Oncol.* **2016**, *5*, 91–105. [CrossRef] [PubMed]
6. Pugh, G.; Hough, R.; Gravestock, H.; Davies, C.; Horder, R.; Fisher, A. The development and user evaluation of health behaviour change resources for teenage and young adult Cancer survivors. *Res. Involv. Engagem.* **2019**, *5*, 9. [CrossRef] [PubMed]

7. Pedersen, C.; Rechnitzer, C.; Andersen, E.A.W.; Kenborg, L.; Norsker, F.N.; Bautz, A.; Baad-Hansen, T.; Tryggvadottir, L.; Madanat-Harjuoja, L.-M.; Holmqvist, A.S.; et al. Somatic Disease in Survivors of Childhood Malignant Bone Tumors in the Nordic Countries. *Cancers* **2021**, *13*, 4505. [CrossRef] [PubMed]
8. Ranft, A.; Seidel, C.; Hoffmann, C.; Paulussen, M.; Warby, A.-C.; Berg, H.V.D.; Ladenstein, R.; Rossig, C.; Dirksen, U.; Rosenbaum, D.; et al. Quality of Survivorship in a Rare Disease: Clinicofunctional Outcome and Physical Activity in an Observational Cohort Study of 618 Long-Term Survivors of Ewing Sarcoma. *J. Clin. Oncol.* **2017**, *35*, 1704–1712. [CrossRef] [PubMed]
9. Tan, P.; Yong, B.; Wang, J.; Huang, G.; Yin, J.; Zou, C.; Xie, X.; Tang, Q.; Shen, J. Analysis of the efficacy and prognosis of limb-salvage surgery for osteosarcoma around the knee. *Eur. J. Surg. Oncol.* **2012**, *38*, 1171–1177. [CrossRef] [PubMed]
10. Pesenti, S.; Peltier, E.; Pomero, V.; Authier, G.; Roscigni, L.; Viehweger, E.; Jouve, J.-L. Knee function after limb salvage surgery for malignant bone tumor: Comparison of megaprosthesis and distal femur allograft with epiphysis sparing. *Int. Orthop.* **2018**, *42*, 427–436. [CrossRef]
11. Mester, B.; Guder, W.; Streitbürger, A.; Schoepp, C.; Nottrott, M.; Podleska, L.; Dudda, M.; Hardes, J. Wiederkehr zu körperlicher Aktivität und Sport in der Tumororthopädie. [Return to Sports and Activity in Tumor Orthopaedics]. *Z. Orthop. Unfall.* **2021**, *online ahead of print*. [CrossRef]
12. Gerber, L.H.; Hoffman, K.; Chaudhry, U.; Augustine, E.; Parks, R.; Bernad, M.; Mackall, C.; Steinberg, S.; Mansky, P. Functional outcomes and life satisfaction in long-term survivors of pediatric sarcomas. *Arch. Phys. Med. Rehabil.* **2006**, *87*, 1611–1617. [CrossRef] [PubMed]
13. Liu, Y.; Hu, A.; Zhang, M.; Shi, C.; Zhang, X.; Zhang, J. Correlation between functional status and quality of life after surgery in patients with primary malignant bone tumor of the lower extremities. *Orthop. Nurs.* **2014**, *33*, 163–170. [CrossRef] [PubMed]
14. Bekkering, W.P.; Vlieland, T.V.; Koopman, H.M.; Schaap, G.R.; Schreuder, H.B.; Beishuizen, A.; Tissing, W.J.; Hoogerbrugge, P.M.; Anninga, J.K.; Taminiau, A.H. Quality of life in young patients after bone tumor surgery around the knee joint and comparison with healthy controls. *Pediatr. Blood Cancer* **2010**, *54*, 738–745. [CrossRef]
15. Müller, D.A.; Beltrami, G.; Scoccianti, G.; Cuomo, P.; Capanna, R. Allograft-prosthetic composite versus megaprosthesis in the proximal tibia-What works best? *Injury* **2016**, *47* (Suppl. S4), S124–S130. [CrossRef] [PubMed]
16. Campbell, K.L.; Winters-Stone, K.M.; Wiskemann, J.; May, A.M.; Schwartz, A.L.; Courneya, K.S.; Zucker, D.S.; Matthews, C.E.; Ligibel, J.A.; Gerber, L.H.; et al. Exercise Guidelines for Cancer Survivors: Consensus Statement from International Multidisciplinary Roundtable. *Med. Sci. Sports Exerc.* **2019**, *51*, 2375–2390. [CrossRef] [PubMed]
17. Patel, A.V.; Friedenreich, C.M.; Moore, S.C.; Hayes, S.C.; Silver, J.K.; Campbell, K.L.; Winters-Stone, K.; Gerber, L.H.; George, S.M.; Fulton, J.E.; et al. American College of Sports Medicine Roundtable Report on Physical Activity, Sedentary Behavior, and Cancer Prevention and Control. *Med. Sci. Sports Exerc.* **2019**, *51*, 2391–2402. [CrossRef]
18. Winter, C.C.; Müller, C.; Hardes, J.; Gosheger, G.; Boos, J.; Rosenbaum, D. The effect of individualized exercise interventions during treatment in pediatric patients with a malignant bone tumor. *Support. Care Cancer* **2013**, *21*, 1629–1636. [CrossRef] [PubMed]
19. Choi, E.; Becker, H.; Kim, S. Unmet needs in adolescents and young adults with cancer: A mixed-method study using social media. *J. Pediatr. Nurs.* **2022**, *64*, 31–41. [CrossRef]
20. Saghaei, M.; Saghaei, S. Implementation of an open-source customizable minimization program for allocation of patients to parallel groups in clinical trials. *JBiSE* **2011**, *04*, 734–739. [CrossRef]
21. Westlake, B.; Pipitone, O.; Tedesco, N.S. Time to Functional Outcome Optimization After Musculoskeletal Tumor Resection. *Cureus* **2022**, *14*, e27317. [CrossRef] [PubMed]
22. Kask, G.; Barner-Rasmussen, I.; Repo, J.P.; Kjäldman, M.; Kilk, K.; Blomqvist, C.; Tukiainen, E.J. Functional Outcome Measurement in Patients with Lower-Extremity Soft Tissue Sarcoma: A Systematic Literature Review. *Ann. Surg. Oncol.* **2019**, *26*, 4707–4722. [CrossRef]
23. Enneking, W.F.; Dunham, W.; Gebhardt, M.C.; Malawar, M.; Pritchard, D.J. A system for the functional evaluation of reconstructive procedures after surgical treatment of tumors of the musculoskeletal system. *Clin. Orthop. Relat. Res.* **1993**, *286*, 241–246. [CrossRef]
24. Davis, A.M.; Wright, J.G.; Williams, J.I.; Bombardier, C.; Griffin, A.; Bell, R.S. Development of a measure of physical function for patients with bone and soft tissue sarcoma. *Qual. Life Res.* **1996**, *5*, 508–516. [CrossRef] [PubMed]
25. Reijers, S.J.; Husson, O.; Soomers, V.L.; Been, L.B.; Bonenkamp, J.J.; van de Sande, M.A.; Verhoef, C.; van der Graaf, W.T.; van Houdt, W.J. Health-related quality of life after isolated limb perfusion compared to extended resection, or amputation for locally advanced extremity sarcoma: Is a limb salvage strategy worth the effort? *Eur. J. Surg. Oncol.* **2022**, *48*, 500–507. [CrossRef] [PubMed]
26. Saebye, C.; Fugloe, H.M.; Nymark, T.; Safwat, A.; Petersen, M.M.; Baad-Hansen, T.; Krarup-Hansen, A.; Keller, J. Factors associated with reduced functional outcome and quality of life in patients having limb-sparing surgery for soft tissue sarcomas—A national multicenter study of 128 patients. *Acta Oncol.* **2017**, *56*, 239–244. [CrossRef] [PubMed]
27. Varni, J.W.; Burwinkle, T.M.; Katz, E.R.; Meeske, K.; Dickinson, P. The PedsQL in pediatric cancer: Reliability and validity of the Pediatric Quality of Life Inventory Generic Core Scales, Multidimensional Fatigue Scale, and Cancer Module. *Cancer* **2002**, *94*, 2090–2106. [CrossRef] [PubMed]

28. Söntgerath, R.; Däggelmann, J.; Kesting, S.V.; Rueegg, C.S.; Wittke, T.-C.; Reich, S.; Eckert, K.G.; Stoessel, S.; Chamorro-Viña, C.; Wiskemann, J.; et al. Physical and functional performance assessment in pediatric oncology: A systematic review. *Pediatr. Res.* **2021**, *91*, 743–756. [CrossRef] [PubMed]
29. Baker, R.; McGinley, J.L.; Schwartz, M.H.; Beynon, S.; Rozumalski, A.; Graham, H.K.; Tirosh, O. The gait profile score and movement analysis profile. *Gait Posture* **2009**, *30*, 265–269. [CrossRef]
30. Schwartz, M.H.; Rozumalski, A. The Gait Deviation Index: A new comprehensive index of gait pathology. *Gait Posture* **2008**, *28*, 351–357. [CrossRef]
31. Kim, S.; Ryu, C.; Jung, S.-T. Differences in Kinematic and Kinetic Patterns According to the Bone Tumor Location after Endoprosthetic Knee Replacement Following Bone Tumor Resection: A Comparative Gait Analysis between Distal Femur and Proximal Tibia. *J. Clin. Med.* **2021**, *10*, 4100. [CrossRef] [PubMed]
32. Rompen, J.C.; Ham, S.J.; Halbertsma, J.P.K.; van Horn, J.R. Gait and function in patients with a femoral endoprosthesis after tumor resection: 18 patients evaluated 12 years after surgery. *Acta Orthop. Scand.* **2002**, *73*, 439–446. [CrossRef]
33. Winter, C.; Müller, C.; Brandes, M.; Brinkmann, A.; Hoffmann, C.; Hardes, J.; Gosheger, G.; Boos, J.; Rosenbaum, D. Level of activity in children undergoing cancer treatment. *Pediatr. Blood Cancer* **2009**, *53*, 438–443. [CrossRef]
34. Bamdad, K.; Hudson, S.; Briggs, T. Factors associated with functional outcome in patients having limb salvage surgery for primary malignant bone sarcoma using TESS. *J. Clin. Orthop. Trauma* **2019**, *10*, 986–990. [CrossRef] [PubMed]
35. Heaver, C.; Isaacson, A.; Gregory, J.J.; Cribb, G.; Cool, P. Patient factors affecting the Toronto extremity salvage score following limb salvage surgery for bone and soft tissue tumors. *J. Surg. Oncol.* **2016**, *113*, 804–810. [CrossRef]
36. Bisschop, C.N.S.; Courneya, K.S.; Velthuis, M.J.; Monninkhof, E.M.; Jones, L.W.; Friedenreich, C.; van der Wall, E.; Peeters, P.H.M.; May, A.M. Control group design, contamination and drop-out in exercise oncology trials: A systematic review. *PLoS ONE* **2015**, *10*, e0120996. [CrossRef]
37. Wilson, P.J.; Steadman, P.; Beckman, E.M.; Connick, M.J.; Carty, C.P.; Tweedy, S.M. Fitness, Function, and Exercise Training Responses after Limb Salvage with a Lower Limb Megaprosthesis: A Systematic Review. *PM&R* **2019**, *11*, 533–547. [CrossRef]
38. Van Egmond-van Dam, J.C.; Bekkering, W.P.; Bramer, J.A.M.; Beishuizen, A.; Fiocco, M.; Dijkstra, P.D.S. Functional outcome after surgery in patients with bone sarcoma around the knee; results from a long-term prospective study. *J. Surg. Oncol.* **2017**, *115*, 1028–1032. [CrossRef] [PubMed]
39. Wurz, A.; McLaughlin, E.; Lategan, C.; Viña, C.C.; Grimshaw, S.L.; Hamari, L.; Götte, M.; Kesting, S.; Rossi, F.; van der Torre, P.; et al. The international Pediatric Oncology Exercise Guidelines (iPOEG). *Transl. Behav. Med. Soc. Behav. Med.* **2021**, *11*, 1915–1922. [CrossRef]
40. Götte, M.; Gauß, G.; Dirksen, U.; Driever, P.H.; Basu, O.; Baumann, F.T.; Wiskemann, J.; Boos, J.; Kesting, S.V. Multidisciplinary Network ActiveOncoKids guidelines for providing movement and exercise in pediatric oncology—Consensus-based recommendations. *Pediatr. Blood Cancer* **2022**, *69*, e29953. [CrossRef] [PubMed]

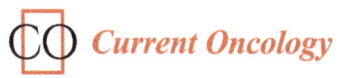 *Current Oncology*

Review

The Impact of Exercise on Cardiotoxicity in Pediatric and Adolescent Cancer Survivors: A Scoping Review

Stephanie J. Kendall [1,2], Jodi E. Langley [2,3], Mohsen Aghdam [1,2], Bruce N. Crooks [2,4], Nicholas Giacomantonio [5], Stefan Heinze-Milne [2,6], Will J. Johnston [1,2], Melanie R. Keats [1,2,7], Sharon L. Mulvagh [5] and Scott A. Grandy [1,2,5,6,7,*]

1 School of Health and Human Performance, Dalhousie University, Halifax, NS B3H4R2, Canada
2 Beatrice Hunter Cancer Research Institute, Halifax, NS B3H4R2, Canada
3 Faculty of Health, Dalhousie University, Halifax, NS B3H4R2, Canada
4 Department of Pediatrics, IWK Health, Halifax, NS B3K6R8, Canada
5 Department of Medicine, Division of Cardiology, Nova Scotia Health, Halifax, NS B3H3A7, Canada
6 Department of Pharmacology, Dalhousie University, Halifax, NS B3H4R2, Canada
7 Department of Medicine, Division of Medical Oncology, Nova Scotia Health, Halifax, NS B3H4R2, Canada
* Correspondence: scott.grandy@dal.ca

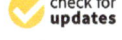

Citation: Kendall, S.J.; Langley, J.E.; Aghdam, M.; Crooks, B.N.; Giacomantonio, N.; Heinze-Milne, S.; Johnston, W.J.; Keats, M.R.; Mulvagh, S.L.; Grandy, S.A. The Impact of Exercise on Cardiotoxicity in Pediatric and Adolescent Cancer Survivors: A Scoping Review. *Curr. Oncol.* **2022**, *29*, 6350–6363. https://doi.org/10.3390/curroncol29090500

Received: 25 July 2022
Accepted: 22 August 2022
Published: 3 September 2022

Publisher's Note: MDPI stays neutral with regard to jurisdictional claims in published maps and institutional affiliations.

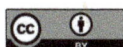

Copyright: © 2022 by the authors. Licensee MDPI, Basel, Switzerland. This article is an open access article distributed under the terms and conditions of the Creative Commons Attribution (CC BY) license (https:// creativecommons.org/licenses/by/ 4.0/).

Abstract: Childhood and adolescent cancer survivors are disproportionately more likely to develop cardiovascular diseases from the late effects of cardiotoxic therapies (e.g., anthracycline-based chemotherapy and chest-directed radiotherapy). Currently, dexrazoxane is the only approved drug for preventing cancer treatment-related cardiac damage. While animal models highlight the beneficial effects of exercise cancer treatment-related cardiac dysfunction, few clinical studies have been conducted. Thus, the objective of this scoping review was to explore the designs and impact of exercise-based interventions for managing cancer treatment-related cardiac dysfunction in childhood and adolescent cancer survivors. Reviewers used Joanna Briggs Institute's methodology to identify relevant literature. Then, 4616 studies were screened, and three reviewers extracted relevant data from six reports. Reviewers found that exercise interventions to prevent cancer treatment-related cardiac dysfunction in childhood and adolescent cancer survivors vary regarding frequency, intensity, time, and type of exercise intervention. Further, the review suggests that exercise promotes positive effects on managing cancer treatment-related cardiac dysfunction across numerous indices of heart health. However, the few clinical studies employing exercise interventions for childhood and adolescent cancer survivors highlight the necessity for more research in this area.

Keywords: exercise; cardiotoxicity; cancer; cancer survivor; pediatric; adolescent

1. Introduction

Antineoplastics are increasingly effective at treating malignancies and minimizing damage to healthy tissues [1]. However, many standard cancer treatments exhibit cardiotoxic effects leading to the development of late or acute cardiovascular complications. Chest-directed radiotherapy and anthracycline treatments are of particular concern as they can cause severe cardiac complications [2–8]. The risk of cancer treatment-related cardiac dysfunction (CTRCD) is related to the dose of cardiotoxic treatment received, and specific populations are at a higher risk.

Childhood and adolescent cancer survivors (CACS) have a remarkably elevated risk of developing CTRCD. The incidence of CTRCD is widely reported in CACS [2,7,8] such that they are two times more likely to develop cardiac abnormalities and have an 11-fold higher cardiovascular disease-related mortality risk than their healthy siblings [9]. Cardiac-related diseases are also the leading cause of non-malignant deaths in CACS [4], likely because CACS often live long into remission, allowing the latent effects of their cancer treatments to manifest. CACS commonly develop left ventricular (LV) systolic dysfunction, heart failure, myocarditis, pericarditis and arrhythmias [2–8]. Such effects can develop acutely, but often do not develop until many years into survivorship [2]. Thus, the high incidence and severity of CTRCD in CACS emphasizes the need to mitigate and manage cases.

Currently, CTRCD prevention methods focus on minimizing radiation exposure and cumulative anthracycline dose. Strategies also include liposomal encapsulated anthracyclines delivery [10] and improvements in radiation therapy that exhibit reduced cardiotoxic properties while maintaining high antineoplastic effects [11]. Unfortunately, these strategies do not apply to all cases [11] and do not fully mitigate CTRCD risk [10]. Dexrazoxane is the only widely used pharmaceutical for preventing anthracycline-induced CTRCD [3,12]. Unfortunately, dexrazoxane's effectiveness is not established in preventing radiation-induced damage as its effects have only been explored in animal models [13], it must be administered concurrently with anthracycline treatment [14], and it may exhibit chronic side effects such as decreased fertility [14]. Other pharmaceuticals, such as conventional heart medications like beta-blockers, statins, and renin-angiotensin-aldosterone system blockades, can be administered upon detecting asymptomatic LV dysfunction to prevent further development of symptomatic heart failure disease [15]. However, conventional heart medications are often not administered timely as routine cardiac imaging is uncommon in CACS and frequently fails to detect asymptomatic LV dysfunction. Consequently, conventional heart medications are often not prescribed until symptomatic, irreversible dysfunction occurs. The severity and high prevalence of CTRCD in CACS and the limitations of the few pharmaceutical treatment options based on symptoms highlights the need for alternative prevention and treatment strategies.

Exercise is a potential solution to mitigate CTRCD. Exercise decreases cardiovascular risk factors, improves cardiovascular fitness, decreases cardiac inflammation, prevents oxidative stress, and preserves cardiac structure and function at the pathophysiological level in animal models [9,16–21]. Notably, the cardiovascular-related benefits of exercise are evident from even light-intensity and voluntary exercise pre-, during, and post-cardiotoxic treatment in mice models [20]. Further, in adult breast cancer survivors, exercise is shown to decrease CTRCD as indicated by significant improvements in aerobic capacity [22–27], cardiac biomarker levels [28,29], strain [23,29], and resting heart rate [22,23,30]. Despite the plethora of evidence in preclinical animal models and adult breast cancer survivors, there is minimal research on other cancer populations, including CACS [10]. While observational studies indicate that low physical activity levels are associated with an increased incidence of cardiac dysfunction in CACS [31,32], few interventional exercise trials have been conducted.

Before conducting future research, it is necessary to understand the extent of the current clinical studies investigating the impact of exercise on CTRCD in CACS. Therefore, the purpose of this review was to summarize the literature regarding exercise interventions aimed at mitigating CTRCD in CACS. Specifically, this review explored the breadth of exercise interventions available to manage CTRCD in at-risk CACS and how the FITT (frequency, intensity, time, and type of exercise) principle is applied to exercise interventions for CACS to manage CTRCD. The review describes the outcomes of the exercise interventions on cardiac health among CACS.

2. Materials and Methods

This review was conducted per Joanna Briggs Institute (JBI) methodology for scoping reviews [33]. There was no patient or public involvement in this research's design, conduct, reporting, or dissemination plans. A full protocol paper was submitted for publication prior to completing the review [34]. The protocol is summarized below.

2.1. Search Strategy

The first author (SJK) developed the search strategy with guidance from a JBI-trained researcher (JEL) and a JBI-trained librarian. This strategy aimed to locate published empirical studies and grey literature. The entire search strategy can be found in Table A1

(Appendix A). The search strategy aimed to identify published primary studies and reviews as well as text and opinion papers.

2.2. Inclusion and Exclusion Criteria

This review included studies whose participants were CACS diagnosed at 19 years of age or younger and received anthracycline treatment and/ or chest-directed radiation therapy. Studies were required to include an exercise intervention aimed at decreasing cardiovascular disease in CACS and needed to employ a measure of cardiac surveillance at a minimum of two different time points. Studies without an exercise intervention (i.e., physical activity recall studies) were excluded.

2.3. Information Sources

The databases searched included MEDLINE, the Cumulative Index to Nursing and Allied Health Literature (CINAHL), Embase, Scopus, PsychINFO and SportDiscus. Sources of unpublished studies and grey literature were searched using the first ten pages of Google Scholar, ProQuest Dissertations, and organizational, governmental and health care association websites, including Children's Oncology Group, PanCare, Canadian Cancer Society, American Cancer Society, National Cancer Society, Cancer Research UK, and National Health Institute (Appendix B).

2.4. Study Selection

Following the search, all identified records were collected and uploaded into Covidence [35], a citation management platform and duplicates were removed. A team of four reviewers (S.J.K., J.E.L., M.A., W.J.J.) screened all titles and abstracts against the inclusion criteria. Potentially relevant papers were retrieved in total, and their full- papers were imported into Covidence. Next, the same four reviews (S.J.K., J.E.L., M.A., W.J.J.) assessed the full text of the selected citations in detail against the inclusion criteria. Reasons for exclusion of full-text articles were recorded and reported. Any disagreements were discussed between two reviewers (S.J.K. & J.E.L.).

2.5. Data Extraction

Data were extracted by a team of 3 extractors (S.J.K., J.E.L., M.A.) with at least two extractors per paper. The extraction tool was initially piloted in five studies, in which any additional aspects were discussed to retrieve from the sources. A complete extraction tool is in Appendix C.

2.6. Data Synthesis and Analysis

All data were combined to provide a complete dataset for analysis and cleaned by one reviewer (S.J.K.). The results were presented to all authors and were discussed regarding the implications.

3. Results

3.1. Study Selection

The reviewers identified 6510 records from the database search. 301, 729, 3866, 132, 160 and 611 reports were found on CINAHL, Medline, Embase, SportDiscus, PsycInfo and Scopus, respectively. All records were loaded into the review management website, Covidence. From the database search, Covidence removed 1891 duplicates, leaving 4616 articles. Two reviewers screened the title and abstract of the 4616 articles against the inclusion and exclusion criteria. Upon completion, the full text of 230 articles was assessed for eligibility, and an exclusion reason was provided for each excluded article. Reviewers identified that 64 reports focused on cardiopulmonary fitness testing, 65 did not have an exercise intervention, 28 were secondary sources, 25 did not focus on cardiotoxicity, ten did not have enough information to extract, nine were measurement validation studies, eight did not have an English full-text version, seven focused on adult cancer survivors, three focused on pharmacological treatments, three were duplicates, two assessed non-human subjects, and one did not assess cancer patients. Thus, six reports were included in the review from the database search. However, two separate papers were written based on the same study cohort and merged during the analysis [36,37]; thus, this review includes five exercise interventions.

Additionally, 80 articles were identified through other search methods, including the grey literature and citation search. A single reviewer screened these articles following the above steps. The reviewer identified that nine reports focused on cardiopulmonary fitness testing, 18 did not have an exercise intervention, five were secondary sources, 32 did not focus on cardiotoxicity, 13 focused on adult cancer survivors, and two did not assess cancer patients. Thus, one record was included in the review through the other search methods. See Figure 1 for the PRISMA flow chart detailing the number of records found at each review stage.

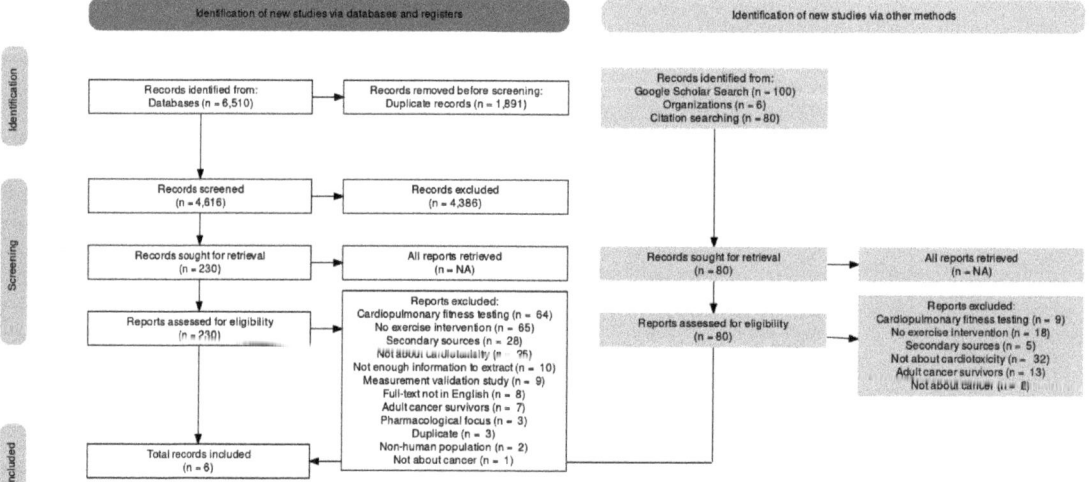

Figure 1. PRISMA flow diagram of included studies.

3.2. Characteristics of Included Studies

Studies were published over 30 years, from 1993 to 2020. Studies were completed in the United States (n = 2), Finland (n = 1), Australia (n = 1), and Spain (n =1). Additionally, the study designs varied and included case series (n = 2), cohort (n = 2), and case-control (n = 1) reports.

Study characteristics are included in Table 1.

3.3. Patient Characteristics of the Included Studies

Morales et al., 2020 was the only study that compared a control group of non-exercising CACS with an intervention group of exercising CACS and conducted a long-term follow-up [41]. The reports from Järvelä et al., 2013 and 2016 included a group of healthy controls to provide a baseline comparison with an exercising group of CACS, but the healthy controls were only assessed at baseline [36,37]. There was no control group in the other three studies [40,42,43].

Patient characteristics varied in the studies included in this review regarding treatment, time since diagnosis, and cancer type. In two studies, all participants were treated with anthracyclines and/ or chest-directed radiation treatment, and in the remaining three studies, most participants were treated with anthracyclines and/or radiation [40,41,43]). All study cohorts analyzed CACS, and various cancer types were included across the study cohorts. Four studies focused on survivors, and one on CACS currently undergoing treatment [41]. Finally, each study included a similar number of males and females, except the Morales et al., 2020 study, whose study sample included more males (n = 124) than females (n = 65) [41].

Table 1. Characteristics of included studies.

Study Identification	Title	Country	Design	Aim	Criteria
Järvelä 2013 [37] & 2016 [36]. Methodologies as cited in [38].	Endothelial function in long-term survivors of childhood ALL: Effects of a home-based exercise program [37]; Home-based exercise training improves LV diastolic function in survivors of childhood ALL: A tissue doppler and velocity vector imaging study [36].	Finland	Case-control study	Assess the effects of a home-based exercise intervention on endothelial structure in survivors of childhood ALL [37]; Determine the effects of an exercise program on anthracycline-induced cardiotoxicity as assessed by tissue doppler imaging and velocity vector imaging in long-term childhood ALL survivors [36].	Age < 16 years at diagnosis, currently age 16–30 years, first continuous remission without hematopoietic bone marrow transplantation, diagnosed in 1986 or later, treated according to the Nordic regimen [39], and no down syndrome diagnosis.
Long 2018 [40]	Exercise training improves vascular function and secondary health measures in survivors of pediatric oncology related cerebral insult.	Australia	Cohort study	Assess the feasibility and effectiveness of a 24-week exercise intervention on cardiovascular health in childhood cancer survivors.	>5-year survivor of pediatric cancer-related cerebral insult, currently aged 15–23, not pregnant and without a current cardiovascular disease diagnosis.
Morales 2020 [41]	Inhospital exercise benefits in childhood cancer: A prospective cohort study.	Spain	Cohort study	Assess the effects of aerobic and resistance training in children with leukemia receiving neoadjuvant or intensive chemotherapy.	Currently aged 4–18 years, received a new cancer diagnosis, diagnosed, treated, and followed at the Hospital Infantil Universitario Nino Jesus, and not currently participating in any other interventional trials.
Sharkey 1993 [42]	Cardiac rehabilitation after cancer therapy in children and young adults.	United States	Case series	Assess childhood cancer survivors using exercise testing before and after a 12-week aerobic exercise program.	Received >100 mg/m^2 of anthracyclines, post-pubertal, ≥1-year post-treatment, and no residual malignancies.
Smith 2013 [43]	Exercise training in childhood cancer survivors with subclinical cardiomyopathy who were treated with anthracyclines.	United States	Case series	Assess the effects of a 12-week exercise program on anthracycline-treated childhood cancer survivors with subclinical cardiomyopathy.	18 years of age, ≥10 years post-diagnosis of childhood cancer, treated with doxorubicin and/or daunorubicin, sedentary (<150 min of moderate-intensity physical activity per week), LVEF ≥ 40 and ≤55%, and not receiving cardiomyopathy treatment or received radiation therapy.

Abbreviations: ALL, acute lymphoblastic leukemia; LV, left ventricle; LVEF, left ventricle ejection fraction; mg/m^2, milligrams per meter squared.

Study patient characteristics are summarized in Table 2.

Table 2. Cancer participant characteristics.

Study ID	Group	Participants (Number)	Anthracyclines Dosage (mg/m^2)	Radiation Field (Gy)	Age (Years)	Time Since Diagnosis (Years)	Cancer Type
Järvelä 2013 & 2016 [36,37]	N/A	M=10 F=11	n = 21 (Med = 240, range: 120–370)	n = 5 (unspecified dosage)	Med = 21.1 (range: 16.0–28.4)	Med = 15.9 (range: 11.3–21.4)	ALL
Long 2018 [40]	N/A	M=6 F=7	n = 4 (unspecified dosage)	n = 8 (unspecified dosage)	Med = 19 (range: 16–23)	Med = 15 (range: 7–22)	Brain = 9, ALL = 3, Other = 1
Morales 2020 [41]	Controls	M=63 F=38	n = 41 (unspecified dosage)	n = 30, (range: 1–≥50)	mean = 11 (range: 4–18)	On treatment	15 various types
Morales 2020 [41]	Exercise	M=61 F=27	n = 27 (unspecified dosage)	n = 27 (range: 1–≥50)	mean = 11 (range: 4–17)	On treatment	15 various types
Sharkey 1993 [42]	N/A	M=5 F=5	n = 10 (mean = 349 ± 69)	n = 9 (range: 18–55)	mean = 19+/−3	mean = 11 (range: 4–18)	5 various types
Smith 2013 [43]	N/A	M=3 F=2	n = 4 (range: 5, 298)	n = 0	Range: 33–41	Range: 25–30	Osteosarcoma = 4, Ewing sarcoma = 1

Abbreviations: N/A, not applicable; M, male; F, female; Med, median; mg/m^2, milligrams per meter squared; Gy, Gray; ALL, acute lymphoblastic leukemia; mean.

3.4. Exercise Intervention Characteristics of the Included Studies

All reviewed exercise interventions included resistance and aerobic exercise training [36,37,40,41,43], except Sharkey et al., 1993, which only included aerobic training [42]. The frequency of exercise in the reviewed studies varied from two to five sessions per week, with most studies asking participants to complete three exercise sessions per week but would allow for two sessions when necessary. For studies including a resistance training component, exercise intensity and time widely varied. However, aerobic training was generally 30 to 45 min of moderate to vigorous-intensity aerobic training, except for Long et al., 2018, which was shorter in duration [40]. Exercise interventions were based out of the participant's home [36,37], the hospital [41], or both [42]. Long et al., 2018 did not state the setting of the exercise intervention [40].

Study exercise intervention characteristics are summarized in Table 3.

The studies used a variety of techniques to determine CACS' heart health. Measurements included echocardiography to assess left ventricular ejection fraction (LVEF) [36,41,43] and tissue doppler imaging to measure mitral annulus valve velocity [36]. Other measurements included velocity vector imaging to assess strain [36], echocardiography using M-mode to assess fractional shortening [36,41], and cardiopulmonary exercise-based testing using a re-breathing technique to estimate cardiac index, defined as the cardiac output divided by body surface area [44], and stroke volume from cardiac output [42].

Three studies investigated the direct impact of the exercise intervention on LV function [36,41,43]. Of these three, only Morales et al., 2020 investigated the impacts of exercise on heart health during treatment in CACS and included a long-term follow-up of the patients [41]. The results of this study indicated that there was not a significant decline in LVEF or fractional shortening in CACS who exercised, while CACS who did not exercise saw a significant decline in LVEF ($p < 0.001$) and fractional shortening ($p < 0.001$). However, LVEF and fractional shortening decreased in CACS who exercised at the 1-year follow-up and after. Similarly, Smith et al., 2013 observed that LVEF markedly improved in all five participants upon completing an exercise intervention (median ΔLVEF = 38.2%, range: 7.6 to 56.9) [43]. In contrast, Järvelä et al., 2016 found that LVEF was not affected by the exercise intervention ($p = 0.82$) [36]. Although, other measures of LV function in this study were affected, including early diastolic mitral inflow velocity ($p < 0.01$) and early diastolic mitral annulus velocity ($p < 0.01$), indicating that the exercise intervention improved LV function.

Table 3. Exercise intervention characteristics for childhood cancer survivors.

Study ID	Mode	Frequency (Sessions/Week)	Intensity	Time (min)	Type	Location	Duration (Weeks)	Instructor
Järvelä 2013 & 2016 [36,37]. Exercise protocol as cited in [38]	Resistance	3–4	3 sets, as many repetitions as possible, no rest stated.	Not stated	Eight exercises to strengthen the gluteal, lower limb, shoulders, upper limb, abdominal, and back muscles.	Home	12	Experts in sports science
	Aerobic	At least 3	Not specified	30	Participant choice (i.e., walking or jogging).			
Long 2018 [40]	Resistance	2 to 3	3 sets, 10 repetitions, 60–70% 3-RM, with 3 to 5 min of rest between exercises.	75–80	Circuit including 6 to 10 exercises targeting the chest, back, shoulders, arms, and legs.	Not stated	24	Exercise physiologist
	Aerobic	2 to 3	40–60% HRmax with individualized progressive increase.	10–15	Three sets of 4 consecutive sprint-rest bouts, with 3 to 5 min of rest between each set. Rowing ergometer, stationary bike, or arm ergometer.			
Morales 2020 [41]	Resistance	2 to 3	1 to 3 sets of 6–15 repetitions, 5% to 10% load increases as needed with 1 min rest between sets.	30	Shoulder, chest and leg press, side-arm rowing extension and flexion, knee extension and flexion and abdominal, lumbar and shoulder adduction.	Hospital	Med duration 22 weeks (IQR: 14, 28)	Exercise physiologist
	Aerobic	2 to 3	65–80% HRreserve with individualized progressive increase.	30–40	Ten minutes each of cycle ergometer leg pedalling, treadmill running, or arm cranking in those missing a lower limb. Ten minutes of aerobic games.			
Sharkey 1993 [42]	Aerobic	Two sessions for weeks 1–6 and 3 sessions for weeks 7–12.	60% to 80% HRmax progressive increase.	45–60	Not stated	Hospital and home	12	Not stated
Smith 2013 [43]	Resistance	3–5	1 set of 12–15 repetitions on 8 to 10 exercises.	Not stated	Not stated	Home	12	Exercise physiologist
	Aerobic	2–3	40–70% HRreserve.	20–45	Not stated			

Abbreviations: min, minutes; Min, minimum; Max, maximum; RM repetitions maximum; reps, repetitions; HR, heart rate; HRR, heart rate reserve; Med, median; IQR, interquartile range.

3.5 Key findings of the included studies relating to heart health.

Sharkey et al., 1993 investigated the impact of the exercise intervention on heart health using cardiac index and stroke volume [42]. This study indicated that the exercise intervention did not significantly change cardiac or stroke volume indices. A summary of the findings related to heart health is presented in Table 4

Table 4. Key cardiovascular health-related findings.

Study ID	LVEF	Valve Velocity	Strain	FS	CI	SV
Järvelä 2013 & 2016 [36,37]	☒	✓↑	✓↑	☒	N/A	N/A
Long 2020 [40]	N/A	N/A	N/A	N/A	N/A	N/A
Morales 2020 [41]	✓↑	N/A	N/A	✓↑	N/A	N/A
Sharkey 1993 [42]	N/A	N/A	N/A	N/A	☒	☒
Smith 2013 [43]	✓↑	N/A	N/A	N/A	N/A	N/A

Abbreviations: ☒, insignificant change; ↑, improvement ✓, significant change; LVEF, left ventricle ejection fraction; FS, fractional shortening; CI, cardiac index; SV, stroke volume; N/A, not applicable.

3.5. Key Findings of the Included Studies Relating to Peripheral Cardiovascular Health

The studies also used various techniques to assess CACS' peripheral cardiovascular health. Measurements included echocardiography for the left common carotid artery intima-media thickness [37], ultrasound to determine flow-mediated dilation of the left brachial artery [37,40], and a cardiopulmonary exercise test to determine peak oxygen pulse [42].

Three studies investigated the impact of the exercise intervention on peripheral cardiovascular health [37,40,43]. Järvelä et al. found that in survivors, the intima-media thickness significantly decreased ($p = 0.02$), and the flow-mediated dilation 40-s time point ($p = 0.01$) increased after the exercise intervention, although the specific flow-mediated dilation values were not reported [37]. Similarly, Long et al. found that in survivors, flow-mediated dilation ($p = 0.008$) significantly increased after the exercise intervention and the change in time to peak brachial diameter ($p = 0.031$) significantly decreased [40]. Smith et al. observed that peak oxygen pulse, defined as peak oxygen consumption divided by the corresponding heart rate, markedly improved in all five of their participants upon completing an exercise intervention (median Δ oxygen pulse = 25.8%, range: 6.3 to 58.6) points [43]. A summary of the findings related to peripheral heart health is presented in Table 5.

Table 5. Key periphery cardiovascular health findings.

Study ID	IMT	FMD	Oxygen Pulse
Järvelä 2013 & 2016 [36,37]	✓↓	✓↑	N/A
Long 2020 [40]	N/A	✓↑	N/A
Morales 2020 [41]	N/A	N/A	N/A
Sharkey 1993 [42]	N/A	N/A	N/A
Smith 2013 [43]	N/A	N/A	✓↑

Abbreviations: ✓, significant change IMT, intima-media thickness; FMD, flow-mediated dilation; NA, not applicable; ↑, increased; ↓, decreased.

4. Discussion

This is the first scoping review exploring the impact of exercise interventions on the development of CTRCD in CACS. The review identified five published studies (six reports) that met this review's inclusion and exclusion criteria. Within these studies, exercise interventions and their impact on CTRCD varied. In brief, exercise interventions included only aerobic [42] or a combination of aerobic and resistance training [36,37,40,41,43]. Most studies (4/5 = 80%) reported positive findings suggesting that exercise may help manage CTRCD in CACS [36,37,40,41,43].

4.1. Impact of Reviewed Exercise Interventions

The impact of exercise on CTRCD were assessed using various measurements across the five studies. All studies but Sharkey et al. [42] found that exercise significantly improved heart [36,41,43] and periphery cardiovascular health [36,40,43]. Such findings align with the current literature on healthy children. A recent interim report from the Cardiovascular Risk in Young Finns Study from 1994 to 2011 indicates that high amounts of physical activity are associated with improved left ventricular function in adulthood, as indicated by echocardiographic measurements [45]. Furthermore, Unnithan et al., 2018 found that child soccer players have significantly greater left ventricular end-diastolic volume than infrequently active controls [46].

Additionally, the findings align with the current literature on adults with cancer. Kirkham et al., 2018 found that a multi-modal exercise intervention administered during adjuvant chemotherapy treatment in early-stage breast cancer patients mitigated CTRCD, specifically exercise prevented increases in resting heart rate, hypotension, tachycardia, and impaired heart rate recovery [30]. Such findings indicate that exercise can prevent cardiac dysfunction by initiating physiological adaptations, including increased cardiac fibre contractility, leading to enhanced cardiac output and a healthier heart [47]. However, in CACS, the benefits of exercise regarding CTRCD are not entirely understood and exhibit inconsistencies. For example, Järvelä et al., 2016 indicated that exercise does not improve LVEF or fractional shortening in CACS [36], while Morales et al., 2020 indicated that exercise significantly maintains LVEF and fractional shortening [41].

Despite the current guidelines from the Children's Oncology Group recommending frequent echocardiograms and cardiovascular monitoring of CACS [48], such intensive screening protocols are challenging to implement because of limited access to cardio-oncology services, infrastructure, interest, and educational opportunities [49]. Moreover, many survivors remain in primary care and do not have access to dedicated survivorship clinics or services. Furthermore, cardiac surveillance measures, such as LVEF, often do not indicate damage until significant and irreversible maladaptation occurs [15,50,51]. Thus, CACS may develop extensive CTRCD before the damage is detected. Additionally, cardiac imaging may not be sensitive enough to detect the positive effects of an exercise intervention on cardiac health in CACS. More in-depth cardiac profiling using biomarkers, such as high sensitivity troponin and natriuretic peptides, combined with cardiac imaging, as proposed by Cardinale et al., may better detect CTRCD and possibly exercise-induced cardiac adaptations [50].

4.2. Exercise Intervention Designs of Reviewed Studies

In this review, exercise intervention designs consisted of aerobic and resistance training, but the specifics of the exercise prescription varied. Most reports investigated CACS four to 30 years after receiving their diagnosis [36,37,40,42,43], while Morales et al., 2020 investigated children receiving treatment [41].

As many exercise guidelines for cancer survivors exist, it is worthwhile to contrast them with the studies reviewed here. The Järvelä 2013 & 2016 [36,37], and Smith et al., 2013 [43] reports aligned with the American College of Sports Medicine Guidelines suggesting that adult cancer survivors complete moderate to vigorous-intensity aerobic training for 75 to 150 min, and resistance training 2 to 3 times, per week [52]. Sharkey et al., 1993 [42] and Long et al.'s, 2018 [40] exercise intervention did not meet the American College of Sports Medicine exercise guidelines. However, Long et al.'s exercise intervention still demonstrated improved brachial artery flow-mediated dilation [40], suggesting the exercise intervention mitigated some CTRCD risk. Furthermore, the Morales et al., 2020 [41] report aligned with the pediatric oncology exercise guidelines that aerobic training should be completed 2 to 5 times per week at a moderate to vigorous intensity for 20 to 70 min and resistance training should be completed 2 to 3 times per week at a high intensity for 20 to 30 min [53]. None of the reviewed studies met the current guidelines for CACS exposed to cardiotoxic treatments. These guidelines indicate that adults should complete 2.5 h per week and children should complete one hour per day of aerobic exercise, and all CACS should also perform strength training twice per week. However, all reviewed reports demonstrated some benefits of exercise in mitigating CTRCD risk, except Sharkey et al., 1993 [42], suggesting that any exercise can mitigate CTRCD. CACS should be encouraged to exercise even if they cannot meet the guidelines and will still reap cardioprotective benefits.

4.3. Limitations

A drawback of this scoping review was that three of the five [40,41,43] reviewed studies did not meet the review's full inclusion and exclusion criteria, which required all participants to have received anthracycline and/or radiation therapy. The reviewers opted to include these three studies as the nature of the review was to map out the literature, and these studies met all other inclusion and exclusion criteria. Further, the few studies to review indicate the importance of more clinical research in this area.

Another limitation of this review was the different methods of the included studies. While most studies indicated that the exercise intervention improved cardiac outcomes, nine measures were used to assess cardiac health across the five included studies. Cardiac surveillance methods of the reviewed studies included measures such as LVEF [36,41,43], strain [36] and fractional shortening [36,41]. Additionally, the reviewed studies used a variety of measures regarding peripheral cardiovascular health, such as brachial artery intima-media thickness [37] and flow-mediated dilation [37,40]. Thus, evaluating the efficacy of the exercise interventions to prevent CTRCD was challenging as no standardized measurements were used.

Furthermore, the reviewed studies included a wide variety of participants. The reviewed study dates occurred within a similar time frame, except Sharkey et al., 1993 [42], published nearly 30 years before Morales et al., 2020 [41]. Compared with 30 years ago, anthracyclines are used with more awareness of cardiotoxicity and better dose limitation, and advancements in radiotherapy techniques allow for decreased exposure of healthy tissues to radiation [11]. Similarly, the studies occurred in four different countries and assessed many different cancer types. As many treatment protocols are not internationally regulated and vary across cancer types, participant heterogeneity was high. Thus, comparing all studies was challenging, and these limitations should be considered when interpreting the results.

5. Conclusions

This review indicates that exercise may be a viable treatment to mitigate/manage CTRCD in CACS. Further, the included studies varied widely concerning exercise intervention design, suggesting that any amount and type of exercise could help manage CTRCD. Finally, very few exercise intervention studies monitoring cardiac health have been conducted in CACS, and thus, extensive clinical research is necessary to increase the homogeneity and applicability of findings.

Notably, the results of this review highlight the importance and benefits of exercise for CACS in preventing and managing the development of CTRCD. As the reviewed exercise interventions for CACS vary, CTRCD can be managed by various forms of physical activity and movement, and CACS should engage in exercise and become more physically active to mitigate CTRCD risk.

Author Contributions: Conceptualization, S.A.G., W.J.J., S.J.K., M.R.K. and J.E.L.; methodology, J.E.L.; investigation, M.A., S.H.-M., W.J.J., S.J.K. and J.E.L.; writing—original draft preparation, S.J.K. and J.E.L.; writing—review and editing, M.A., B.N.C., N.G., S.A.G., S.H.-M., W.J.J., M.R.K., S.J.K., J.E.L., S.L.M. and S.A.G.; supervision, S.A.G. All authors have read and agreed to the published version of the manuscript.

Funding: This paper was not funded. However, the following authors are students supported in their programs via the stated funders. Stephanie Kendall is a trainee in the Cancer Research Training Program of the Beatrice Hunter Cancer Research Institute, with funds provided by Saunders Matthey. Jodi Langley is supported by the Beatrice Hunter Cancer Research Institute, funding provided by the Canadian Cancer Society's Carol Ann Cole Graduate Studentship, and is a trainee in the Cancer Research Training Program. William Johnston is a trainee in the Cancer Research Training Program of the Beatrice Hunter Cancer Research Institute, with funds provided by CIBC.

Acknowledgments: Shelley McKibbon from Dalhousie University's W. K. Kellogg Health Sciences Library provided extensive knowledge and generous assistance with the search protocol.

Conflicts of Interest: The authors declare no conflict of interest.

Appendix A

Table A1. Search Strategy for database search.

1	(Cancer* OR Neoplas* OR Leukemia* OR Leukaemia* OR Tumor* OR Tumour* OR Lymphoma* OR Chemotherap* OR Malignanc* OR anthracycline* OR 'Antineoplastic Agent*' OR Immunotherap* OR 'Monoclonal Antibod*' OR 'Tyrosine Kinase Inhibitor*' OR Radiation OR Radiology)
2	Child* OR Adolescent* OR Teen* OR 'Young Adult*' OR 'Early Child*' OR Pediatric* OR Paediatric* OR Infant* OR Toddler* OR Bab* OR Juvenile* OR 'Pre Pubescent*'
3	1 AND 2
4	Exercise* OR 'Resistance Training*' OR Aerobic* OR 'Motor Activity' OR 'Exercise Therap*' OR 'Physical Activit*' OR Training OR 'Physical Fitness' OR Exertion OR Yoga OR Pilates OR 'Dance Therap*' OR 'Tai Ji' OR Qigong
5	Exp Exercise/
6	4 OR 5
7	3 AND 6
8	Myocarditis* OR 'Heart Failure' OR Cardiotoxic* or Cardiomyopath* OR Heart* OR 'Radiation Injury*'
9	7 AND 8

Appendix B

Grey Literature Check

Google Scholar

- Cancer AND Child AND Exercise AND Cardio*
- Cancer AND Pediatric AND Exercise AND Cardio*
- Cancer AND Child AND "Physical Activity" AND Cardio*

ProQuest

- cancer AND child AND exercise AND cardiotoxicity
- cancer AND pediatric AND exercise and cardiotoxicity
- cancer AND child AND 'Physical Activity' AND cardiotoxicity

Websites

- Canadian cancer society
- American Cancer Society
- Cancer Research UK
- National Health Institute
- American College of Sports Medicine
- Canadian Society for Exercise Physiologies
- Canadian Cardiology Society

Appendix C

Data Extraction Instrument

- Title
- Contact
- Year
- Country
- Aim
- Design
- Start date
- End date
- Inclusion criteria
- Exclusion criteria
- Method of recruitment
- Cancer type
- Cancer stage
- Time since diagnosis
- Control group details
- Age of participants
- Chemotherapy treatment
- Radiotherapy
- Exercise program
    - Setting
    - Frequency
    - Intensity
    - Time
    - Type
    - Duration
    - Location
    - Instructor
    - Adherence
- Measure of cardiac health
- Other outcome measures
- Results
- Key findings
- Limitations
- Implications

References

1. Arruebo, M.; Vilaboa, N.; Sáez-Gutierrez, B.; Lambea, J.; Tres, A.; Valladares, M.; González-Fernández, Á. Assessment of the Evolution of Cancer Treatment Therapies. *Cancers* **2011**, *3*, 3279–3330. [CrossRef] [PubMed]
2. Lipshultz, S.E.; Adams, M.J.; Colan, S.D.; Constine, L.S.; Herman, E.H.; Hsu, D.T.; Hudson, M.M.; Kremer, L.C.; Landy, D.C.; Miller, T.L.; et al. Long-Term Cardiovascular Toxicity in Children, Adolescents, and Young Adults Who Receive Cancer Therapy: Pathophysiology, Course, Monitoring, Management, Prevention, and Research Directions. *Circulation* **2013**, *128*, 1927–1995. [CrossRef] [PubMed]
3. Chow, E.J.; Leger, K.J.; Bhatt, N.S.; Mulrooney, D.A.; Ross, C.J.; Aggarwal, S.; Bansal, N.; Ehrhardt, M.J.; Armenian, S.H.; Scott, J.M.; et al. Paediatric Cardio-Oncology: Epidemiology, Screening, Prevention, and Treatment. *Cardiovasc. Res.* **2019**, *115*, 922–934. [CrossRef] [PubMed]
4. Armenian, S.H.; Armstrong, G.T.; Aune, G.; Chow, E.J.; Ehrhardt, M.J.; Ky, B.; Moslehi, J.; Mulrooney, D.A.; Nathan, P.C.; Ryan, T.D.; et al. Cardiovascular Disease in Survivors of Childhood Cancer: Insights Into Epidemiology, Pathophysiology, and Prevention. *J. Clin. Oncol.* **2018**, *36*, 2135–2144. [CrossRef]
5. Ryan, T.D.; Nagarajan, R.; Godown, J. Pediatric Cardio-Oncology: Development of Cancer Treatment-Related Cardiotoxicity and the Therapeutic Approach to Affected Patients. *Curr. Treat. Options Oncol.* **2019**, *20*, 56. [CrossRef]
6. Mulrooney, D.A.; Yeazel, M.W.; Kawashima, T.; Mertens, A.C.; Mitby, P.; Stovall, M.; Donaldson, S.S.; Green, D.M.; Sklar, C.A.; Robison, L.L.; et al. Cardiac Outcomes in a Cohort of Adult Survivors of Childhood and Adolescent Cancer: Retrospective Analysis of the Childhood Cancer Survivor Study Cohort. *BMJ* **2009**, *339*, b4606. [CrossRef]
7. Lipshultz, S.E.; Colan, S.D.; Gelber, R.D.; Perez-Atayde, A.R.; Sallan, S.E.; Sanders, S.P. Late Cardiac Effects of Doxorubicin Therapy for Acute Lymphoblastic Leukemia in Childhood. *N. Engl. J. Med.* **1991**, *324*, 808–815. [CrossRef]

8. Tan, C.; Tasaka, H.; Yu, K.-P.; Murphy, M.L.; Karnofsky, D.A. Daunomycin, an Antitumor Antibiotic, in the Treatment of Neoplastic Disease. Clinical Evaluation with Special Reference to Childhood Leukemia. *Cancer* **1967**, *20*, 333–353. [CrossRef]
9. Chao, C.; Xu, L.; Bhatia, S.; Cooper, R.; Brar, S.; Wong, F.L.; Armenian, S.H. Cardiovascular Disease Risk Profiles in Survivors of Adolescent and Young Adult (AYA) Cancer: The Kaiser Permanente AYA Cancer Survivors Study. *J. Clin. Oncol.* **2016**, *34*, 1626–1633. [CrossRef]
10. Kang, D.-W.; Wilson, R.L.; Christopher, C.N.; Normann, A.J.; Barnes, O.; Lesansee, J.D.; Choi, G.; Dieli-Conwright, C.M. Exercise Cardio-Oncology: Exercise as a Potential Therapeutic Modality in the Management of Anthracycline-Induced Cardiotoxicity. *Front. Cardiovasc. Med.* **2022**, *8*, 2194. [CrossRef]
11. Chow, E.J.; Antal, Z.; Constine, L.S.; Gardner, R.; Wallace, W.H.; Weil, B.R.; Yeh, J.M.; Fox, E. New Agents, Emerging Late Effects, and the Development of Precision Survivorship. *J. Clin. Oncol.* **2018**, *36*, 2231–2240. [CrossRef] [PubMed]
12. Kopp, L.M.; Womer, R.B.; Schwartz, C.L.; Ebb, D.H.; Franco, V.I.; Hall, D.; Barkauskas, D.A.; Krailo, M.D.; Grier, H.E.; Meyers, P.A.; et al. Effects of Dexrazoxane on Doxorubicin-Related Cardiotoxicity and Second Malignant Neoplasms in Children with Osteosarcoma: A Report from the Children's Oncology Group. *Cardio-Oncology* **2019**, *5*, 15. [CrossRef] [PubMed]
13. Li, L.; Nie, X.; Zhang, P.; Huang, Y.; Ma, L.; Li, F.; Yi, M.; Qin, W.; Yuan, X. Dexrazoxane Ameliorates Radiation-Induced Heart Disease in a Rat Model. *Aging* **2021**, *13*, 3699–3711. [CrossRef]
14. Eneh, C.; Lekkala, M.R. Dexrazoxane. In *StatPearls*; StatPearls Publishing: Treasure Island, FL, USA, 2022.
15. Saleh, Y.; Abdelkarim, O.; Herzallah, K.; Abela, G.S. Anthracycline-Induced Cardiotoxicity: Mechanisms of Action, Incidence, Risk Factors, Prevention, and Treatment. *Heart Fail. Rev.* **2021**, *26*, 1159–1173. [CrossRef] [PubMed]
16. Chicco, A.J.; Schneider, C.M.; Hayward, R. Voluntary Exercise Protects against Acute Doxorubicin Cardiotoxicity in the Isolated Perfused Rat Heart. *Am. J. Physiol. -Regul. Integr. Comp. Physiol.* **2005**, *289*, R424–R431. [CrossRef]
17. Guo, S.; Wong, S. Cardiovascular Toxicities from Systemic Breast Cancer Therapy. *Front. Oncol.* **2014**, *4*, 346. [CrossRef]
18. Hayward, R.; Lien, C.-Y.; Jensen, B.T.; Hydock, D.S.; Schneider, C.M. Exercise Training Mitigates Anthracycline-Induced Chronic Cardiotoxicity in a Juvenile Rat Model. *Pediatr. Blood Cancer* **2012**, *59*, 149–154. [CrossRef] [PubMed]
19. Hofmann, U.; Frantz, S. How Can We Cure a Heart "in Flame"? A Translational View on Inflammation in Heart Failure. *Basic Res. Cardiol.* **2013**, *108*, 356. [CrossRef]
20. Hydock, D.S.; Lien, C.-Y.; Jensen, B.T.; Parry, T.L.; Schneider, C.M.; Hayward, R. Rehabilitative Exercise in a Rat Model of Doxorubicin Cardiotoxicity. *Exp. Biol. Med.* **2012**, *237*, 1483–1492. [CrossRef]
21. Jones, L.W.; Fels, D.R.; West, M.; Allen, J.D.; Broadwater, G.; Barry, W.T.; Wilke, L.G.; Masko, E.; Douglas, P.S.; Dash, R.C.; et al. Modulation of Circulating Angiogenic Factors and Tumor Biology by Aerobic Training in Breast Cancer Patients Receiving Neoadjuvant Chemotherapy. *Cancer Prev. Res.* **2013**, *6*, 925–937. [CrossRef]
22. Hornsby, W.E.; Douglas, P.S.; West, M.J.; Kenjale, A.A.; Lane, A.R.; Schwitzer, E.R.; Ray, K.A.; Herndon, J.E.; Coan, A.; Gutierrez, A.; et al. Safety and Efficacy of Aerobic Training in Operable Breast Cancer Patients Receiving Neoadjuvant Chemotherapy: A Phase II Randomized Trial. *Acta Oncol.* **2014**, *53*, 65–74. [CrossRef] [PubMed]
23. Kirkham, A.A.; Virani, S.A.; Bland, K.A.; McKenzie, D.C.; Gelmon, K.A.; Warburton, D.E.R.; Campbell, K.L. Exercise Training Affects Hemodynamics Not Cardiac Function during Anthracycline-Based Chemotherapy. *Breast Cancer Res. Treat.* **2020**, *184*, 75–85. [CrossRef] [PubMed]
24. Howden, E.J.; Bigaran, A.; Beaudry, R.; Fraser, S.; Selig, S.; Foulkes, S.; Antill, Y.; Nightingale, S.; Loi, S.; Haykowsky, M.J.; et al. Exercise as a Diagnostic and Therapeutic Tool for the Prevention of Cardiovascular Dysfunction in Breast Cancer Patients. *Eur. J. Prev. Cardiol.* **2019**, *26*, 305–315. [CrossRef]
25. Foulkes, S.; Costello, B.T.; Howden, E.J.; Janssens, K.; Dillon, H.; Toro, C.; Claus, P.; Fraser, S.F.; Daly, R.M.; Elliott, D.A.; et al. Exercise Cardiovascular Magnetic Resonance Reveals Reduced Cardiac Reserve in Pediatric Cancer Survivors with Impaired Cardiopulmonary Fitness. *J. Cardiovasc. Magn. Reson.* **2020**, *22*, 64. [CrossRef] [PubMed]
26. Mijwel, S.; Backman, M.; Bolam, K.A.; Olofsson, E.; Norrbom, J.; Bergh, J.; Sundberg, C.J.; Wengström, Y.; Rundqvist, H. Highly Favorable Physiological Responses to Concurrent Resistance and High-Intensity Interval Training during Chemotherapy: The OptiTrain Breast Cancer Trial. *Breast Cancer Res. Treat.* **2018**, *169*, 93–103. [CrossRef] [PubMed]
27. Lee, K.; Kang, I.; Mack, W.J.; Mortimer, J.; Sattler, F.; Salem, G.; Lu, J.; Dieli-Conwright, C.M. Effects of High Intensity Interval Training on Vascular Endothelial Function and Vascular Wall Thickness in Breast Cancer Patients Receiving Anthracycline-Based Chemotherapy: A Randomized Pilot Study. *Breast Cancer Res. Treat.* **2019**, *177*, 477–485. [CrossRef]
28. Ansund, J.; Mijwel, S.; Bolam, K.A.; Altena, R.; Wengström, Y.; Rullman, E.; Rundqvist, H. High Intensity Exercise during Breast Cancer Chemotherapy—Effects on Long-Term Myocardial Damage and Physical Capacity—Data from the OptiTrain RCT. *Cardio-Oncology* **2021**, *7*, 7. [CrossRef]
29. Kirkham, A.A.; Eves, N.D.; Shave, R.E.; Bland, K.A.; Bovard, J.; Gelmon, K.A.; Virani, S.A.; McKenzie, D.C.; Stöhr, E.J.; Waburton, D.E.R.; et al. The Effect of an Aerobic Exercise Bout 24 h Prior to Each Doxorubicin Treatment for Breast Cancer on Markers of Cardiotoxicity and Treatment Symptoms: A RCT. *Breast Cancer Res. Treat.* **2018**, *167*, 719–729. [CrossRef]
30. Kirkham, A.A.; Lloyd, M.G.; Claydon, V.E.; Gelmon, K.A.; McKenzie, D.C.; Campbell, K.L. A Longitudinal Study of the Association of Clinical Indices of Cardiovascular Autonomic Function with Breast Cancer Treatment and Exercise Training. *Oncologist* **2019**, *24*, 273–284. [CrossRef]

31. Meacham, L.R.; Chow, E.J.; Ness, K.K.; Kamdar, K.Y.; Chen, Y.; Yasui, Y.; Oeffinger, K.C.; Sklar, C.A.; Robison, L.L.; Mertens, A.C. Cardiovascular Risk Factors in Adult Survivors of Pediatric Cancer—A Report from the Childhood Cancer Survivor Study. *Cancer Epidemiol. Biomark. Prev.* **2010**, *19*, 170–181. [CrossRef]
32. Jones, L.W.; Liu, Q.; Armstrong, G.T.; Ness, K.K.; Yasui, Y.; Devine, K.; Tonorezos, E.; Soares-Miranda, L.; Sklar, C.A.; Douglas, P.S.; et al. Exercise and Risk of Major Cardiovascular Events in Adult Survivors of Childhood Hodgkin Lymphoma: A Report from the Childhood Cancer Survivor Study. *J. Clin. Oncol.* **2014**, *32*, 3643–3650. [CrossRef] [PubMed]
33. Peters, M.D.; Godfrey, C.; McInerney, P.; Munn, Z.; Tricco, A.C.; Khalil, H. Chapter 11: Scoping Reviews (2020 Version). In *JBI Manual for Evidence Synthesis*; Aromataris, E., Munn, Z., Eds.; JBI: Adelaide, Australia, 2020.
34. Kendall, S.J.; Langley, J.E.; Crooks, B.; Giacomantonio, N.; Heinze-Milne, S.; Johnston, W.J.; Mulvagh, S.L.; Grandy, S.A. The Impact of Exercise on Cardiotoxicity in Pediatric Cancer Survivors: A Scoping Review Protocol. *Healthy Popul. J.* **2022**; *in press*.
35. *Covidence Systematic Review Software*; Veritas Health Innovation: Melbourne, Australia, 2022.
36. Järvelä, L.S.; Saraste, M.; Niinikoski, H.; Hannukainen, J.C.; Heinonen, O.J.; Lähteenmäki, P.M.; Arola, M.; Kemppainen, J. Home-Based Exercise Training Improves Left Ventricle Diastolic Function in Survivors of Childhood ALL: A Tissue Doppler and Velocity Vector Imaging Study. *Pediatr. Blood Cancer* **2016**, *63*, 1629–1635. [CrossRef] [PubMed]
37. Järvelä, L.S.; Niinikoski, H.; Heinonen, O.J.; Lähteenmäki, P.M.; Arola, M.; Kemppainen, J. Endothelial Function in Long-Term Survivors of Childhood Acute Lymphoblastic Leukemia: Effects of a Home-Based Exercise Program. *Pediatr. Blood Cancer* **2013**, *60*, 1546–1551. [CrossRef] [PubMed]
38. Järvelä, L.S.; Kemppainen, J.; Niinikoski, H.; Hannukainen, J.C.; Lähteenmäki, P.M.; Kapanen, J.; Arola, M.; Heinonen, O.J. Effects of a Home-Based Exercise Program on Metabolic Risk Factors and Fitness in Long-Term Survivors of Childhood Acute Lymphoblastic Leukemia. *Pediatr. Blood Cancer* **2012**, *59*, 155–160. [CrossRef] [PubMed]
39. Gustafsson, G.; Schmiegelow, K.; Forestier, E.; Clausen, N.; Glomstein, A.; Jonmundsson, G.; Mellander, L.; Mäkipernaa, A.; Nygaard, R.; Saarinen-Pihkala, U.M. Improving Outcome through Two Decades in Childhood ALL in the Nordic Countries: The Impact of High-Dose Methotrexate in the Reduction of CNS Irradiation. Nordic Society of Pediatric Haematology and Oncology (NOPHO). *Leukemia* **2000**, *14*, 2267–2275. [CrossRef]
40. Long, T.M.; Rath, S.R.; Wallman, K.E.; Howie, E.K.; Straker, L.M.; Bullock, A.; Walwyn, T.S.; Gottardo, N.G.; Cole, C.H.; Choong, C.S.; et al. Exercise Training Improves Vascular Function and Secondary Health Measures in Survivors of Pediatric Oncology Related Cerebral Insult. *PLoS ONE* **2018**, *13*, e0201449. [CrossRef]
41. Morales, J.S.; Santana-Sosa, E.; Santos-Lozano, A.; Baño-Rodrigo, A.; Valenzuela, P.L.; Rincón-Castanedo, C.; Fernández-Moreno, D.; González Vicent, M.; Pérez-Somarriba, M.; Madero, L.; et al. Inhospital Exercise Benefits in Childhood Cancer: A Prospective Cohort Study. *Scand. J. Med. Sci. Sports* **2020**, *30*, 126–134. [CrossRef]
42. Sharkey, A.M.; Carey, A.B.; Heise, C.T.; Barber, G. Cardiac Rehabilitation after Cancer Therapy in Children and Young Adults. *Am. J. Cardiol.* **1993**, *71*, 1488–1490. [CrossRef]
43. Smith, W.A.; Ness, K.K.; Joshi, V.; Hudson, M.M.; Robison, L.L.; Green, D.M. Exercise Training in Childhood Cancer Survivors with Subclinical Cardiomyopathy Who Were Treated with Anthracyclines. *Pediatr. Blood Cancer* **2013**, *61*, 942–945. [CrossRef]
44. Patel, N.; Durland, J.; Makaryus, A.N. Physiology, Cardiac Index. In *StatPearls*; StatPearls Publishing: Treasure Island, FL, USA, 2022.
45. Heiskanen, J.S.; Ruohonen, S.; Rovio, S.P.; Pahkala, K.; Kytö, V.; Kähönen, M.; Lehtimäki, T.; Viikari, J.S.A.; Juonala, M.; Laitinen, T.; et al. Cardiovascular Risk Factors in Childhood and Left Ventricular Diastolic Function in Adulthood. *Pediatrics* **2021**, *147*, e2020016691. [CrossRef]
46. Unnithan, V.B.; Rowland, T.W.; George, K.; Lord, R.; Oxborough, D. Left Ventricular Function during Exercise in Trained Pre-Adolescent Soccer Players. *Scand. J. Med. Sci. Sports* **2018**, *28*, 2330–2338. [CrossRef] [PubMed]
47. Nystoriak, M.A.; Bhatnagar, A. Cardiovascular Effects and Benefits of Exercise. *Front. Cardiovasc. Med.* **2018**, *5*, 135. [CrossRef] [PubMed]
48. Children's Oncology Group. *Long-Term Follow-Up Guidelines for Survivors of Childhood, Adolescent and Young Adult Cancer*; Children's Oncology Group: Birmingham, UK, 2018.
49. Barac, A.; Murtagh, G.; Carver, J.R.; Chen, M.H.; Freeman, A.M.; Herrmann, J.; Iliescu, C.; Ky, B.; Mayer, E.L.; Okwuosa, T.M.; et al. Cardiovascular Health of Patients with Cancer and Cancer Survivors. *J. Am. Coll. Cardiol.* **2015**, *65*, 2739–2746. [CrossRef] [PubMed]
50. Cardinale, D.; Colombo, A.; Bacchiani, G.; Tedeschi, I.; Meroni, C.A.; Veglia, F.; Civelli, M.; Lamantia, G.; Colombo, N.; Curigliano, G.; et al. Early Detection of Anthracycline Cardiotoxicity and Improvement with Heart Failure Therapy. *Circulation* **2015**, *131*, 1981–1988. [CrossRef]
51. Zamorano, J.L.; Lancellotti, P.; Rodriguez Muñoz, D.; Aboyans, V.; Asteggiano, R.; Galderisi, M.; Habib, G.; Lenihan, D.J.; Lip, G.Y.H.; Lyon, A.R.; et al. 2016 ESC Position Paper on Cancer Treatments and Cardiovascular Toxicity Developed under the Auspices of the ESC Committee for Practice Guidelines. *Eur. J. Heart Fail.* **2017**, *19*, 9–42. [CrossRef] [PubMed]
52. American College of Sports Medicine. *ACSM's Guidelines for Exercise Testing and Prescription*, 10th ed.; Wolters Kluwer: Philadelphia, PA, USA, 2018; ISBN 978-1-4963-3906-5.
53. Chamorro Viña, C.; Keats, M.R.; Culos-Reed, S.N. *POEM for Professionals: Pediatric Oncology Exercise Manual*, 1st ed.; Health & Wellness Lab., Faculty of Kinesiology, University of Calgary: Calgary, AB, Canada, 2014; ISBN 978-0-88953-380-6.

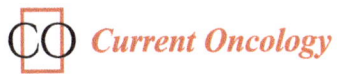 *Current Oncology*

Article

Utilization, Delivery, and Outcomes of Dance/Movement Therapy for Pediatric Oncology Patients and their Caregivers: A Retrospective Chart Review

Karolina Bryl [1], Suzi Tortora [1,2], Jennifer Whitley [1,2], Soo-Dam Kim [1], Nirupa J. Raghunathan [1,3], Jun J. Mao [1,*] and Susan Chimonas [4]

1. Department of Medicine, Integrative Medicine Service, Memorial Sloan Kettering Cancer Center, New York, NY 10065, USA; brylk@mskcc.org (K.B.)
2. MSK Kids, Memorial Sloan Kettering Cancer Center, New York, NY 10065, USA
3. Department of General Internal Medicine, Memorial Sloan Kettering Cancer Center, New York, NY 10065, USA
4. Department of Epidemiology and Biostatistics, Memorial Sloan Kettering Cancer Center, New York, NY 10065, USA
* Correspondence: maoj@mskcc.org

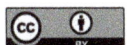

Citation: Bryl, K.; Tortora, S.; Whitley, J.; Kim, S.-D.; Raghunathan, N.J.; Mao, J.J.; Chimonas, S. Utilization, Delivery, and Outcomes of Dance/Movement Therapy for Pediatric Oncology Patients and their Caregivers: A Retrospective Chart Review. *Curr. Oncol.* **2023**, *30*, 6497–6507. https://doi.org/10.3390/curroncol30070477

Received: 22 May 2023
Revised: 30 June 2023
Accepted: 4 July 2023
Published: 6 July 2023

Copyright: © 2023 by the authors. Licensee MDPI, Basel, Switzerland. This article is an open access article distributed under the terms and conditions of the Creative Commons Attribution (CC BY) license (https://creativecommons.org/licenses/by/4.0/).

Abstract: Children with cancer and their caregivers face physical and psychosocial challenges during and after treatment. Dance/movement therapy (DMT) has been used to improve well-being, promote healthy coping, and mitigate the impact of illness, but limited knowledge exists regarding DMT utilization, delivery, and outcomes in pediatric oncology. This retrospective study aimed to identify reasons for referral to DMT, DMT visit characteristics, key DMT techniques and processes, and clinician-reported outcomes. We examined the electronic medical records of 100 randomly selected pediatric patients (resulting in 1160 visits) who received DMT services between 2011 and 2021. Sociodemographic, clinical, and visit characteristics, referral reasons, and clinician-reported outcomes were reported as frequency and proportions. Qualitative thematic analysis was used to identify key DMT techniques and processes. Among 100 patients (63% female, aged 0–27 years), 77.9% were referred for psychological distress and 19.6% for pain. Two distinct DMT approaches were used during visits: a traditional DMT approach (77%) and a multisensory DMT approach (23%). The most common visit length was 15–25 min (41.6%), followed by sessions of 30–45 min (22.5%) and ≤10 min (18.1%). A total of 61.9% of DMT visits were inpatient and 38.1% outpatient. Of all visits, 8.8% were new and 91.2% were follow-ups. Caregivers were engaged in treatment in 43.7% of visits, and 5.5% of visits focused entirely on the work with the caregiver. DMT intervention focused on self-expression, emotional self-regulation, coping strategies, socialization, and caregiver–child interaction. Clinician-reported outcomes included enhanced coping with hospital experience (58%), improved pain management (27%), improved self-regulation (21%), and increased physical activation (13.2%). The results suggest DMT as a supportive intervention for psychological distress and pain management in pediatric oncology patients and provide insights into DMT practices and outcomes to guide intervention development and future research.

Keywords: dance/movement therapy; pediatric oncology; creative arts therapies; psychological distress; pain management

1. Introduction

Pediatric cancer, with an incidence of approximately 400,000 children and adolescents, is the leading cause of death in children worldwide [1,2]. In the United States, approximately 15,780 children (1 in 285) are diagnosed with cancer each year [3]. With pediatric oncology advances, survival rates for most childhood cancers have improved [4], but the psychosocial (e.g., anxiety, depression, difficulties in interpersonal relationships, noncompliance with treatment) and physical (e.g., fatigue, sleep disturbances, pain) burdens of cancer on patients remain high [5–7]. Furthermore, pediatric cancer also substantially affects the emotional and physical functioning of parents and caregivers [8–12]. Thus, standard supportive care plans should include interventions to manage cancer-related side effects and symptoms and to provide socio-emotional support [13].

Dance/movement therapy (DMT) is defined by the American Dance Therapy Association (ADTA) as "the psychotherapeutic use of movement to promote emotional, social, cognitive and physical integration of the individual" [14]. This therapeutic approach, grounded within a biopsychosocial framework, aims to support well-being and physical and social/emotional development, improve healthy coping, and decrease the impact of illness for children living with cancer and their caregivers. DMT therapists are master's degree-level clinicians and licensed providers who utilize components of dance, improvised or structured movement, and creative and emotional expression, as well as other (psycho)therapeutic techniques (e.g., symbolism, metaphor), in a supportive therapeutic relationship within individual therapy sessions or group settings [14,15]. Movement and non-verbal behaviors are considered the primary mediums of assessment, interaction, and therapeutic interventions [16]. Several qualitative and theoretical contributions suggest that DMT can be implemented to support psychological adjustment [17,18], body image [19], and communication of difficult feelings and emotions [17,19]. DMT can also increase participation in therapeutic activities by reducing movement limitations in children and adolescents with cancer [19]. Results from two pilot studies suggest that DMT improves body image in adolescents with cancer [20] and quality of life for children receiving chemotherapy for brain tumors [21].

In medical settings, a distinct Multisensory Dance Movement Psychotherapy (MSDMT) approach is often incorporated to support the youngest patients during painful medical procedures [22–24]. This pain management approach to DMT is the application of pediatric medical dance/movement therapy with an added emphasis on the role of the body and multisensory experience to support physiologic and psychological coping, specifically related to medical illness. Within this approach, therapists provide children with a variety of activities that redirect focus away from pain and towards pleasurable sensory sensations [22,23]. These activities include the use of movement, music, touch, breath awareness, hypnosis, imagery, and meditation to augment pain control. One exploratory study examined pain control responses to MSDMT among pediatric neuroblastoma patients receiving an antibody therapy called 3F8 [25]. The study found that patients who were engaged, enthusiastic, had a capacity to develop coping skills, and were earlier in their treatment tended to have a positive pain control response to MSDMT. As such, MSDMT could be a noninvasive method that complements pharmacological and medical treatments.

Despite DMT's long presence and great promise in medical settings, including oncology [23], little is known about DMT utilization, delivery, and outcomes I n pediatric oncology patients and their caregivers. Beyond two pilot studies [20,21] and several theoretical contributions [17–19,22–24,26,27], no data describe the therapeutic provisioning of DMT in this context. To address this critical knowledge gap, this study aimed to identify: (1) reasons for referral to DMT; (2) visit characteristics: DMT approach, session length, setting, visit type, and caregiver involvement; (3) key techniques and processes of DMT intervention; and (4) clinician-reported outcomes.

2. Materials and Methods

2.1. Study Setting

The Integrative Medicine (IM) Service at Memorial Sloan Kettering Cancer Center (MSK) has offered DMT since 2003, averaging 1000 inpatient and outpatient pediatric visits per year (approximately 42,120 visits since the program's inception). Through dance and movement within a safe therapeutic environment DMT encourages patients to express their feelings and experiences, helps them to develop new coping and effective communication skills, supports child–caregiver relationships, and promotes body awareness, self-esteem, and socialization [22–24]. Dance/movement therapists also provide counseling, education (e.g., psychoeducation, education on services, development of coping strategies), and support to caregivers [23]. Within an inpatient setting, dance/movement therapists provide DMT individually to patients, together with caregivers, at the bedside, or in weekly group sessions in the pediatric recreation center. Within the outpatient setting, dance/movement therapists attend to patients and their caregivers while they are receiving or waiting for treatment. All IM services are offered free of charge.

2.2. Data Sources

Data were obtained from the electronic medical records (EMR) of pediatric in- and out-patients who received DMT services between January 2011 and December 2021. We employed a simple random sampling technique using a random number generator to randomly select 100 unique patients. Abstraction of 100 patient charts resulted in 1160 DMT visit notes, from which the following data were abstracted: sociodemographic characteristics (i.e., gender, date of birth, race, ethnicity), clinical variables (i.e., age at appointment, cancer type), referral reasons, DMT visit characteristics (i.e., intervention type, session length, setting, visit type), clinician-reported outcomes (as noted as clinical observations of change pre–post session in the visit notes), and key features and specific processes of DMT intervention. MSK's institutional review board (IRB) approved the retrospective study protocol (IRB #17-481).

2.3. Data Analysis

To describe the sociodemographic and clinical patient characteristics, we calculated descriptive statistics, such as means and medians for continuous data and frequencies and percentages for categorical data. We used age-at-appointment categories for patients based on the Centers for Disease Control (CDC) Child Developmental Milestones [28]: "infants and toddlers" (0- to 2-year-olds), "preschoolers" (3- to 5-year-olds), "middle childhood" (6- to 11-year-olds), "adolescents" (12- to 17-year-olds), and "young adults" (18- to 39-year-olds). For race and ethnicity, we followed the Office of Management and Budget (OMB) standards [29]. All analyses were performed using SPSS version 29 [30].

To identify key features and specific processes of DMT intervention, we analyzed DMT visit notes using an inductive approach to thematic analysis [31,32]. To ensure inter-coder agreement, the first 10 visit notes were coded independently by 2 coders (KB and SDK), who then discussed and resolved discrepancies. This procedure was repeated 5 times, after which a formal codebook was developed to ensure the validity and consistency of the results. The remaining notes were coded by SDK, with the senior coder (KB) providing supervision for every 10 visit notes. After coding all 1160 visit notes, codes were grouped into themes, which were defined and reviewed with the study team.

3. Results

3.1. Sociodemographic and Clinical Characteristics

As shown in Table 1, the mean age of patients in our sample was 8.24 ± 6.26 years, and most were female (63%). Among 100 patients, the majority were White (64%) and not Hispanic or Latino (83%). In terms of age, receipt of DMT services was almost equally distributed among preschoolers, middle childhood, and adolescent groups (26.1% vs. 27.4% vs. 22.3%, respectively), with fewer DMT visits delivered to infants and toddlers (16.5%) and young adults (7.7%). The most common pediatric cancer types were neuroblastomas (45%), followed by sarcomas (16%), leukemias (13%), and lymphomas (11%). Patients with blood and immune disorders received the most DMT visits (37 per patient, on average), followed by those with brain tumors, neuroblastomas, lymphomas, and leukemias (15, 12, 12, and 10 visits per patient, on average, respectively).

Table 1. Patients' demographic and clinical characteristics.

Characteristics	Number of Patients/Inpatient	Number of Visits/Inpatient	Average Visit per Patient
Total	n	n (%)	n
	100	1160	
Gender			
Female	63	685 (59.1)	-
Male	37	475 (40.9)	-
Age at Appointment (years)			
Mean (SD)	8.24 (6.26)	-	-
Median	7	-	-
Age at Appointment categories (years)			
Infants & Toddlers (birth–2 years)	25/15	191 (16.5)/141 (12.1)	9
Preschoolers (3–5 years)	26/14	303 (26.1)/124 (10.7)	12
Middle Childhood (6–11 children)	22/8	318 (27.4)/191 (16.5)	14
Adolescents (12–17 years)	18/11	259 (22.3)/163 (14)	12
Young adults (18–39 years)	9/6	89 (7.7)/71 (6.1)	10
Race			
White	64	656 (56.6)	-
Black	12	89 (7.7)	-
Asian	7	89 (7.7)	-
American Indian or Alaska Native	3	124 (10.7)	-
Other and Unknown	14	202 (17.4)	-
Ethnicity			
Not Hispanic or Latino	83	926 (79.8)	-
Hispanic or Latino	16	177 (15.3)	-
Unknown	1	57 (4.9)	-
Cancer type			
Adrenal tumors	2	8 (0.7)	4
Blood and Immune Disorders	5	129 (11.1)	37
Liver tumors	1	7 (0.6)	7
Neuroblastoma	45	534 (46)	12
Brain tumors	3	45 (3.9)	15
Leukemias	13	132 (11.4)	10
Lymphomas	11	159 (13.7)	12
Sarcomas	16	124 (10.7)	8
Sacrococcygeal Teratoma	1	2 (0.2)	2
Wilms' tumor and other kidney tumors	3	20 (1.7)	7
Treatment type			
Chemotherapy	48	635 (54.7)	-
Immunotherapy	21	233 (20.1)	-
Surgery	16	63 (5.4)	-
Chemoimmunotherapy	9	136 (11.7)	-
Bone Marrow Transplant	6	93 (8.0)	-

3.2. Reasons for Referral to DMT

Table 2 shows the most common referral reasons by visit type (new vs. follow-up) and setting (in- vs. outpatient). Psychological distress was the most common referral reason overall ($n = 904$, 77.9%) and across visit types (new visit: $n = 74$, 72.5%; follow-up: $n = 830$, 78.4%) and settings (inpatient: $n = 670$, 93.3%; outpatient: $n = 234$, 52.9%). Pain was the second most common referral reason overall ($n = 227$, 19.6%) and across visit types (new visit: $n = 21$, 20.6%; follow-up: $n = 206$, 19.5%) and settings (inpatient: $n = 25$, 3.5%; outpatient: $n = 202$, 45.7%). Other reasons included psychological and/or developmental support ($n = 8$, 0.7%), Enhanced Recovery After Surgery (ERAS) ($n = 7$, 0.6%), end-of-life care (n = 4, 0.3%), and fatigue (n = 2, 0.2%). No referral reason was specified in eight cases (0.7%).

Table 2. Referral reason.

Referral Reason	Total n (%)	New Visit n (%)	Follow-Up n (%)	Inpatient n (%)	Outpatient n (%)
Psychological Distress	904 (77.9)	74 (72.5)	830 (78.4)	670 (93.3)	234 (52.9)
Pain	227 (19.6)	21 (20.6)	206 (19.5)	25 (3.5)	202 (45.7)
Other [1]	29 (2.5)	7 (6.9)	22 (2.1)	23 (3.1)	6 (1.4)

[1] "Other" included: psychological and/or developmental support; Enhanced Recovery After Surgery; end-of-life care; fatigue; and not specified.

3.3. Visit Characteristics: DMT Approach, Session Length, Setting, Visit Type, and Caregiver Involvement

Visit characteristics are presented in Table 3. Of 1160 visits, 102 (8.8%) were new visits, and 1058 (91.2%) were follow-ups. The most common session length was 15–25 min (n = 483, 41.6%), followed by 30–45 min (n = 261, 22.5%), and ≤10 min (n = 210, 18.1%). DMT was provided 718 times (61.9%) in the inpatient setting and 442 times (38.1%) in the outpatient setting. Caregivers were present 507 (43.7%) times during visits, and 64 (5.5%) sessions focused on caregivers (e.g., education, support). Traditional DMT (n = 893, 77%) was offered almost four times as often as MSDMT (n = 267, 23%).

Table 3. Visit characteristics.

Visit Characteristics	Total n (%)	Inpatient n (%)	Outpatient n (%)
DMT approach			
DMT *	893 (77)	698 (60)	195 (17)
MSDMT **	267 (23)	20 (2)	247 (21)
Session length			
≤10 min	210 (18.1)	151 (13)	59 (5.1)
15–25 min	483 (41.6)	352 (30.3)	131 (11.3)
30–45 min	261 (22.5)	168 (14.5)	93 (8)
60 min	168 (14.5)	39 (3.4)	129 (11.1)
75 min	22 (1.9)	3 (0.3)	19 (1.6)
≥90 min	12 (1)	2 (0.1)	10 (0.9)
Unspecified	4 (.3)	3 (0.3)	1 (>0.1)
Setting			
Inpatient	718 (61.9)	-	-
Outpatient	442 (38.1)	-	-
Visit type			
New Visit	102 (8.8)	60 (5.2)	42 (3.6)
Follow-up	1058 (91.2)	658 (56.7)	400 (34.5)
Caregiver involvement			
Work with caregiver	64 (5.5)	44 (3.8)	20 (1.7)
Caregiver engaged in session	507 (43.7)	226 (19.5)	281 (24.2)

* DMT—Dance/Movement Therapy. ** MSDMT—Multisensory Dance/Movement Psychotherapy.

3.4. Key Techniques and Specific Processes of DMT Intervention

Qualitative analysis, focusing on key techniques and processes of DMT, elicited four main themes. These themes are discussed below.

Theme 1. Self-expression and meaning-making. Dance/movement therapists create a safe therapeutic environment and encourage children to express themselves primarily through natural movement, employing techniques such as metaphorical representation, symbolism, or play. To support a sense of agency, therapists follow the child's lead and tailor session activities (e.g., physical role-play, physical imagine-play, free dance, and choreographed dance) to their individual needs. Dance and movement offer a creative outlet for emotional release, and physicality provides a sense of control.

Theme 2. Emotional self-regulation, feeling identification, processing, and validation. Dance/movement therapists use techniques such as: (1) mirroring (e.g., embodiment or reflection) of the child's physical expression or non-verbal communications; (2) attunement and rhythmic synchronizing to the child's verbal and non-verbal physical and emotional state; and (3) other kinesthetic–sensory techniques (e.g., touch, sound) to assist children who under- or over-regulate to identify, physically express, process, and validate suppressed or difficult feelings.

Theme 3. Embodied coping strategies. Dance/movement therapists focus on embodied activities that increase children's body awareness and help them recognize, understand, and respond to physical signs of distress. These activities include: (1) grounding techniques to slow down stress responses and emotional or physiological dysregulation; (2) anchoring to bring the patient's attention to the present moment or shift sensations from anxious to calm (e.g., dancing to a favorite song); (3) auditory cues (e.g., entrainment) to redirect energy and attention toward positive, calm, and self-empowered emotional states; and (4) anxiety reducing activities (e.g., breathing exercises, embodied meditation, guided imagery) tailored to developmental and cultural preferences.

Theme 4. Socialization and caregiver-child interaction. Therapists teach caregivers how to read and respond to non-verbal (e.g., muscular tension, facial expression) and verbal cues (e.g., gurgling, babbling, crying) through movement (e.g., rocking) and use of props (e.g., toys, shakers) to support bonding and dyadic regulation with the youngest patients. With older patients, therapists engage caregivers in movement-based games, creative dance, expressive movement, or role-playing to help build responsive caregiver–child interactions and improve communication.

3.5. Clinician-Reported Outcomes

Clinician-reported pediatric outcomes are presented in Table 4. These included outcomes related to the treatment of psychological distress, such as enhanced coping with the hospital experience (n = 663, 58%) and improved self-regulation (n = 241, 21%), as well as improved pain management (n = 311, 27%) and increased physical activization (n = 151, 13.2%). Caregiver outcomes included decreased burden (n = 183, 16%) and enhanced parent–child relationship (n = 10, 0.9%).

Table 4. Clinician-reported outcomes.

Outcomes	N * (%)
Pediatric	
Psychological Distress	
Enhanced coping with hospital experience	663 (58)
Increased social interaction	372 (32.5)
Reduced anxiety/stress/fear	169 (14.7)
Decreased levels of depression	117 (10.2)
Comfort/End of life care	5 (0.4)
Improved self-regulation	241 (21)
Feeling calm and relaxed	199 (17.4)
Improved self-regulation skills	42 (3.7)
Pain	
Improved pain management **	311 (27)
Other	
Increased physical activization	151 (13.2)
Active physical engagement	78 (6.8)
Supported developmental milestones (developmental and sensory stimulation)	73 (6.4)

Table 4. *Cont.*

Outcomes	N * (%)
Caregiver	
Decreased caregiver burden	183 (16)
Caregiver education	73 (6.4)
Psychological needs and disease-related issues assessment	39 (3.4)
Caregiver counseling (e.g., coping with emotional distress, parental adjustment support)	71 (6.2)
Enhanced parent–child relationship	10 (0.9)

* N reflects the number of times the outcome was reported in visit notes. Note that for each visit note analyzed, multiple outcomes could be reported. Outcomes reported were not always in line with referral reasons; e.g., a patient could have been referred for pain, but during the visit the patient could also report feeling depressed, and the therapeutic activities would be focused on alleviating feelings of depression in addition to pain management.
** Improved pain management was reported in 98% of the MSDMT visits (263 of 267 total visits).

4. Discussion

In this retrospective chart review, we used quantitative and qualitative methods to analyze 1160 pediatric DMT treatments across 100 randomly selected patients. To the authors' knowledge, this is the largest pediatric DMT study reported to date. We found that DMT can be successfully used across pediatric age groups, cancer types, and treatment settings to help treat psychological distress and improve pain management.

In our study, the most common reason for referral to DMT services was psychological distress, including anxiety, stress, and depression. This finding highlights the psychological and psychosocial effects of cancer diagnosis, hospitalization, and treatment on children [33]. These symptoms can significantly impact the quality of life, psychosocial development, symptom management, and treatment compliance [34], ultimately leading to lasting negative effects on patients' physical and psychological health [35,36].

To target psychological distress, DMT therapists use dance and movement to help children express thoughts, emotions, and body sensations that are often difficult for them to verbalize. Movement used in sessions encompasses body postures, gestures, breathing exercises, natural and spontaneous movement, improvised dance, and various movement and dance sequences [37]. Movement also stimulates the imagination, enabling the creation and living of new experiences, promoting self- and body awareness, and enhancing self-efficacy. This is particularly important for cancer patients, as increased self-efficacy is linked to decreased psychological symptoms and increased self-care behaviors [38]. Furthermore, therapists use dance and movement to support the development of emotional self-regulation, which enables patients to recognize, name, and express a broad range of emotions and experiences [22–24]. As a result, patients can improve their psychological outcomes, such as anxiety, depression, or stress. Among older patients, this increased self-awareness can also lead to changes in habitual response patterns and a better understanding of their impact on themselves and their relationships with others [23]. Moreover, movement and dance in DMT promote physical activity and vitalization and therefore target anhedonia, apathy, and underactivity, which are common symptoms in children living with cancer.

In our study, we also found that DMT services were requested for pain almost as often as for psychological distress among pediatric outpatients, indicating that these patients often experience pain not only as a result of their illness but also due to diagnostic and therapeutic procedures often performed in outpatient settings [39,40]. Anxiety and depression are also significant factors contributing to ongoing pain in patients after cancer treatment [41]. Pain experienced by children with cancer can vary in type and severity [42,43], but is understood to be both a sensory and emotional experience [41]. In addition, unmanaged pain during cancer treatment can cause more psychological distress and post-traumatic stress for patients and their families [43].

DMT, and MSDMT specifically, can provide a non-invasive and complementary pain management treatment for pain and physical discomfort in pediatric patients [24]. These therapies teach children embodied coping strategies, such as relaxation, redirection from the experience of pain, and self-regulation, through dance and movement. Techniques used in these therapies also include breathing, working with muscular tension, and attunement to somato-sensorial sensations. Furthermore, we also found that the MSDMT approach was offered almost 25% of the time and resulted in improved pain management among 98% of outpatients, suggesting that, for younger children, more sophisticated therapeutic approaches may be needed to help with pain coping. MSDMT may be particularly beneficial for children who might lack the comprehension and ability to effectively respond to verbal interventions when experiencing pain. This therapeutic approach recognizes that children, irrespective of their age, inherently absorb information through multiple senses. Moreover, this sensitivity to multisensory input becomes more pronounced during challenging medical situations. During visits, activities are administered by layering specific sensory experiences through playful engagements, which, at first, distract the patient, then ultimately support them to reach a meditative state when in heightened arousal or perceiving pain [23,24]. Within MSDMT, therapists help the youngest patients achieve a self-regulatory state by attuning to the child's multisensory input and co-regulating their reactions to the painful experience. This is achieved through a variety of activities that are conducted by gradually incorporating various sensory experiences into playful interactions. Initially, these experiences serve as distractions for the patient, but eventually they help the patient attain a state of meditation when they are experiencing heightened arousal or perceiving pain [24]. As such, DMT results in enhanced coping with the hospital experience, improved pain management, and improved self-regulation.

Caregivers also play a crucial role in children's pain experiences and are often included in pain treatments [44]. Studies have shown that there is a connection between how caregivers respond to their child's pain and the severity of pain, functional disability, and other somatic complaints that the child experiences [45–47]. Depending on the child's developmental stage, parents may also be essential to the treatment process, as their support is necessary for children to improve their adaptive pain management skills. Without their targeted support, it can be more difficult for children and adolescents to make progress in this area. DMT not only facilitates socialization but also caregiver–child interaction through creative dance-play with their children during treatment, procedure, or hospital stay. Notably, in our study, caregivers were present and engaged in almost 44% of DMT visits. In addition, 5.5% of visits focused solely on caregiver support, resulting in decreased caregiver burden and enhanced parent–child relationship support. The inclusion of caregivers in therapeutic interventions should be strongly considered while developing treatment and research protocols.

We acknowledge several study limitations. First, the retrospective nature of this study limits our ability to examine other factors that may be associated with utilization and delivery of DMT (e.g., patient/caregiver feedback, perception of treatment benefits, outcomes/symptomatic relief). Second, this study was conducted at a single academic cancer center; therefore, our sample may not be representative of other populations, so the generalizability of our findings may be limited. Third, in our study, patients were specifically referred to DMT services by their health care providers; therefore, clinician referral bias might confound our results. Fourth, we assessed outcomes as reported by the clinicians; therefore, it is possible that, while highly trained, the two DMT therapists in our study may have personal biases that influenced their treatment approaches and reported outcomes. Finally, our DMT program is supported by specific institutional support that may not be available in other settings, and therefore it may be difficult to implement in less supportive contexts. Despite these limitations, our study represents an important step towards understanding pediatric DMT utilization, delivery, and outcomes.

5. Conclusions

In this retrospective study of over 1000 treatments among 100 pediatric cancer patients, we found that DMT is commonly offered to patients who experience psychosocial and physical difficulties related to cancer treatment and hospitalization. We also discerned specific patterns of utilization (e.g., session length, average follow-up visits) and described key features and specific processes of DMT (e.g., how DMT is delivered and the ways dance and movement are used in a therapeutic context) and clinician-reported pediatric and caregiver outcomes (e.g., enhanced coping with hospital experience, improved pain management, decreased caregiver burden). Our results suggest that DMT can be successfully used across pediatric age groups, cancer types, and treatment settings to treat psychological distress and improve pain management. This knowledge is instrumental in intervention development and will help formulate hypotheses for future research aiming to enhance the effectiveness of DMT for children living with cancer.

Author Contributions: Conceptualization, K.B. and J.J.M.; methodology, K.B. and J.J.M.; validation, K.B.; formal analysis, K.B. and S.-D.K.; investigation, K.B. and S.-D.K.; data curation, K.B.; writing—original draft preparation, K.B.; writing—review and editing, K.B., S.-D.K., S.T., J.W., N.J.R., J.J.M. and S.C.; visualization: K.B.; supervision, J.J.M. and S.C.; project administration, K.B. All authors have read and agreed to the published version of the manuscript.

Funding: This work was funded, in part, by the National Institutes of Health's Cancer Center Support Grant (P30-CA008748), the Andrea Rizzo Foundation, and the Memorial Sloan Kettering Translational and Integrative Medicine Research Fund.

Institutional Review Board Statement: The study was conducted in accordance with the Declaration of Helsinki and approved by the Institutional Review Board at Memorial Sloan Kettering Cancer Center (Protocol #17-481; Approval Date: 26 September 2017).

Informed Consent Statement: Patient consent was waived due to research involving existing data, with minimal risk to the participants, and authorization was granted by the Institutional Review Board at Memorial Sloan Kettering Cancer Center (Protocol #17-481; Approval Date: 26 September 2017).

Data Availability Statement: Data sharing is not applicable to this article.

Conflicts of Interest: J.J.M. reports grants from Tibet CheeZheng Tibetan Medicine Co., Ltd. and from Zhongke Health International LLC outside the submitted work. K.B., S.D.K., S.T., J.W., N.J.R. and S.C. declare no conflict of interest. The funders had no role in the design of the study; in the collection, analysis, or interpretation of data; in the writing of the manuscript; or in the decision to publish the results.

References

1. Steliarova-Foucher, E.; Colombet, M.; Ries, L.A.G.; Moreno, F.; Dolya, A.; Bray, F.; Hesseling, P.; Shin, H.Y.; Stiller, C.A.; IICC-3 contributors. International incidence of childhood cancer, 2001–2010: A population-based registry study. *Lancet Oncol.* **2017**, *18*, 719–731. [CrossRef] [PubMed]
2. Siegel, R.L.; Miller, K.D.; Fuchs, H.E.; Jemal, A. Cancer Statistics, 2021. *CA Cancer J. Clin.* **2021**, *71*, 7–33. [CrossRef] [PubMed]
3. Howlader, N.; Noone, A.M.; Krapcho, M.; Miller, D.; Brest, A.; Yu, M.; Ruhl, J.; Tatalovich, Z.; Mariotto, A.; Lewis, D.R.; et al. (Eds.) SEER Cancer Statistics Review, 1975–2018. National Cancer Institute: Bethesda, MD. Based on November 2020 SEER Data Submission, Posted to the SEER Web Site, April 2021. Available online: https://seer.cancer.gov/csr/1975_2018/ (accessed on 19 May 2023).
4. Jemal, A.; Ward, E.M.; Johnson, C.J.; Cronin, K.A.; Ma, J.; Ryerson, B.; Mariotto, A.; Lake, A.J.; Wilson, R.; Sherman, R.L.; et al. Annual Report to the Nation on the Status of Cancer, 1975–2014, Featuring Survival. *J. Natl. Cancer Inst.* **2017**, *109*, djx030. [CrossRef] [PubMed]
5. Li, H.C.; Chung, O.K.; Chiu, S.Y. The impact of cancer on children's physical, emotional, and psychosocial well-being. *Cancer Nurs.* **2010**, *33*, 47–54. [CrossRef] [PubMed]
6. Wakefield, C.E.; McLoone, J.; Goodenough, B.; Lenthen, K.; Cairns, D.R.; Cohn, R.J. The Psychosocial Impact of Completing Childhood Cancer Treatment: A Systematic Review of the Literature. *J. Pediatr. Psychol.* **2009**, *35*, 262–274. [CrossRef]
7. Brinkman, T.M.; Recklitis, C.J.; Michel, G.; Grootenhuis, M.A.; Klosky, J.L. Psychological Symptoms, Social Outcomes, Socioeconomic Attainment, and Health Behaviors Among Survivors of Childhood Cancer: Current State of the Literature. *J. Clin. Oncol.* **2018**, *36*, 2190–2197. [CrossRef]
8. Steele, R.G.; Long, A.; Reddy, K.A.; Luhr, M.; Phipps, S. Changes in maternal distress and child-rearing strategies across treatment for pediatric cancer. *J. Pediatr. Psychol.* **2003**, *28*, 447–452. [CrossRef]
9. Ahmadi, M.; Rassouli, M.; Karami, M.; Abasszadeh, A.; Poormansouri, S. Care burden and its Related Factors in Parents of Children with Cancer. *Iran J. Nurs.* **2018**, *31*, 40–51. [CrossRef]

10. Greenzang, K.A.; Kelly, C.A.; Al-Sayegh, H.; Ma, C.; Mack, J.W. Thinking ahead: Parents' worries about late effects of childhood cancer treatment. *Pediatr. Blood Cancer* **2021**, *68*, e29335. [CrossRef]
11. Sulkers, E.; Tissing, W.J.E.; Brinksma, A.; Roodbol, P.F.; Kamps, W.A.; Stewart, R.E.; Sanderman, R.; Fleer, J. Providing care to a child with cancer: A longitudinal study on the course, predictors, and impact of caregiving stress during the first year after diagnosis. *Psycho-Oncology* **2015**, *24*, 318–324. [CrossRef]
12. van Warmerdam, J.; Zabih, V.; Kurdyak, P.; Sutradhar, R.; Nathan, P.C.; Gupta, S. Prevalence of anxiety, depression, and posttraumatic stress disorder in parents of children with cancer: A meta-analysis. *Pediatr. Blood Cancer* **2019**, *66*, e27490. [CrossRef]
13. Grassi, L.; Spiegel, D.; Riba, M. Advancing psychosocial care in cancer patients. *F1000Research* **2017**, *6*, 2083. [CrossRef] [PubMed]
14. American Dance Therapy Association. What Is Dance/Movement Therapy? Available online: https://adta.memberclicks.net/what-is-dancemovement-therapy (accessed on 26 June 2023).
15. American Dance Therapy Association. Become a Dance Movement Therapist! Available online: https://adta.memberclicks.net/become-a-dance-movement-therapist (accessed on 26 June 2023).
16. Bryl, K. The three pillars of movement observation and analysis. A brief introduction to the LMA, KMP and MPI. In *The Art and Science of Embodied Research Design*; Tantia, J.F., Ed.; Routledge: New York, NY, USA, 2020; pp. 101–112.
17. Goodill, S.; Morningstar, D. The role of dance/movement therapy with medically ill children. *Int. J. Arts Med.* **1993**, *2*, 24–27.
18. Cohen, S.O.; Walco, G.A. Dance/movement therapy for children and adolescents with cancer. *Cancer Pract.* **1999**, *7*, 34–42. [CrossRef] [PubMed]
19. Mendelsohn, J. Dance/Movement therapy with hospitalized children. *Am. J. Dance Mov. Ther.* **1999**, *21*, 65–80. [CrossRef]
20. Madden, J.R. Dance/Movement Therapy and Body Image in Adolescents with Cancer. Master's Thesis, Yale University, New Haven, CT, USA, 1999.
21. Madden, J.R.; Mowry, P.; Gao, D.; Cullen, P.M.; Foreman, N.K. Creative arts therapy improves quality of life for pediatric brain tumor patients receiving outpatient chemotherapy. *J. Pediatr. Oncol. Nurs.* **2010**, *27*, 133–145. [CrossRef]
22. Tortora, S. Dance movement psychotherapy in early childhood treatment and pediatric oncology. In *The Art and Science of Dance/Movement Therapy: Life is Dance*; Chaiklin, S., Wengrower, H., Eds.; Routledge: New York, NY, USA, 2015.
23. Tortora, S. Children are born to dance! Pediatric Medical Dance/Movement Therapy: The view from Integrative Pediatric Oncology. *Children* **2019**, *6*, 14. [CrossRef]
24. Tortora, S.; Keren, M. *Dance/Movement Therapy for Young Children with Medical Illness: Treating Somatic and Psychic Distress*; Routledge: New York, NY, USA, 2023.
25. Ehrmann, B.; Tailor, D.; Tortora, S.; Mao, J.J.; Coleton, M.; Deng, G. Predictors of Success of Multisensory Dance/Movement Therapy In Improving Pain Control Among Children Treated with 3F8 Immunotherapy for Advanced Neuroblastoma. In Proceedings of the 13th International Conference of the Society for Integrative Oncology, Miami, FL, USA, 5–7 November 2016.
26. Vincent, S.R.; Tortora, S.; Shaw, J.; Basiner, J.; Devereaux, C.; Mulcahy, S.; Ponsini, M.C. Collaborating with a Mission: The Andréa Rizzo Foundation Spreads the Gift of Dance/Movement Therapy. *Am. J. Dance Ther.* **2007**, *29*, 51–58. [CrossRef]
27. Zilius, M.N. Dance/Movement Therapy in Pediatrics: An Overview. *Altern. Compliment. Ther.* **2010**, *16*, 87–92. [CrossRef]
28. Centers for Disease Control and Prevention (CDC). Child Development. Available online: https://www.cdc.gov/ncbddd/childdevelopment/index.html (accessed on 1 March 2023).
29. Executive Office of the President; Office of Management and Budget; Office of Information and Regulatory Affairs. Revisions to the Standards for the Classification of Federal Data on Race and Ethnicity. *Fed. Regist.* **1997**, *62*, 58782–58790.
30. IBM Corp. *IBM SPSS Statistics for Windows*; Version 28.0; IBM Corp: Armonk, NY, USA, 2021.
31. Braun, V.; Clarke, V. Using thematic analysis in psychology. *Qual. Res. Psychol.* **2006**, *3*, 77–101. [CrossRef]
32. Braun, V.; Clarke, V. Can I use TA? Should I use TA? Should I not use TA? Comparing reflexive thematic analysis and other pattern-based qualitative analytic approaches. *Couns. Psychother. Res.* **2020**, *21*, 37–47. [CrossRef]
33. American Cancer Society. Emotional, Mental Health, and Mood Changes. Available online: https://www.cancer.org/treatment/treatments-and-side-effects/physical-side-effects/emotional-mood-changes.html#:~:text=A%20cancer%20diagnosis%20can%20affect,and%20get%20help%20when%20needed (accessed on 1 March 2023).
34. Malbasa, T.; Kodish, E.; Santacroce, S.J. Adolescent Adherence to Oral Therapy for Leukemia: A Focus Group Study. *J. Pediatr. Oncol. Nurs.* **2007**, *24*, 139–151. [CrossRef] [PubMed]
35. Sandeberg, M.A.; Johansson, E.; Björk, O.; Wettergren, L. Health-Related Quality of Life Relates to School Attendance in Children on Treatment for Cancer. *J. Pediatr. Oncol. Nurs.* **2008**, *25*, 265–274. [CrossRef] [PubMed]
36. Coughtrey, A.; Millington, A.; Bennett, S.; Christie, D.; Hough, R.; Su, M.T.; Constantinou, M.P.; Shafran, R. The Effectiveness of Psychosocial Interventions for Psychological Outcomes in Pediatric Oncology: A Systematic Review. *J. Pain Symptom Manag.* **2018**, *55*, 1004–1017. [CrossRef]
37. Pędzich, Z.; Wiśniewska, M. Psychoterapia tańcem i ruchem. Podstawowe założenia, czynniki leczące i zastosowania. In *Psychoterapia Tańcem i Ruchem. Teoria i Praktyka*; Pędzich, Z., Ed.; GWP: Warsaw, Poland, 2014.
38. Lev, E.L. Bandura's theory of self-efficacy: Applications to oncology. *Sch. Inq. Nurs. Pract.* **1997**, *11*, 21–37; discussion 39–43. [PubMed]
39. National Cancer Institute. Side Effects of Cacner Treatment. Available online: https://www.cancer.gov/about-cancer/treatment/side-effects/pain (accessed on 4 April 2023).

40. Jibb, L.A.; Nathan, P.C.; Stevens, B.J.; Seto, E.; Cafazzo, J.A.; Stephens, N.; Yohannes, L.; Stinson, J.N. Psychological and Physical Interventions for the Management of Cancer-Related Pain in Pediatric and Young Adult Patients: An Integrative Review. *Oncol. Nurs. Forum.* **2015**, *42*, E339–E357. [CrossRef]
41. Uhl, K.; Burns, M.; Hale, A.; Coakley, R. The Critical Role of Parents in Pediatric Cancer-Related Pain Management: A Review and Call to Action. *Curr. Oncol. Rep.* **2020**, *22*, 37. [CrossRef]
42. Mertens, R. Pain therapy in pediatric oncology: Pain experience, drugs and pharmacokinetics. *Anasthesiol Intensiv. Notfallmed Schmerzther* **2011**, *46*, 736–742. [CrossRef]
43. Tutelman, P.R.; Chambers, C.T.; Stinson, J.N.; Parker, J.A.; Fernandez, C.V.; Witteman, H.O.; Nathan, P.C.; Barwick, M.; Campbell, F.; Jibb, L.A.; et al. Pain in Children With Cancer: Prevalence, Characteristics, and Parent Management. *Clin. J. Pain* **2018**, *34*, 198–206. [CrossRef]
44. Olarte-Sierra, M.F.; Rossell, N.; Zubieta, M.; Challinor, J. Parent Engagement and Agency in Latin American Childhood Cancer Treatment: A Qualitative Investigation. *JCO Glob. Oncol.* **2020**, *6*, 1729–1735. [CrossRef] [PubMed]
45. Claar, R.L.; Simons, L.E.; Logan, D.E. Parental response to children's pain: The moderating impact of children's emotional distress on symptoms and disability. *Pain* **2008**, *138*, 172–179. [CrossRef] [PubMed]
46. Eccleston, C.; Crombez, G.; Scotford, A.; Clinch, J.; Connell, H. Adolescent chronic pain: Patterns and predictors of emotional distress in adolescents with chronic pain and their parents. *Pain* **2004**, *108*, 221–229. [CrossRef] [PubMed]
47. Eccleston, C.; Fisher, E.; Law, E.; Bartlett, J.; Palermo, T.M. Psychological interventions for parents of children and adolescents with chronic illness. *Cochrane Database Syst. Rev.* **2015**, *4*, Cd009660. [CrossRef]

Disclaimer/Publisher's Note: The statements, opinions and data contained in all publications are solely those of the individual author(s) and contributor(s) and not of MDPI and/or the editor(s). MDPI and/or the editor(s) disclaim responsibility for any injury to people or property resulting from any ideas, methods, instructions or products referred to in the content.

MDPI
St. Alban-Anlage 66
4052 Basel
Switzerland
www.mdpi.com

Current Oncology Editorial Office
E-mail: curroncol@mdpi.com
www.mdpi.com/journal/curroncol

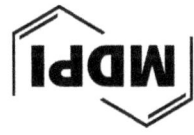

Disclaimer/Publisher's Note: The statements, opinions and data contained in all publications are solely those of the individual authors(s) and contributor(s) and not of MDPI and/or the editor(s). MDPI and/or the editor(s) disclaim responsibility for any injury to people or property resulting from any ideas, methods, instructions or products referred to in the content.

www.ingramcontent.com/pod-product-compliance
Lightning Source LLC
LaVergne TN
LVHW070401100526
83820ZLV000148/1366